W9-BUY-322

Psychology of Sport Injury

John Heil, DA
Lewis-Gale Clinic, Roanoke, VA

Human Kinetics Publishers

Library of Congress Cataloging-in-Publication Data

Heil, John.
 Psychology of sport injury / John Heil.
  p. cm.
 Includes index.
 ISBN 0-87322-463-9
 1. Sports--Accidents and injuries--Psychological aspects.
 I. Title.
 RD97.H45 1993
 617.1'027--dc20   92-35854
                                                  CIP

ISBN: 0-87322-463-9

Developmental Editor: Rodd Whelpley; **Assistant Editors**: Moyra Knight, and Julie Swadener, and Valerie Rose Hall; **Copyeditor**: Julie Anderson; **Proofreader**: Kathy Bennett; **Indexer**: Theresa Schaefer; **Production Director**: Ernie Noa; **Typesetting and Text Layout**: Yvonne Winsor; **Text Design**: Keith Blomberg; **Cover Design**: Jack Davis; **Interior Art**: Tim Offenstein and Gretchen Walters; **Author Photo**: David Youngblood; **Printer**: Edwards Brothers

Printed in the United States of America   10 9 8 7 6 5 4 3 2 1

Human Kinetics Publishers
Box 5076, Champaign, IL 61825-5076
1-800-747-4457

Canada: Human Kinetics Publishers, P.O. Box 2503, Windsor, ON N8Y 4S2
1-800-465-7301 (in Canada only)

Europe: Human Kinetics Publishers (Europe) Ltd., P.O. Box IW14,
Leeds LS16 6TR, England
0532-781708

Australia: Human Kinetics Publishers, P.O. Box 80, Kingswood 5062,
South Australia
618-374-0433

New Zealand: Human Kinetics Publishers, P.O. Box 105-231,
Auckland 1
(09) 309-2259

The poem "To an Athlete Dying Young" on p. 17 is from *The Collected Poems of A.E. Housman* by A.E. Housman. Copyright 1940, © 1965 by Holt, Rinehart and Winston. Copyright © 1967, 1968 by Robert E. Symons. Reprinted by permission of Henry Holt and Company, Inc.

For Ethan, Eliz, and Carm

Contents

About the Author

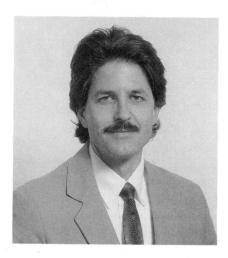

John Heil is a psychologist with the Lewis-Gale Clinic and the coordinator of psychological services for the Lewis-Gale Hospital Pain Center in Roanoke, Virginia. He experienced the problems and frustrations of sport injuries during his college career as a long-distance runner. This personal perspective has motivated him to concentrate on the psychology of sport injuries and helps him balance his professional psychologist's perspective with that of the injured athlete.

Dr. Heil received his doctor of arts degree from Lehigh University in 1982. In 1987, he completed a postdoctoral fellowship in the Division of Pain and Behavioral Medicine at the University of Utah School of Medicine. He developed a special counseling program for athletes at Radford University and a behavioral medicine consultation service for athletes at the University of Utah.

Dr. Heil provides psychological services for athletes and coaches through his private practice with Lewis-Gale Clinic and through consultation with the United States Fencing Association, the Commonwealth Games of Virginia, and the Lewis-Gale Foundation's Sports Wellness Committee. He is a member of the Association for the Advancement of Applied Sport Psychology and the American Psychological Association's Division of Exercise and Sport Psychology.

About the Contributors

Mark B. Andersen, PhD, is a licensed psychologist in the School of Physical and Health Education at the University of Wyoming. He has published in the areas of athletic injury, perception, and gender roles. His interests also include the supervision of sport psychology services. In his free time he enjoys sailing and cross-country skiing.

Bill Bean, ATC, PT, MS, is the head athletic trainer at the University of Utah. His academic interests are focused on sports medicine and physical therapy. His favorite leisure activities include fly fishing and skiing.

John J. Bowman, PhD, is the director of the Mind Plus Muscle Institute for Applied Sport Psychology in Port Jefferson Station, New York, where he conducts programs in performance enhancement and injury management for athletes. Bowman is on the teaching faculty of the Department of Physical Education, SUNY at Stony Brook, and is a member of the clinical faculty of the Department of Psychiatry at University Hospital in Stony Brook.

Perry G. Fine, MD, is an associate professor in the Department of Anesthesiology and an instructor of advanced cardiac life support at the University of Utah Medical Center, an attending physician at the University of Utah Pain Management Center, and medical director at the Hospice of Salt Lake. He is also a team physician for the University of Utah football team.

Juergen Froehlich, MD, has a professional background in internal medicine and sports medicine in Germany. He has done regular physical examinations and performance tests of world-class athletes in many sports, particularly swimming, triathlon, and water polo. His research has focused on energy metabolism, sport immunology, and issues of overtraining. He recently accepted a position as senior research physican in clinical research at Genentech, Inc., in South San Francisco and is continuing in California his successful career as a master swimmer.

Keith Henschen, PED, is a professor in exercise and sport science at the University of Utah. He has published more than 150 articles and 11 book chapters and has made over 200 presentations on sport psychology. He has worked with numerous national governing bodies of sport and with world-class and professional athletes. His leisure interests include travel, reading, jogging, and watching sporting activities.

Arthur G. Lipman, PharD, is a professor of clinical pharmacy at the University of Utah and is on staff with the Pain Management Center at University Hospital in Salt Lake City. He sits on two panels for the U.S. Department of Health and Human Services, the Acute Pain Management Guideline Panel and the Cancer-Related Pain Management Guideline Panel. Lipman is also editor of the *Journal of Pharmaceutical Care in Pain Symptom Control*.

Geoff Petrie is senior vice president of operations for the Portland Trail Blazers. He has been a player, an assistant coach, and a radio broadcaster in the NBA.

J. Richard Steadman, MD, is a partner at the Steadman Hawkins Clinic in Vail, Colorado, and chairman of the Steadman Sports Medicine Foundation, a center where orthopedists from around the world come to learn and practice new surgical techniques. Steadman is involved in the American Academy of Orthopaedic Surgeons, the American Orthopaedic Society for Sports Medicine, the Herodicus Society, and the ACL Study Group. Currently a member of the Sports Medicine Committee for the U.S. Alpine Team, he also served as team physician for the 1976, 1984, and 1988 Winter Olympics.

Jean M. Williams is a professor in the Department of Exercise and Sport Sciences at the University of Arizona. She has edited two books and has published numerous articles in refereed journals. Her primary research areas are psychology of injury, group dynamics, and the relationship of psychological states to performance. She is president-elect of the Association for the Advancement of Applied Sport Psychology.

Preface

Injury is one of the most significant obstacles to successful athletic performance. Because injury is virtually a daily concern in sport, its scope as a problem is broad and far-reaching. Injury downtime and career termination are the most salient aspects of this problem. However, the effects on the psychological well-being of the athlete and on subsequent performance are noteworthy as well, although less readily apparent. The ability to resist injury and to rehabilitate well when injury occurs is fundamental to longevity in sport and to the full realization of athletic potential.

I was first exposed to sport injury as a competitive athlete. Although fortunate to receive quality medical care and support from my coaches, I was impressed by the sense of uncertainty about the eventual outcome as well as by my limited understanding of how injury was caused and treated. I came to realize that I had a significant role to play in the management of my injury despite my limited understanding. Subsequent experience as a coach and physical educator reinforced my initial impressions about sport injury. As my experiential knowledge base grew, so did my awareness of the varied ways in which injury influences the athlete's ability to perform.

As a health professional, my initial experience with injured athletes was in the role of a sport psychologist. I quickly realized that the performance-enhancement approaches typically used with the healthy athlete were also effective with the injured athlete, although some modification was necessary. However, it was also apparent that in some cases additional intervention was needed. Subsequently, I completed training in clinical psychology as a behavioral medicine specialist focusing on injury and illness management. I was surprised to see that so little had been done to apply this well-developed base of knowledge and practice to the special needs of athletes. The recognition of this void prompted the writing of this text.

The goal of this work is to present a practical applied guide to the psychology of sport injury that is comprehensive, systematic, and coherent. While focused ostensibly on the sport participant, this work applies generally to anyone for whom effective performance relies on physical and mental prowess. To accomplish this, the book integrates the largely applied and anecdotal work in sport psychology with the more formal literature of behavioral medicine and sports medicine. Key principles and practices from these disciplines are synthesized and presented in a way that is relevant to the distinct needs of the athlete. In so doing, I have relied heavily on my own personal experience and the experiences shared with me by colleagues, many of whom have contributed to this text.

This work is equally directed to the sport psychologist and the clinical psychologist, with the assumption that those working with athletes within either of these specialties should be prepared to treat injury. Prior knowledge of both sport psychology and clinical psychology is helpful, and readers are encouraged to cross over disciplines and extend their knowledge base. Literature referenced in the text may be used to extend what the reading of this work begins. This book is also written for the physician and the sports medicine specialist (i.e., sport physical therapist or athletic trainer), based on the assumption that medical treatment and rehabilitation have an important psychological impact on the athlete. Given the straightforward and practical approach with which this book is written, I believe that athletes and coaches can also benefit from a selected reading, especially where this is done in consultation with a psychologist.

My strong impression is that the physician and the sports medicine specialist have unique roles to play in the psychological management of the athlete. Injury is most effectively managed with a team approach between physicians, sports medicine specialists, and psychologists, which provides better continuity of care and better quality of care. The team approach works best when each member's knowledge base extends beyond his or her own discipline. Thus, this book encompasses not just psychology but also medical information of use to the psychologist. The book also includes specific recommendations regarding psychological intervention in a format that is of practical value to the physician and sports medicine specialist.

To accomplish these objectives, I found it necessary to create a text of substantial breadth, as reflected in content and authorship. There are 19 chapters organized into six parts that examine psychological perspectives on injury, behavioral risk factors, the assessment of injury, the treatment of injury, the sports medicine team, and biomedical issues. There are three chapters written by physicians, and one each by a pharmacologist, an athlete, and a sports medicine specialist. To provide a sense of continuity and coherence, 12 chapters are authored by the editor. To offer a diversity of opinion, contributions are provided by nine other psychologists, primarily in a case review format.

The foundations of a psychology of sport injury are presented in an introductory chapter. This is followed by Part I, a series of differing perspectives on injury that includes chapters by an athlete, a physician, and a psychologist. Part II contains chapters on psychosocial risk factors and overtraining syndrome. Part III is introduced with a chapter that reviews a general framework for psychological assessment. This is followed by more practically oriented chapters on the use of methods and measures and on matching the diagnostic approach to the athlete's injury. Part IV, which discusses the treatment of injury, is the most lengthy one. Its five chapters present strategies for intervention in routine injuries as well as in those for which severity or problems in rehabilitation necessitate specialized treatment. This section concludes with a case study review that includes input from a variety of practitioners. Part V, which discusses the sports medicine team, includes chapters on patient management and on the referral and coordination of care. In Part VI, which presents biomedical issues, chapters discuss the biology of pain and the use of medications in the treatment of pain and injury. A final chapter summarizes key concepts and looks at the future of the psychology of sport injury.

It is my hope that this book will stimulate interest in the psychology of sport injury within both medicine and psychology and will lead to more frequent and effective psychological treatment for the injured athlete.

Acknowledgments

I would like to express my appreciation to those who have directed and assisted me in the preparation of this text.

For their review and critical comments I wish to thank my Lewis-Gale Clinic colleagues, Ed Waybright of neurology, Bert Spetzler of orthopedics, Darrell Powledge of occupational medicine, and Steve Strosnider of counseling and psychology.

Special thanks go to the clerical and secretarial staff of Lewis-Gale Clinic, especially Sherry Robertson, and to the staff of the Lewis-Gale Hospital Library.

I also wish to express my appreciation to Olle Larsson of Rowmark Ski Academy, Salt Lake City; Doug Fonder of Sport Design Associates, Roanoke, Virginia; Scot Russell of the University of Utah; Jim Lanter of the Veterans Administration Medical Center, Salem, Virginia; Jim Schmidt of Scandia Centrum, Charlottesville, Virginia; George Kish of Roanoke, Virginia; and Lewis Armistead of Roanoke Memorial Hospital.

For their counsel, I express my gratitude to David Shapiro of Safety First and Less Stress, Colmar Manor, Maryland; and Tommy Spencer of Spencer & Filson, Lexington, Virginia.

My appreciation also goes to the many athletes and coaches with whom I have had the pleasure to work—for sharing with me their enthusiasm and desire for excellence.

I would like to thank my family and friends for their patience and understanding.

For my earliest lessons in the psychology of sport injury, I offer my heartfelt thanks to Jim Matthews.

Credits

Table 4.1 is adapted with permission from "Coping With the Stresses of Illness" by F. Cohen and R.S. Lazarus. In *Health Psychology: A Handbook: Theories, Applications, and Challenges of a Psychological Approach to the Health Care System* (pp. 217-255) by G.C. Stone, F. Cohen, N.E. Adler, and Associates (Eds.), 1979, San Francisco: Jossey-Bass. Copyright 1979 by Jossey-Bass.

Figure 4.2 is adapted with permission from "Concepts of Pain" by J. Loeser. In *Chronic Low Back Pain* (p. 146) by M. Stanton-Hicks and R.A. Boas (Eds.), 1982, New York: Raven. Copyright 1982 by Raven Press.

Figure 5.1 is adapted with permission from "A Model of Stress and Athletic Injury: Prediction and Prevention" by M.B. Andersen and J.M. Williams, 1988, *Sport and Exercise Psychology*, **10**(3), pp. 294-306. Copyright 1988 by Human Kinetics Publishers, Inc.

Figures 8.1-8.7 are adapted with permission from "Psychological Characterization of the Elite Distance Runner" by W.P. Morgan and P.J. O'Conner, 1977, *Annals of the New York Academy of Science*, **301**, pp. 382-403. Copyright 1977 by the *Annals of the New York Academy of Science*.

Figures 8.8 and 8.9 are adapted with permission from "The Pain Drawing as an Aid to the Psychologic Evaluation of Patients with Low-Back Pain" by A.O. Ransford, D. Cairns, and V. Mooney, 1976, *Spine*, **1**, pp. 127-134. Copyright 1976 by J.B. Lippincott.

Table 10.3 is adapted with permission from "Examining Social Support Networks Among Athletes: Description and Relationship to Stress" by L.B. Rosenfeld, J.N. Richman, and C.J. Hardy, 1989, *The Sport Psychologist*, **3**, pp. 23-33. Copyright 1989 by Human Kinetics Publishers.

Table 11.2 is adapted with permission from "Overall and Relative Efficacy of Cognitive Strategies in Attenuating Pain" by E. Fernandez and D.C. Turk, 1986, August, in a paper presented at the 94th annual convention of the American Psychological Association, Washington, DC.

Table 13.1 was developed by Heil, Wakefield, Reed, Knuppel, Kay, and Minter at the Lewis-Gale Pain Center, Roanoke, VA, 1990. Requests to use Table 13.1 should be forwarded to the aforementioned authors at the Lewis-Gale Pain Center.

Figure 16.1 is adapted with permission from *Sport in Society: Issues and Controversies* (p. 303) by J.J. Coakley, 1986, St. Louis: Mosby. Copyright 1986 by Mosby-Year Book.

Table 16.1 is reprinted with permission from *Guidelines in Children's Sports* by R. Martens and V. Seefeldt (Eds.), 1979, Washington, DC: American Alliance for Health, Physical Education, and Recreation. Copyright 1979 by AAHPERD.

Table 16.2 is adapted with permission from *Parenting Your Superstar* (pp. 169-179) by R.J. Rotella and L.K. Bunker, 1987, Champaign, IL: Leisure Press. Copyright 1987 by R.J. Rotella and L.K. Bunker.

Figures 17.1-17.3 are adapted with permission from "The Pathways and Mechanisms of Pain and Analysis: A Review and Clinical Perspective" by P.G. Fine and B.D. Hare, 1985, *Hospital Formulary*, 20, pp. 973-976. Copyright © 1985 by Advanstar Communications.

1
CHAPTER

Sport Psychology, the Athlete at Risk, and the Sports Medicine Team

John Heil

The threat of injury is ever-present in sport. The ability to remain relatively injury-free and to recover rapidly when injured is important to any athlete's longevity and success. Given the frequency of injury and its often devastating impact, we need greater understanding of the role of psychological forces in injury and the value of psychological rehabilitation methods.

The groundwork for a psychology of sport injury has been laid by a series of developments in sport, including

- a growing appreciation of the scope, severity, and underlying causes of injury,
- the development of sports medicine as a multidisciplinary specialty,
- the emergence of a psychology for performance enhancement in sport, and
- the growth of a behavioral medicine.

I have two general objectives for this introductory chapter. The first is to identify athletes as a special population at tremendous risk for injury. Psychological predispositions and consequences play a critical role in determining the ultimate impact of injury. My second objective is to trace the emergence of psychological intervention in sport performance and in injury management and to clarify the role of the psychologist on the sports medicine team.

Special Considerations in the Treatment of Athletes

A thorough and systematic approach to the psychological treatment of injury is based on an understanding of the challenges, pressures, and hazards that shape the athlete's world. This understanding begins with an appreciation of sport as a subculture where rules that are implicitly understood but seldom spoken guide behavior. Consistent expectations for high performance are nowhere more present than in sport. Concepts of behavior change as reflected in the clinical and research concepts of "within normal limits" and "statistical significance" lose meaning in the world of sport, where small differences in behavior can be of great importance.

The subtle interplay of psychological and physiological factors is acutely evident in sport, requiring a multidisciplinary approach to managing sport injury and related problems in athlete functioning. This team approach is part of a growing trend with special populations and one that is natural to the sport environment. Psychological services, in particular, need to be offered along a continuum of care that incorporates both a health-oriented psychology of performance and a clinical psychology of behavior disorder.

Sport as Subculture

Sport is a world unto itself, especially for the serious competitor. It is marked by the pursuit of excellence, emotional intensity, and expectations regarding risk taking. It is useful to think of sport as a subculture in which behavior is guided by a unique set of principles, which are implicitly observed and fundamental to acceptance and success. Subtleties of language and behavior distinguish the insider from the outsider. Special privileges and recognition are accorded to the elite competitor. The path to elite status involves "survival of the fittest." From youth sport through high school and college sport and on to varying degrees of professional sport, the climb up the ladder of competitive excellence becomes steeper and more challenging, leaving room for fewer and fewer athletes. Injury figures significantly influencing who will survive.

The idea of athleticism as heroism is woven into the very fabric of sport and dates to the dawn of competitive sport. It is reported that following an important victory by the Greek army over a Persian invasion force, Pheidippides ran from the battle site at Marathon to Athens to announce the victory. As he delivered this news he collapsed and died. His effort is emulated in today's marathon, and more importantly, his behavior reflects the importance long placed on intensity, determination, and sacrifice in sport. In modern sport athletes are reminded "no pain, no gain, no fame." They are encouraged to play with pain, to give 110%, to be mentally tough. The expectation for high performance and maximal effort permeates the world of sport. In high-visibility sports, the fans and media join the athlete and coach in evaluating performance by these standards. As a consequence, the athlete is implicitly encouraged to take risks that potentially impact both physical and mental well-being.

Athletes are also encouraged to seek the ideal body for performance, and the relationship between body type and sport success is evident. Pursuit of the ideal body type can lead to extremes of behavior, such as the use of ergogenic drugs and extreme weight-control measures, that carry substantial health risks as well as increased injury risk.

The importance of large muscle mass in sports such as football has led to increasing use of anabolic steroids and related substances. Concerns regarding long-term medical side effects and short-term effects on mood as well as withdrawal-like symptoms have fueled the controversy that surrounds steroid use (Lubell, 1989b; Tricker & Cook, 1990; Wadler & Hainline, 1989). There is evidence that steroid-using athletes are more prone to soft-tissue injury that occurs during routine activity.

Dancers, as well as women who compete in sports where attractiveness of physical form can influence scoring (e.g., gymnastics and figure skating), are most at risk for eating disorders. Among the array of medical problems that can arise from eating disorders are changes that render the athlete more prone to stress fractures (Lloyd et al., 1986; "Repeated stress fractures," 1989). In that large muscle mass for men and a slender form for women reflect prevailing cultural sex stereotypes, the pursuit of the ideal body is a reflection of a more broadly based societal problem. However, the added pressures of competitive sport render the athlete all the more vulnerable to these patterns of behavior. Attitudes and expectations in sport combined with the inherent risk of sport itself make injury a common event.

The Performing Artist as Athlete

Legendary ballet master Joffrey referred to his dancers as artistic athletes, reflecting the fundamental athleticism of ballet. However, because aesthetics is the final standard of quality in the performing arts, the importance of underlying physical prowess often goes unrecognized. The need for finely developed motor skill as well as emotional intensity and the need to cope effectively with the stress of performance are shared by the athlete and the performing artist. The worlds of visual art and sport inasmuch as the mental preparation and attitudes regarding the pursuit of excellence are quite similar in these endeavors (Koesters & Heil, 1986).

In an evaluation of the physical skills necessary for optimal performance of a variety of athletic activities, prepared at the Institute of Sportsmedicine and Athletic Trauma (Nicholas, 1976), ballet and other forms of dance were judged comparable to sports in terms of depth and diversity of athletic skill.

The physical aspects of actor training and theatrical performance also often go unappreciated. Theatrical performance does at times require displays of physical prowess in the form of stunts, sword play, and other forms of stage combat. Various physical techniques are typically incorporated into actor training (Spolin, 1963).

Physical injury is equally devastating to the athlete and the artist. Dancers and musicians, like sport participants, commonly suffer from overuse syndromes. Dancers are prone to acute injury as well, which is related to the intense athletic demands of practice and performance. Among musicians, lengthy practice often in awkward positions is a significant factor contributing to injury. For musicians, injury may arise not only as a direct consequence of overuse but also indirectly due to compensatory posture changes that occur as a consequence of fatigue or persistent pain.

Sports medicine should, therefore, be considered a medicine for the arts (Strauss, 1989). In fact, the development of a dance-oriented sports medicine is well underway (Shell, 1986). For all performers, medical care is governed by an overriding concern: expedient return to play. The vigorous use of restorative surgical approaches and rehabilitation for the performer, whether athlete, dancer, or musician, is advocated (Cross, Pinczewski, & Bokor, 1989).

Excellence: Not "Within Normal Limits"

Those devoted to the pursuit of excellence (in sport and other endeavors) will inevitably judge performance by a standard more lofty and stringent than that reflected in normative behavior. A distinctive element of sport is the tremendous importance of what in day-to-day life might amount to trivial differences in time and distance. The motto "citius, altius, fortius" ("faster, higher, stronger") emphasizes this. Exquisite physical and mental prowess is the hallmark of sport performance, and even slight decrements in physical and mental skills can affect performance. In essence, variations in psychological and physical functions that are "within normal limits" for daily behavior may be of critical significance in the highly demanding arena of sport. Even subtle or transient disruptions in mental and emotional state may impact physical performance. These can be precipitated by a number of factors including pain, fear of injury, and dysphoria.

Despite the inherently stressful nature of injury, athletes generally tend to rehabilitate well and return to play without evident complication. However, the speed of physical recovery from injury and related mental recovery varies. Hastening an athlete's recovery to optimal form by a few days or even a week can significantly impact the success of the athlete as well as the team. Factors that influence performance during competition (e.g., pain or fear of injury) can also affect the process of injury rehabilitation. Consequently the management of "within normal limits" variations in the psychological factors that bear upon the effectiveness of rehabilitation is an important aspect of injury treatment. This is consistent with the basic goal of sports medicine: speedy and safe return to play. Even when recovery from injury is successful, psychological intervention is justified if treatment leads to a faster or less stressful rehabilitation or to a better understanding of pain and injury management.

The Athlete at Risk

An estimated 17 million sport injuries occur yearly among American athletes (Booth, 1987). The estimated 1 million yearly injuries in high school football include about 10 fatalities (Mueller & Blyth, 1987). Almost one in two collegiate football players suffers an injury severe enough to lose playing time (Zemper, 1989). A third of the nation's 15 million joggers sustain a musculoskeletal injury each year (Booth, 1987). Nearly half of habitual runners experience lower extremity injury every year (Macera et al., 1989). And each year, 1,000 spinal cord injuries occur when swimmers dive into pools and other bodies of water (Samples, 1989). In addition to physical injury, athletes risk medical and psychological "injuries" as a consequence of sport participation. Overtraining syndrome, eating disorders, and drug abuse are prime examples. These have a direct impact on health and performance and in turn increase the risk of physical injury.

These details on sport injury are drawn from the growing body of sport epidemiology research and injury surveillance (systematic attempts to monitor injury occurrence on an ongoing basis in selected sports; Damron, Hoerner, & Shaw, 1986). Although these developments in data collection are relatively new, they have already proven their worth. Work by the National Center for Catastrophic Sports Injury Research (Mueller & Cantu, 1990) in identifying the frequency and circumstances of serious injury has prompted effective injury-reducing changes in some sports. Also, recognizing the tremendous emotional and financial costs of sport injuries, the National Institute of Arthritis and Musculoskeletal and Skin Diseases has designated sport injuries as a major health issue (Booth, 1987).

The Psychophysiological Mechanism of Risk

Many psychological and physical factors interact to influence the risk of injury and the effectiveness of rehabilitation. The loss of playing time and its potential impact on success as well as pain and the rigors of rehabilitation are significant sources of psychological distress arising from physical injury. Psychological distress can also sensitize the athlete to pain, especially when recovery from injury is prolonged due to severity or reinjury. Psychological factors also appear to be involved in the muscular guarding that occurs as a sequela to injury.

Interacting psychological and physical factors are intensified during competition. Psychological stressors, such as fear of injury or reinjury, may elicit a cycle of physical and psychological effects that result in worsened performance (Nideffer, 1983). Fear may diminish concentration and self-confidence and produce physiological changes such as increased muscle tension and overarousal. In conjunction with this, the athlete also tends to become preoccupied with physical sensations arising from the site of injury or with slight decrements in performance (e.g., momentary loss of balance). These sensations may be intensified by the psychophysiological dynamics of the fear response, and the athlete may perceive them as signs of injury. These perceptions affect performance through decreased efficiency in the biomechanics of skill execution, poor use of energy resources, and decreased attention to performance-related factors. The athlete's sense of poor performance may then exacerbate the initial precipitating physiological and psychological factors, which leads to a mutually reinforcing, self-perpetuating cycle (see Figure 1.1). For example, awareness of autonomic changes such as accelerated heart rate may distract the athlete. Increased pain awareness, or a decrease in self-confidence, may lead to further acceleration of heart rate. Furthermore, there also appears to be a potentiating effect among physiological mechanisms as well as among psychological ones. For example, muscle tension and autonomic changes may perpetuate one another as may the skill-based and interpretive psychological mechanisms.

This phenomenon may be manifested acutely, as described previously, or in a more chronic form, in which the same general pattern of physiological and psychological changes takes place but is more subtle and prolonged. This is best conceived of in the context of the general adaptation syndrome described by Selye (1956), which explains the influence of stress on health. The chronic form is more insidious in its etiology, more difficult to detect, and less readily modified. Consequently, early identification of such changes and timely treatment are quite important.

The Subclinical Psychological Adjustment Syndrome

Jean-Claude Killy, the premier Alpine skier of his time, has told of an injury that left him unable to practice as an important competition approached (Suinn, 1976). He has reported that his only preparation for this race was to rehearse it mentally. His performance proved to be outstanding, attesting to the importance of mental readiness for performance. Although few athletes possess Killy's combination of resourcefulness and sheer talent, all hope for fast and remarkably effective recoveries from

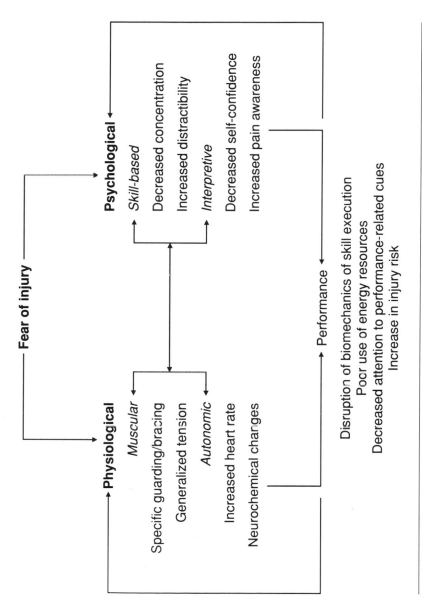

Figure 1.1   The mind-body connection: a psychophysiological model of risk.

injury. This anecdote raises questions as to when psychological intervention is appropriate. Typically, it is used to alleviate psychological suffering and disorder. However, sports medicine promises more—specifically, as speedy a recovery (physical and psychological) as possible. It follows that psychological intervention need not be limited to clearly defined cases of overt adjustment problems. Although not feasible or desirable for all injuries, psychological intervention is clearly beneficial in many situations even where the need is not readily apparent. The subclinical syndrome, subsequently described, identifies those likely to benefit significantly from psychological treatment in the absence of clear-cut behavioral disorder.

Traditional medical and psychological approaches to disorder are notable for their focus on disease and disorder manifested in large deviations from the norm; from this, treatment follows. Smaller deviations from the norm are less likely to be immediately disruptive to the person, and thus they receive less attention, either resolving naturally or continuing for long periods without notice by others (Bortz, 1984). The subclinical syndrome is identified by these relatively small deviations that predict diminished performance and health but fall short of disorder as traditionally defined (Kerlan, 1978).

The subclinical psychological adjustment syndrome is most likely to occur where injury is severe, requires surgery or a long period of rehabilitation, or is perceived as a threat to the athlete's career. The underlying mechanism is a relatively slowed process of emotional reorganization following injury. This may result in a delay in mental readiness for return to play, ongoing psychological distress, and slowed physical recovery. The magnitude of emotional distress may be obvious only under careful scrutiny. This occurs when the athlete either intentionally refuses to acknowledge the distress for fear of appearing weak or denies his or her distress so strongly at a personal level that he or she is unaware of the emotional impact of injury—even though it may be apparent to others. To identify this syndrome, the practitioner should look carefully for a subset of the following behavioral signs that may be only subtly manifested:

- Unusual pain complaints
- Sleep disturbance
- Fatigue
- Moodiness
- Situational anxiety
- Compliance problems
- Rehabilitation setbacks
- Excessive or awkward optimism
- Poor understanding of rehabilitation

Most who suffer subclinical syndromes will recover effectively but slowly. Others will appear to recover well but will never quite return to their prior levels of ability. Some will go on to develop full-blown clinical syndromes. Timely psychological intervention will hasten recovery and prevent the development of more significant adjustment problems.

Historical Foundations of a Sports Medicine of the Mind

All those involved in sports readily recognize the critical role of the mental game. Although it is most significant where competitors are well matched on physical ability, it is an important factor at all levels of sport. Simultaneous developments in sports medicine, behavioral medicine, and sport psychology have paved the way for the emergence of a sports medicine team that treats mind and body.

Sports Medicine

Sports medicine is a relatively new discipline. Its roots are uncertain, but it appears to date at least as far back as the era of the formal duel of honor (Baldick, 1985). It was common practice during the heyday of dueling to have a physician available to deliver medical care promptly at the conclusion of the duel. Looking backward even further in time, Galen treated the athletic injuries of gladiators in the 2nd century (Gayuna & Hoerner, 1986).

Since the late 1960s, sports medicine has emerged as a specialized area of study. Sports medicine and the related sport sciences focus on the benefits and the demands of athletic participation and on the special needs of athletes. The scope of sports medicine is broad, involving not only diagnosis and treatment but also prevention and performance enhancement.

The diagnosis and treatment of injury have been improved substantially through interrelated developments in special techniques and technology. For example, the development of arthroscopy, which allows a surgeon to see into and operate upon the knee and other joints through a small incision, has led to more rapid recovery from injury following surgery. New computerized muscle-testing devices allow more accurate determination of rehabilitation progress and of the athlete's readiness to return to play. The development of improved conditioning techniques and special protective equipment as well as other preventive measures is also noteworthy. Speedy, safe return to play has emerged as the hallmark of sports medicine.

Behavioral Medicine

Behavioral medicine involves the application of the practices and principles of clinical psychology to the management of medical problems

(Blanchard, 1982; Pomerleau, 1982). Its emergence in the 1970s began with the application of behavioral techniques (that were initially designed for the treatment of mental health problems) to medical disorders. The development of behavioral medicine was encouraged by the growing recognition of the roles of exercise, diet, and other behaviors in illness and injury. There was also an increasing awareness that chronic diseases need to be managed in lieu of a cure. Further impetus was provided by the development of biofeedback as an applied technology allowing precise measurement and control of changes in the psychophysiological substrates of behavior. The initial areas of application included obesity, smoking, hypertension, and headache. This was followed by work with insomnia, chronic pain, asthma, peripheral vascular disease, and coronary prone behavior. More recently work has been directed toward gastrointestinal disorders, arthritis, diabetes, and cancer.

Behavioral medicine encompasses not only evaluation and treatment but also prevention. Systematic approaches to manage compliance with prescribed medical regimens have been developed. There is also growing interest in the role of exercise in the management of medical problems. Practitioners of behavioral medicine attempt to achieve specific change in target behaviors through programs that are goal oriented, that are time limited, and that place the client/patient in an active, skill-based role.

Initial research on the cost-effectiveness of behavioral medicine has been encouraging. Timely psychological interventions appear to decrease the use of medical services by the "worried well," who constitute a large proportion of those seeking outpatient medical treatment (Cummings, 1985). It has been demonstrated that psychological services in conjunction with medical treatment for physical disorders decrease hospital costs. Provision of behavioral medicine services to sufferers of chronic disease has resulted in improved quality of care and lower overall costs (Schlesinger, Mumford, Glass, Patrick, & Sharfstein, 1983). Psychological intervention also has been shown to reduce length of hospitalization following surgery and heart attack (Mumford, Schlesinger, & Glass, 1982).

Sport Psychology

Since the late 1960s sport psychology has emerged as an interdisciplinary stepchild of psychology and the biologically based sport sciences (Browne & Mahoney, 1984). As an academic discipline it is broadly concerned with the relationship between psychological behavior and sport and exercise. Its three related focal areas of study—social issues (e.g., aggression, sex roles), health and well-being, and performance enhancement—are reflected in the organizational structure of the Association for the Advancement of Applied Sport Psychology. The most distinctive focus is the applied science of performance enhancement, which deals with motivation, leadership, team building, group cohesion, and mental training. The use of mental training methods has captured the interest of growing numbers of athletes and coaches and is part of a trend toward specialization in sport. Like the strength and conditioning coach who works with the basics of physical ability, the sport psychologist works with the basics of mental ability.

Sport psychology and behavioral medicine share much in common including a strong goal orientation, an active role for the patient/client in the treatment, and application of self-directed skill-based approaches to change in specific target behaviors. Distinct elements of sport psychology are the recognition of the coach's important role in athlete management and the importance of providing services on site at practices and competition. Initial empirical evidence of the effectiveness of the use of sport psychology as a means of enhancing athletic performance is promising (Druckman & Bjork, 1991). The greatest boost to continued use of performance-enhancement approaches in general, and mental training in particular, is the enthusiasm of the players and coaches who feel they have benefited.

Although the initial and distinctive focus of sport psychology has been on enhancing performance in the healthy, well-adjusted athlete, the need for a clinical psychology of sport has become increasingly evident. The growing involvement of the sport psychologist with the athlete has led to a greater understanding of the pressures of sport performance and the unique hazards that athletes face. Injury is but one example; alcohol and drug use, eating disorders, overtraining, and psychological stress are others. These problems interact with injury, functioning as predisposing risk factors and as sequelae to injury. Consequently, a psychology of sport injury must be developed to address these problems.

The Sports Medicine Team

There is increasing use of team-based approaches in health care services. In the multidisciplinary team approach, a better quality of care can be provided because of greater breadth of services, broader bases for treatment decision making, and improved continuity of care. The importance of a sports medicine for the mind as well as the body is increasingly recognized (Munnings, 1987). Because of the many risks that sport presents to the medical and psychological well-being of the athlete, a team approach is necessary, and psychologists are an important part of the team. However, a team approach to sport injury that includes routine psychological intervention is far more often the exception than the rule. Four fundamental assumptions guide the comprehensive team-based approach recommended here:

- Sports medicine is a multispecialty discipline amenable to a team approach.

- The interventions of all members of the sports medicine team have a psychological impact.
- Psychological recovery is an essential element in injury rehabilitation.
- Optimal treatment outcomes are based on the careful coordination of care.

The treatment team is composed of the sport physician, the sports medicine specialist (e.g., physical therapist or athletic trainer), the sport psychologist, and the clinical psychologist (Heil, 1987). The natural alliance between the athletic trainer and the sports medicine physician based on a common medical perspective of injury is already well established. However, the relationships among other specialists in this team need further definition and direction for development. Collaborative interactions between the athletic trainer and the sport psychologist and between the physician and the clinical psychologist have grown with the development of sport psychology and behavioral medicine.

The relationship between the sport psychologist and the clinical psychologist is currently being scrutinized by both professional groups (Monahan, 1987). The sport psychologist tends to draw upon a broad background in sport sciences that is usually oriented specifically toward performance enhancement. The clinical psychologist is trained in the treatment of clinical syndromes and adjustment problems. Because the sport psychologist and clinical psychologist offer overlapping domains of expertise, there are roles to be played by each in the psychological management of injury.

It is useful to think of the athlete, the coach, and in some circumstances the parents as an extended treatment team. The athlete is far from a passive observer in the rehabilitation process. Involving the athlete more actively motivates the athlete and makes rehabilitation a learning experience. Because the coach is the overall sports team leader, sports medicine will work best with his or her cooperation. The coach can contribute special knowledge of the athlete and the sport to the rehabilitation process. As caretakers of the minor athlete, parents need to be involved in treatment for practical as well as legal and ethical reasons. The younger the athlete, the more important the role of the parents.

Challenges to a team-based approach are substantial. Communication and coordination of care require a greater outlay of time, especially from the core team, and issues such as shared decision making and confidentiality can become quite complex. Nonetheless, the benefits far outweigh the potential problems.

Concluding Comments

This chapter has laid the groundwork for an understanding of issues that are of particular relevance to the injured athlete. A thorough approach to the psychology of sport injury rests upon an awareness of a number of factors. These include the significant impact of subtle decrements in psychological skills on sport performance, an appreciation of the interrelationships between psychological and physical factors, and sensitivity to the prevailing attitudes that shape sport performance. This chapter has presented a team-oriented approach to treatment and has emphasized the importance of a continuum of care from healthy to disordered behavior which incorporates medical and psychological interventions.

I
PART

Perspectives on Injury

Injury presents not only a physical problem but also a challenge to the maintenance of emotional equilibrium and to the athlete's mental game. It is widely recognized that typically the athlete is powerfully driven to return to play quickly. Related to this drive are implicit expectations that an athlete should be mentally tough, maintain a positive attitude, and play with pain. These expectations can discourage athletes from acknowledging emotional distress and can thus impair identification of injury adjustment problems.

Views on the nature of injury and treatment are presented in the following three chapters. In "Injury From the Athlete's Point of View," Geoff Petrie offers a candid and analytic view of injury based on his experiences as an athlete, a perspective enriched by his continued involvement with basketball in a variety of roles. Personal commentary on living with injury, the doctor-patient relationship, coping with surgery, decision making about return to play, and injury-forced retirement contributes a practical understanding of the meaning of injury to the athlete. He emphasizes the complexity and critical importance of the decision to return to play and provides recommendations for guiding athletes' participation in this process.

In "A Physician's Approach to the Psychology of Injury," Richard Steadman, an orthopedic surgeon, provides a clinical perspective on the psychology of the injured athlete. He proposes a multistage model of rehabilitation encompassing the preinjury period through return to play. He emphasizes the importance of psychological factors in treatment and identifies the psychological challenges of rehabilitation relative to his rehabilitation model. The chapter emphasizes a strong goal orientation as well as the importance of the athlete's taking an active role in rehabilitation, a role that includes input into decision making regarding surgery and return to play.

In "A Psychologist's View of the Personal Challenge of Injury," I present a formal psychological perspective on injury, describing the emotional and cognitive concomitants of injury and the roles of denial and pain and emphasizing their interrelationship and mutually reinforcing natures. The emotional reaction to injury is presented as a grief process triggered by injury that unfolds as the athlete progresses through the stages of rehabilitation. The chapter develops a cognitive schema of injury that provides a conceptual basis from which to understand certain pitfalls of injury.

2
CHAPTER

Injury From the Athlete's Point of View

Geoff Petrie

To an Athlete Dying Young

The time you won your town the race
We chaired you through the marketplace;
Man and boy stood cheering by,
And home we brought you shoulder-high.

To-day, the road all runners come,
Shoulder-high we bring you home,
And set you at your threshold down,
Townsman of a stiller town.

Smart lad, to slip betimes away
From fields where glory does not stay
And early though the laurel grows
It withers quicker than the rose.

Eyes the shady night has shut
Cannot see the record cut,
And silence sounds no worse than cheers
After earth has stopped the ears:

Now you will not swell the rout
Of lads that wore their honours out,
Runners whom renown outran
And the name died before the man.

So set, before its echoes fade,
The fleet foot on the sill of shade,
And hold to the low lintel up
The still-defended challenge cup.

And round that early-laurelled head
Will flock to gaze the strengthless dead,
And find unwithered on its curls
The garland briefer than a girl's.

Even though A.E. Housman's classic 1895 poem (Nims, 1983) refers to the premature death of a young athlete, it is included here because the specter of serious injury in modern-day athletics can spell almost immediate competitive athletic death in amateur and professional sports. The diagnosis, treatment, and rehabilitation of sport injuries have become a major growth industry, which is fueled by the tremendous social and economic emphasis that we place on competitive sport. The ongoing fitness boom has led more and more of the general population to seek the type of medical care that was once reserved for only the elite world-class athlete, and the demand for competent professional care will no doubt continue to increase. The major force propelling millions of people to engage in athletics is the health-related benefits that have been documented through many varied areas of research. A common thread of experience shared by all athletes from the weekend warrior to the professional is that when injury strikes, each is denied the opportunity to train or compete and is denied access to the benefits sport provides.

As a basketball player for the Portland Trailblazers I underwent five surgeries for recurrent knee problems, which eventually forced my retirement. Since retiring I have remained involved in basketball as a coach and instructor, broadcaster, and manager. Currently, I am a vice president in the Portland Trailblazers organization. From my days as an athlete to the present I have seen similar injury situations repeated and have seen athletes face similar challenges in coping with injury. While my initial response to my serious injury was emotional, I gradually developed a more analytic approach. I found it essential to differentiate between things that were within my control and things that were beyond it and to deal with each accordingly. The ability to do this and to develop an analytic problem solving style is important to success as an athlete. Drawing on my personal experience, I hope to provide some insight into the medical and psychological battleground that surrounds sport injuries.

The Meaning of Injury

Serious injury is one of the most emotionally and psychologically traumatic things that can happen to an athlete. Injury can take away an athlete's career at any time, and it threatens the feelings of invincibility and immortality that all young people have to some degree. Because athletes are so dependent upon their physical skills and because their identities are so wrapped up in their sport, injury can be tremendously threatening to them. There are some injuries from which a highly competitive athlete simply cannot recover, at least not to the point where he or she can return to a prior level of competition. In comparison, someone not involved in sports who sustains the same injury may be able to rehabilitate to the point of maintaining normal physical activity, and thus his or her life is relatively unchanged. The sense of loss is potentially greatest for top-level athletes at the peak of their competitive skills. The more time invested in sport and the greater the athlete's success, the harder it is ultimately to face serious injury. As the athlete ages, it becomes more difficult to recover effectively.

One of the saddest things to see is an injured athlete who attempts to compete, only to do so poorly. Some athletes refuse to give up sport and keep searching for a solution to the limits posed by injury, a solution that unfortunately does not exist. In the process they experience tremendous frustration.

Dealing with minor injury presents special problems as well. Pushing oneself to the limit is an expectation that is very much a part of the heritage of sport. This means not only playing well but also playing through pain and tolerating injury. How effectively each athlete deals with pain and injury varies a great deal and relates to his or her psyche.

Whether injury is minor or serious, the challenge it presents goes beyond the physical aspect of rehabilitation. It is complicated by the expectations and reactions of others, including teammates, coaches, medical staff, and media. With the strong media presence in top level sport, player behavior inadvertently becomes a part of the public domain. A negative reaction by the media, to a slow recovery from injury, for example, can be a cruel blow to a player.

Living With Injury

Injury is an everyday problem in sport. If every time athletes got a bump or a bruise they stopped playing, they would never achieve their maximum potential. Adding to the stress of injury is the cold reality that there are many people available to replace an injured player. It is just the nature of the game. In the NBA very few professional athletes who get a lot of playing time do not have some kind of physical complaint. This is true of pro athletes in general and occurs to a lesser but significant degree at other levels of competition. Athletes tend to be highly motivated to compete and have a strong desire to continue to do so in spite of injury. Most successful athletes are so driven to excel that they do whatever they can to return to play as quickly as possible. This may mean opting for radical or aggressive treatment approaches that provide the possibility of a quicker return to play, even though such approaches carry greater risk of reinjury. Many times the best treatment strategy is a conservative approach. Because of the many options available, it is important that the athlete be advised by coaches and physicians who can provide an objective point of view.

For some injured players, remaining close to teammates and other people in the sport organization and having their encouragement is a real benefit. To accomplish this the injured athlete can attend practices and team meetings and thus remain in some way a part of the team. However, some athletes will find it painful to watch other people compete at a sport they love when they cannot. That is why players should be allowed the freedom to exercise their own judgment in this area.

Dealing with injury is a very personal thing. Healing processes vary, as well as the amount of pain people experience. Two athletes can have the same injuries yet one will be able to play and the other will not. This is most evident in an injury that carries low risk of reinjury yet is very painful. Many athletes have the mental discipline to push pain aside and still concentrate on the job at hand, but others can't handle both. I think basketball great Bill Russell summed it up best when he said that you expect athletes to play hurt, you just don't want them to play injured.

The Doctor-Patient Relationship

The doctor-patient relationship is of great importance especially when the athlete has to make difficult decisions about treatment. Athletes need to feel confident that they are going to recover fully, and physicians need to remain positive yet realistic about rehabilitation.

Aside from providing purely medical services, the sport physician has a number of roles to play. The willingness to function as an educator, clearly and carefully laying out all the options in a given situation, is of great help. This enables athletes, who obviously do not have medical backgrounds, to make decisions that are in their best interest. At times the physician may have to protect the athlete's right to make decisions and help prevent others from putting pressure on the athlete to compete. At other times, it may be necessary to rein in an athlete who wants to compete and protect him or her from danger of reinjury. The bond that is the basis of the relationship between the physician and the athlete is built around the immediate and obvious needs of the injured athlete and the ability of the physician to meet these needs.

The success of a psychologist in a sport setting is also based on establishing a similar bond, and the athlete needs to understand how sport psychology can meet her or his needs. For example, the use of psychological testing can pose problems with trust if players don't understand the purpose and benefits of the testing or if players sense that testing is for the benefit of management and not necessarily for themselves. In contrast there are a lot of advantages to performance-enhancement techniques, which focus on goal setting and concentration. In general, athletes relate best to approaches that have been shown to lead to better personal performance statistics. It can be quite difficult to approach a player about seeing a sport psychologist, because this implies the presence of a problem that the player may not acknowledge. Athletes must feel that their interaction with the sport psychologist is for their benefit and not management's. When dealing with a personal emotional problem, it is critical that it all remain strictly between the player and the sport psychologist.

Surgery

Looking back at my first surgery, I realize that I had a tremendous amount of concern, which was based on a fear of the unknown. I found myself asking questions that had no clear answers: What are they going to find? Am I ever going to be able to play again? How much is it going to hurt?

I found a number of things very helpful, such as knowing what to expect at each stage of treatment, trust and confidence in my physician, and a positive attitude from the medical staff. My physician did a great job of explaining all the options to me, so I understood the potential risks and benefits of each possibility. With that information, I was able to make the choice that was best for me. Making a decision about surgery can be really complicated, and a player who wants to "comparison shop" can go to five different physicians and get five different opinions, which won't make the decision any easier. This is where a good relationship between the player and his or her personal physician is so important. It is much easier for an athlete to think through the possibilities with someone who knows the player personally and has special medical knowledge.

I ended up having five surgeries in all. Because I had reasonable success with my first surgery, the following surgeries did not scare me as much. I found that I could get accustomed to the regimen and know what to expect. I knew what I would have to do after surgery and what rehabilitation would be like. My experience is that knowing what to expect and trust in one's physician are both of great importance.

Return to Play

Making the decision about return to play is as important as it is complicated. There are three types of injury situations. The first type includes "self-limiting" injuries; an athlete with such an injury is physically unable

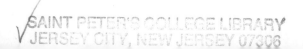

to play, so there are no difficult decisions to make. The second type of injury involves a great deal of pain but little danger of reinjury; there is a potential problem for some athletes. The third type of injury falls into a "gray" area where there is no clear best decision about whether to compete.

The coach, physician, and player need to share in the decision-making process. When the coach's judgment of the player's competitive status and the physician's determination of his or her medical status coincide with the athlete's sense of readiness, the decision is relatively straightforward. However, in most cases the athlete will want to compete before either the physician or coach thinks the athlete is ready. The physician's concern for the player's safety is obvious. No matter what athletes say about being ready to play, there are some situations where the coach knows that the athlete is not going to be able to compete. The athlete should not return to play until all three agree that he or she is ready.

When injury occurs at a particularly critical time in the competitive season or in an athlete's career, the decision whether to play or rehabilitate is especially difficult. If a player is in the seventh game of an NBA Championship and has an injury in the "gray" area, what should he do? This is a very tough decision to make. The player may feel able to play one more game, yet there is the risk that something will go wrong and the player will end up with a more serious injury. In this situation, all the options must be put on the table and the associated benefits and risks examined as well as they can be. When a significant medical risk is involved, the final decision about returning to play should be purely between the player and the medical people. It is not right for the team, the organization, or anyone else to put pressure on the athlete to perform while injured.

Sometimes a player does not feel ready to return to play even though the coach and medical people believe differently. When players do not think that they are ready to play, they should not be pressured to do so. Coaches must realize that such a reluctance may reflect the makeup of a particular athlete. Unfortunately, a public perception may develop that the player does not really care about competing or cannot play with pain. Sportswriters and fans who follow highly competitive levels of sport can be very opinionated, and it's easy for a negative (and damaging) image of the athlete to develop. Coaches must protect players from that kind of situation as much as possible by supporting the players' decisions.

Injury-Forced Retirement

Retirement from sport is difficult, especially when it is caused by injury, and it is something for which the serious athlete is seldom prepared. I imagine the emotions are very similar to what a lot of people experience when they retire at age 60 or 65. It is my impression that many people go through at least a temporary loss of self-esteem and self-confidence, because so much of their lives have revolved around sport. The more time invested and the greater the success, the harder it is to deal with retirement. With sudden, unexpected retirement due to injury, adjustment is more difficult still and can take as long as 2 years.

When top-level athletes retire, they have most of their adult lives still ahead of them. Unlike the runner in Housman's poem, they must face the prospect of swelling "the rout/Of lads who wore their honours out." Sometimes they need counseling to help them adjust to a new lifestyle and cope with emotional trauma. Counseling should focus on helping the athlete learn to apply sport skills such as concentration, goal setting, and teamwork to career pursuits. Some athletes are so physically gifted and their sport has come so naturally to them that they do not really realize how difficult it is to make the transition to other "work." It is not that they are unfamiliar with these principles, it is just that it is more difficult for them to apply them outside of sport. Physical activity should continue after an athlete retires, especially given the tremendous amount of information we now have about its effect on wellness and health. Since retirement, I have enjoyed working out just for the pleasure of it, not having to push myself to the limit.

Counseling can benefit athletes even before retirement. Counseling can help athletes keep their lives in balance and encourage them to develop other interests so they do not become wrapped up in a one-dimensional existence.

Concluding Comments

For weekend warriors and professional athletes, injury is an ever-present concern. Mostly this involves everyday aches and pains but it also includes serious injury. When injury challenges the committed athlete's ability to play, it can be traumatic. For the highly successful athlete, dealing with injury can be all the more difficult because of the greater degree of personal investment in sport.

I appreciate having good medical care and advice during my competitive career. But it is difficult to deal with the fact that I could have had a longer competitive career had sports medicine developed to the point where it is today. Arthroscopic surgery was not available when I was having my problems, nor was the current rehabilitation strategy for my particular knee injury. But this is the nature of science, and I am pleased to see continued growth and new developments in the rehabilitation of sport injuries.

3

CHAPTER

A Physician's Approach to the Psychology of Injury

J. Richard Steadman

The appropriate application of psychology is one of the cornerstones of success in treatment of the injured athlete. Rehabilitation can be divided into three areas: psychological rehabilitation, general physiological rehabilitation (aerobic conditioning, overall strength, and flexibility), and specific rehabilitation of the injured area (Steadman, 1982). Without appreciating the psychological aspects of injury and recovery, the injured athlete is unlikely to attain optimum healing, conditioning, and early return to function.

Our society has shown a marked increase in the active search for health and fitness. Exercise is now perceived as an important factor in improving the quality and longevity of life. People of all ages and occupations consider health and fitness to be important parts of their identities, and these people must therefore be ranked with professional athletes in terms of their seriousness about sport activities.

The professional athlete and the intense recreational athlete are equally eager to return from injury to the performance levels achieved prior to injury. Thus, in this chapter, the word *athlete* refers to both. Admittedly, the athlete who needs to return to sport in order to earn $3 million experiences a different type of stress than the one who wants to return to jogging 3 to 5 miles per day at a 10 min per mile pace. Sport injuries, however, seem to be the greatest equalizer, bringing these two athletes together toward a common goal.

Goal Orientation and Rehabilitation

The athlete is goal oriented. Throughout an athletic career, the emphasis is on better times, better scores, and longer shots. This focus on achieving goals can be harnessed in rehabilitation if the physician, sports medicine specialist, and athlete are innovative in their approaches. Goals give the athlete something concrete to reach for and actively engage the athlete in the rehabilitation process.

Goals must be achievable. For example, in the early postoperative period, a goal of full motion may be unrealistic, yet the athlete may be able to achieve partial motion. Setting a goal that the athlete can achieve helps him or her reestablish self-esteem and allows the patient to begin charting a course toward recovery. In general, early rehabilitation stages should focus on short-term goals, yet long-term goals can be helpful in mental training techniques, such as visualization (see chapter 11). As recovery progresses toward the specificity period, goals regarding return to play and sport performance can be brought into progressively greater focus. For more information on goal setting see chapter 10.

Process of Injury and Rehabilitation

When organizing a rehabilitation program, the rehabilitation team will find it helpful to identify and observe the interplay between specific time periods extending from preinjury to return to sport. These time periods compose the process of injury and rehabilitation:

1. Preinjury
2. Immediate Postinjury
3. Treatment decision and implementation
4. Early postoperative/rehabilitation
5. Late postoperative/rehabilitation
6. Specificity
7. Return to play

During each of these periods there is an intense psychological demand on the patient. A treatment approach that addresses key psychological issues according to this stage theory will optimize both the surgical and rehabilitative outcome. As illustrated in Figure 3.1, a similar process is followed for injury that requires surgery and for injury that is severe but does not require surgery. In relatively minor injury, rehabilitation moves more directly from treatment decision and implementation toward the specificity period and return to play.

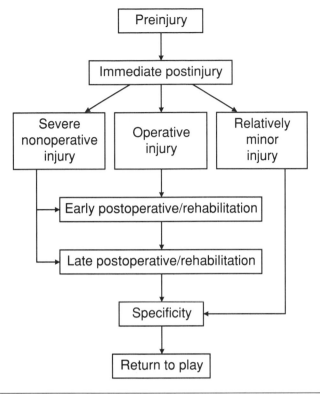

Figure 3.1   The process of rehabilitation.

Preinjury Period

Several studies have indicated that injury is frequently not purely an accident but is a culmination of a number of factors, including loss of concentration, pressures of performance, and fatigue. (See chapters 5 and 6 for more detailed information on injury risk.) When an injured athlete begins treatment, it is helpful for the practitioner to examine factors that created the environment in which the injury occurred. If identified, pre-injury factors may be addressed through psychological counseling during the course of treatment and rehabilitation.

Immediate Postinjury Period

This is the phase of fear and denial, accompanying the immediate pain and disability that have been described by Rotella and Heyman (1986) and others. At this point, the patient will need an accurate diagnosis, a complete explanation of this diagnosis, a proposed course of treatment, and an estimate of the duration of treatment (Steadman, 1981). This esti-mate will be approximate, but it will give the athlete an idea of what is in store. Most athletes, particularly successful ones, are aware that injury is often a part of athletics. However, clinicians sometimes assume that athletes know more than they do about injury, treatment, and rehabilitation. A patient's denial and fear can deter healing, though this can be countered by a plan that lays out the severity of injury, duration of disability, and expected recovery level. Such a plan allows the patient to take control and become an important part of the recovery team. For more about denial, see chapter 4.

Treatment Decision and Implementation

The decision-making process is easier if the first two phases are managed satisfactorily, that is, if the patient has dealt with the injury and is mentally able to assume an analytical role in helping decide on appropriate treatment. Treatment may be easily selected in some cases, but when many issues are involved the decision can be difficult to make. For instance, treatments may affect a patient's career or a team's performance and the physician should be aware of such factors, which necessarily affect the final decision on a treatment course.

In some cases, injury at a critical point in a career may force an athlete to make a decision that may be hazardous to future physical well-being. This seemingly irresponsible decision may nonetheless be a good one for the athlete, especially one who feels strongly that an additional year's salary or other benefits may provide financial stability for life. Also, some athletes may perceive the psychological gratification experienced by playing one more game or one more year as worth any risk. In these instances, it is necessary for the athlete, agent, management, and family to understand the hazards involved before accepting or rejecting a treatment course. The patient's input can only be truly effective if she or he has been apprised of the choices available and understands the risks involved.

Early Postoperative/Rehabilitation Period

In the immediate postoperative phase, the rehabilitation team must consider more than the surgical event and its sequelae. The patient is affected in varying degrees by important psychological factors that can influence the final outcome of treatment (Chapman & Turner, 1986).

If surgery is performed, the patient is transformed from an active, athletic person with the high humoral levels associated with activity to a bedridden, disabled patient. From both a physical and psychological standpoint, it is necessary to initiate a program of rehabilitation goals (Fordyce, Brockway, Bergman, & Spengler, 1986). Thus, for example, providing an athlete with well-leg aerobic workouts following knee surgery encourages a goal-seeking orientation and helps the athlete maintain aerobic conditioning. In addition, setting appropriate goals for the injured area—for example, achieving a certain range of motion or level of exercise intensity—permits the patient to take an active part in treatment and assume a level of control over the postoperative environment (Steadman, 1980).

Late Postoperative/Rehabilitation Period

During this phase, the drudgery of rehabilitation takes its toll. The physician must help the patient and the sports medicine specialist continue on a direct course to recovery. Continued goal orientation, provided by steadily increasing levels of activity, allows sustained patient input and permits the patient to feel in control throughout rehabilitation. This emphasis on setting and achieving goals parallels the patient's preinjury mind-set. For example, the athlete's preinjury goal may have been to run 5 miles in 30 minutes, and if he or she achieved this, confidence was boosted. During rehabilitation it is necessary to redirect goals, so that, for example, three sets of one-third knee bends become the mark of achievement. If goals are met, the patient feels control over the environment and a sense of accomplishment.

Achieving rehabilitation goals requires several elements. First, the milestones should be challenging but realistic and should be designated by the combined input of the physician, sports medicine specialist, and patient. Second, goals should stretch the limits of what the injured area can tolerate (without causing deformation or further injury) but should not extend beyond these limits, which requires a thorough understanding of the physiology and biomechanics of the injured area. Third, the patient should use noninjured parts in aerobic training, which prevents reinjury while providing more goal orientation. In the case of a leg injury, this training can include well-leg biking or swimming with or without float. The positive psychological effects of aerobic training are an important aspect of treatment during this period (Morgan & O'Conner, 1988).

Specificity Period

This period is less challenging psychologically, because at this point the end is in sight. Exercise should become more specific for the sport, which entails a greater emphasis on patterns and muscle recruitment mimicking those used in the sport.

During this period the athlete needs to be reassured that she or he will return to sport and once again achieve success. The patient may fear that success will not occur and thus may need psychological reinforcement, which can be readily provided through continued emphasis on achievable goals (Danish, 1986). Psychological counseling may be required if the athlete's subconscious fears of failure become manifest and seem obsessive.

Return to Play

This period may require psychological counseling for several reasons. First, the athlete's prolonged absence from sport can produce fears, especially if success has not been reinforced in earlier stages of rehabilitation. Second, the athlete may feel that peers have passed him or her by. Third, even though the rehabilitation program has been designed to return the athlete to a preinjury level, absence from regular participation in a sport can create other realistic concerns.

However, if the road to recovery has been successfully covered and the team (athlete, sports medicine specialist, physician, and psychologist) has provided appropriate standards for achievement at each level of rehabilitation, then the experience will have served a useful psychological purpose. The athlete's ability to overcome the obstacles of injury and to gain a level of performance equal to or higher than preinjury levels can create a confidence that will enhance performance. It is unlikely that this success can be achieved, however, without application of each element of the rehabilitation program.

Concluding Comments

This approach represents a physician's clinical perspective on the psychology of injury rehabilitation. The opportunities I have had to observe numerous world-class and intense recreational athletes have reinforced my appreciation for the role of psychological factors in active rehabilitation. In some cases, patients intuitively apply the principles discussed in this chapter. This ability to structure rehabilitation reasonably is probably a reflection of their preinjury success.

In treating numerous athletes, I have observed many who have returned to their sports at higher levels than those achieved at the time of injury. This can be partially explained by the possibility that these athletes were on an ascending curve of performance at the time of the accident, but this cannot be the entire explanation. Nor can good surgery and rehabilitation alone account for such successful recoveries. A comprehensive approach to rehabilitation provides a learning opportunity and helps create psychological momentum that the athlete can carry beyond rehabilitation.

To summarize, the psychological program includes the following:

1. The patient's complete understanding of the injury, the treatment, and the phases of treatment. This allows the patient to feel a part of the team guiding the recovery process.
2. Establishment of attainable goals at each stage in rehabilitation. These are simple but demanding goals that allow an immediate focus but do not look too far ahead.

3. Prompt initiation of an aerobic program to help avoid the depression associated with the immediate postinjury period. In addition, this counters other stress-related psychological changes that occur due to the abrupt transition from intense physical activity to no activity at all. (See chapter 4 for more information on psychological changes in injury.)
4. Psychological counseling to help the patient deal with his or her altered status as an athlete, especially during extended periods of inactivity.

Although this program seems simple, it requires careful judgment calls by the rehabilitation team at each phase of treatment.

This approach to treatment is based on over 15 years of clinical experience with most of the major world-class competitive skiers and with top-level athletes from virtually all other competitive sports, as well as work with large numbers of recreational athletes. The careful use of standardized treatment methods along with personal attention to the athlete's needs given his or her injury rehabilitation phase has proven effective. Our treatment team has contributed to some outstanding postinjury success stories. The return of several of our patients to top world-class performance after potentially career-ending accidents is eloquent testimony to the validity of this approach as well as to the intensity of their motivation.

4
CHAPTER

A Psychologist's View of the Personal Challenge of Injury

John Heil

By age 30 Andre Dawson, Montreal Expos center fielder, had won four Gold Gloves for outstanding defensive play and three Silver Slugger awards for excellence in hitting. He was also suffering from progressive worsening of a high school football injury that was threatening his ability to perform. Sportswriter Harry Stein (1984), in a close-up of the impact of this injury on Dawson, stated, "Dawson was obviously working hard to keep the self-doubts at bay. The predominant mood he showed the world was an almost dogged positivism" (p. 66). As much as Dawson tried to hide his pain and suffering, they were apparent to people close to him, leading his best friend on the club to comment, "He doesn't ever complain . . . but it is heartbreaking to see what he is going through" (p. 63). Stein (1984) also observed that in addition to the threat to Dawson's career and his constant pain, continual questioning about his health became a problem. Dawson is quoted as saying, "[It's] gotten kind of old. I mean I try and block it out of my mind, but it's tough when I've got to talk about it every day" (p. 64). One news story that quoted Dawson suggested that he had been exploited by the team. This upset Dawson as well as team management, prompting the club president to comment, "It's hard not to believe that those quotes were not in some way elicited from Andre in a period of depression" (p. 64). In the midst of the chaos and controversy, Dawson continually looked for the bright spots, one of which was provided when the team physician indicated that Dawson would be able to play with limited restrictions. To this Dawson responded, "I really needed to know that . . . I needed the reassurance that I'm not damaging myself by playing the rest of the year. Now I can concentrate on playing ball" (p. 64). When asked whether he would ever be able to return to top form Dawson responded, "I feel there is going to be a miracle in my life. I don't think this will hinder my career in the least" (p. 67). Andre Dawson's situation highlights the thoughts and feelings, pain and frustration, hope and uncertainty that can come with injury. He was able to continue his career, but others are not so fortunate. Sometimes an athlete can fall prey not just to the injury itself but to the emotional trauma that surrounds it.

The Stresses of Injury: An Introduction

Minor aches and pains are a routine part of sport. They may be frustrating and aggravating but are generally accepted as part of the game. More serious injury resulting in downtime is another matter. In this case, the disrupting influence of injury on the athlete's life is evident. Initial theoretical and applied perspectives on the psychological impact of injury (Little, 1969; Nideffer, 1983; Ogilvie & Tutko, 1966; Rotella, 1982) are supported by more recent research (McDonald & Hardy, 1990; Smith, Scott, O'Fallon, & Young, 1990). There is temporary loss of the ability to participate in a highly valued activity as well as a significant threat to continued success at sport. This can challenge the athlete's sense of self at a very fundamental level. Both self-esteem (perception of worth as a person) and self-efficacy (perception of one's self as competent and effective) are influenced. The stresses of injury as they influence physical, social, and emotional well-being, as well as underlying self-concept, are described in Table 4.1.

Ultimately the impact of injury is the net effect of the stress of the injury itself and the athlete's coping resources. How these balance out determines how traumatic injury will be. Preliminary research supports the long-held assumption that athletes with similar injuries often recover at different rates (Ievleva, 1988; Ievleva & Orlick, 1991). Thus recovery appears to be a function of the athlete's personal response to injury.

Injury is more than an event. It is a process played out over days or months—or even years. Attempts have been made to describe this process by a stage theory of emotion. Although this approach is of important conceptual value, the variability of emotional response and the difficulty in assessing emotional status with precision limit the practical usefulness of this approach. In chapter 3, Steadman offered a pragmatic stage theory based on the chronology of injury, treatment, rehabilitation, and return to play. This chapter introduces an affective cycle of injury that complements Steadman's model. The chapter describes cognitive response to injury

---

Table 4.1
The Stresses of Injury

Physical well-being

Physical injury
Pain of injury
Physical rigors of treatment and rehabilitation
Temporary physical restriction
Permanent physical changes

Emotional well-being

Psychological trauma at injury occurrence
Feelings of loss and grief
Threats to future performance
Emotional demands of treatment and rehabilitation

Social well-being

Loss of important social roles
Separation from family, friends, and teammates
New relationships with treatment providers
Necessity of depending upon others

Self-concept

Loss of sense of control
Dealing with altered self-image
Threat to life goals and values
Necessity for decision making under stressful circumstances

---

and a maladaptive cognitive schema of injury and discusses the role of pain and denial in coping with injury.

A Stage Theory of Emotional Response to Injury

Personal reaction to the experience of trauma may be viewed as a grieving process that occurs in stages. Kubler-Ross (1969) in *On Death and Dying* provided seminal thinking on this process of adaptation to loss. Drawing on her work with terminally ill patients, she described a series of stages that patients typically face: disbelief, denial, and isolation; anger; bargaining; depression; and acceptance and resignation. Her model provides a simple yet intuitively meaningful strategy for conceptualizing a complex set of emotional responses without the assumption of underlying pathology. The model constitutes a strong statement for the dynamic nature of affective response and is sensitive to the sometimes puzzling concurrent existence of contradictory emotions and to the transformation of emotional experience. It defines a "logic of emotion" in response to significant loss. Kubler-Ross's theoretical perspective has been applied to a wide variety of trauma including surgery, chronic illness, and spinal cord injury (McDonald & Hardy, 1990).

Kubler-Ross's stage theory has also been applied to athletic injury (e.g., Rotella, 1982). The wisdom of this is evident given that injury can mean the instant death of an athletic career cultivated by years of work. Rotella suggests that athletes often respond to injury initially by underplaying its severity, believing that they will soon be back to competition. Upon realizing the true impact of the injury they initially feel isolated and lonely. Anger and irritability with themselves and others follow as they work with the process of recovery. This is followed by a true sense of loss and depression. Eventually, the athlete accepts the injury and hopes for return to competition. The intuitive appeal of this argument for linking the typical emotional response to injury to the Kubler-Ross model of grief has led to its continued support by sport psychologists. However, others have offered variations on the model as proposed initially. McDonald and Hardy (1990) suggested a simplified two-stage process characterized simply as "reactive" and "adaptive," downplaying the importance of denial. Given the obvious and important differences between terminally ill patients and injured athletes, work on understanding emotional response to injury needs continued development. To what extent this emotional response is characteristic of all athletic injury, or alternately is limited to severe or psychologically traumatic injury, has not been clarified by proponents of stage theory.

The Affective Cycle of Injury

An alternative to a stage theory is the affective cycle of injury; the fundamental assumption of which is that movement through stages is not a one-time linear process but is a cycle that may repeat itself. This model retains three important ideas from the initial work of Kubler-Ross (1969) and Rotella (1982): the dynamic transformational nature of emotional experience, the patient's active "work of recovery," and the importance of denial. Figure 4.1 illustrates a three-element repeating cycle of affective response to injury that includes distress, denial, and determined coping.

Distress recognizes the inherently disrupting and disorganizing impact of injury on emotional equilibrium. It includes shock, anger, bargaining, anxiety, depression, isolation, guilt, humiliation, preoccupation, and helplessness. The psychologist (or other member of the sports medicine team)

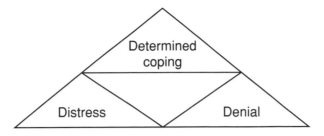

Figure 4.1   The affective cycle of injury.

should assess the magnitude of this distress and how appropriate it is relative to the severity of the injury. *Denial* includes a sense of disbelief as well as varying degrees of outright failure to accept the severity of injury. Denial may be reflected in the athlete's rather transparent assurances to health providers, teammates, and others about plans to quickly return to top form. It can range on a continuum from mild to profound and vary across time or circumstances. Given the specifics of its manifestation it may serve an adaptive purpose or may interfere with rehabilitation progress. Denial is described in detail in a subsequent section. *Determined coping* implies acceptance (to varying degrees) of the severity of injury and its impact on the athlete's short-term and long-term goals. It is characterized by the purposeful use of coping resources in working through the process of recovery.

In the early stages of injury, distress and denial will tend to be at their peak. There is a general trend toward determined coping as rehabilitation proceeds. However, shifts in emotional response from denial to distress to determined coping can occur at any time. This is not a random process but is tied to specific experiences or events. One element will tend to dominate at a given stage in the rehabilitation process; however, any given element will seldom dominate 24 hr a day. Even during a period primarily characterized by determined coping, denial or distress may resurface for varying periods of time and with varying degrees of impact. Something as simple as a review of game films that show any injury can elicit this. Setbacks during the treatment process and pain flare-ups are the most likely triggers of a shift from determined coping to distress or denial. To the extent that these situations make the athlete feel that he or she is making no progress, they will tend to be a problem. Difficulties may also occur at natural transitions in the rehabilitation process as described by Steadman (chapter 3). Generally, an athlete's emotional well-being will vary predictably with her or his subjective sense of progress through rehabilitation.

The Affective Cycle and the Chronology of Injury

A synthesis of Steadman's stage theory and the affective cycle of injury provides a perspective that is practical and conceptually rich. The athlete's emotional status most typically varies according to severity of injury and the related degree of psychological trauma. However, a psychological approach to injury management will minimize distress and optimize determined coping.

The immediate postinjury period is one of maximum emotional disorganization. In conjunction with injury there may be a shocklike response. The athlete may make unrealistic statements about speed of recovery and return to play, and specific fears and generalized anxiety may be evident. Denial is most adaptive during this phase of injury and need not be challenged by the psychologist (or other member of the sports medicine team) as long as it does not jeopardize the athlete's safety. This is also a time of uncertainty, especially if surgery is to follow. Establishing rapport and moving the athlete toward realistic expectations regarding recovery will prompt determined coping.

The treatment decision and implementation period is a direct extension of the immediate postinjury period and is marked by a similar emotional profile. Because time has allowed the athlete to emotionally reorganize somewhat, reactive anxiety to injury may begin to resolve, but anticipatory anxiety regarding surgery may replace this. Determined coping rests on the athlete's ability to shift from an emotionally reactive mind-set to one of careful, calculated decision making. It is important that denial not interfere with this process.

At the beginning of the early postoperative/rehabilitative period, the athlete is severely limited physically, which with a related sense of helplessness, can set up acute depression. The athlete may seize upon surgery as a quick cure, reeliciting denial. Treatment complications following surgery may lead to renewed anxiety as well as questions of trust in treatment providers. The athlete will be prone to loneliness and isolation during this period, especially if away from his or her home environment. Presenting the athlete with achievable short-term goals will guide determined coping and facilitate emotional reorganization around productive activity.

The late postoperative/rehabilitative period is an extension of the early postoperative/rehabilitative period. Well on the road to recovery, the athlete may feel an enhanced sense of self-control or may struggle to maintain emotional equilibrium. Treatment setbacks may elicit transitory anxiety or depression during this period as well as throughout the remainder of rehabilitation. The drudgery of rehabilitation may begin to take its toll, sapping motivation and setting up irritability and anger. If acting out behavior results in significant guilt or alienation from others, it may contribute to depression. Continued consistent support and encouragement are essential.

By the time the athlete reaches the specificity period, success at rehabilitation should diminish depression, and an improving level of fitness should enhance vitality. As the athlete anticipates return to play, fear of failure or reinjury may arise, and self-confidence may be further threatened if confidence in the athlete is not expressed by significant others (e.g., the coach). A continuing goal orientation and emphasis on treatment gains cue determined coping.

Return to play is a natural extension of the specificity period; participation replaces anticipation. Heightened anxiety and fear will resolve with success, but problems with return to play can reelicit anxiety, depression, and irritability. If denial is still present it will be challenged directly by the sport environment itself. By reinforcing success and by developing specific problem-solving strategies for difficulties that are encountered, treatment providers can guide the athlete in developing effective coping strategies.

Understanding Denial and Pain

Pain and denial are complex phenomena that figure importantly in successful rehabilitation. Both have positive adaptive value; however, each is capable of playing a potentially confounding role during rehabilitation. An overly simplified approach to the understanding and management of these phenomena will interfere with effective rehabilitation of the injured athlete, especially one with adjustment problems. Denial, an integral part of the affective cycle of injury, is described in detail next. Pain—which is often the most salient physical manifestation of injury, influencing not only the athlete's physical perception of injury and rehabilitation but also the athlete's emotional and cognitive understanding of (and response to) injury—will be introduced in this section and dealt with in greater detail in subsequent chapters.

Denial

Denial may be viewed as both a clinically significant intrapsychic defense mechanism and an ordinary process of selective attention. Denial itself is neither good nor bad, but how a person uses it is important. It is an ever-present aspect of daily life. Our bad moments and worst fears forever lurk in the recesses of our mind, and dwelling on these would be devastating, interfering with our abilities to maintain productive lives. Alternately, should we fail to recognize these hard facts of life it would be difficult to keep the normal ups and downs of daily living in perspective. Without the ability to selectively focus our attention, we would be unable to play with pain or perform unencumbered by the potential negative outcomes of poor performance. Our abilities to put distressing thoughts out of our minds and keep them from distracting us call into operation the same psychological mechanism of selective attention upon which denial is based. Events of potentially traumatic proportions tend to awaken our deepest fears and at the same time call upon our abilities to use selective attention.

The greater the trauma, the greater the potentially adaptive role of repression and denial (Ford, 1983). Denial is the psyche's way of protecting the athlete, like a floodgate holding back the flow of negative emotions. Its beneficial effect is that it delays the task of processing a sudden and large emotional flood of experience, allowing these emotions to be processed slowly and systematically over time. Within limits denial is useful, allowing the athlete to maintain a positive attitude and cope with the situation at hand. Denial becomes potentially problematic when it allows the athlete to avoid the emotional work of recovery. In such a case the process of denial can consume significant energy itself and lock the athlete into a self-defeating cycle. And there is the ever-present prospect that the floodgate holding back the emotions may be suddenly and unpredictably released at a time of subsequent distress.

Some of the athlete's worst fears regarding injury will be dispelled with good progress in rehabilitation and so need not be dealt with at all. In this situation denial has worked constructively. Where recovery is not prompt and trouble-free, the athlete must acknowledge, experience, and resolve the physical and emotional impact of an injury. Persistent denial can interfere with the process of recovery, and when this happens, denial clearly is a problem and must be dealt with as such. Profound denial is easy to see, but in its more subtle manifestations denial can be quite elusive to the observer. It can subside only to recur again. Although strong emotional reactions and denial most often occur at the time of injury, they may also occur in conjunction with treatment setbacks as well as at transitions in the rehabilitation process. Denial may also be at work when the athlete perceives rehabilitation progress to be more favorable than do treatment providers.

Systematic therapeutic attempts to counter this defense mechanism are most productive when treatment providers can give the athlete a positive and adaptive future focus. Because the most subtle manifestation of denial in injury may be in the form of poor setting of limits and the resultant risk of reinjury, systematic goal setting effectively challenges denial. Where denial is more blatant and persistent, a direct challenge of denial by the sports medicine team may be necessary. The implicit goal of sport performance, to exceed what appear to be one's limits (and, if possible, to surpass all others' performances), may subtly encourage the use of denial. Without his eventual remarkable recovery Andre Dawson's statement—"I feel there is going to be a miracle in my life" (Stein, 1984, p. 67)—could well be interpreted as denial. Similar statements by other injured athletes are clearly the result of denial.

Pain

Pain is an integral part of the athletic experience both in sport performance and in injury. It is a complex phenomenon that is often grossly oversimplified. Pain begins as a biological event (nociception) that gives rise to psychological awareness (perception). From this follows a search for meaning rooted in cognitive and affective processes, which subsequently serves as a guide for action (see Figure 4.2).

One of the problems with understanding pain is that the word *pain* describes many things. The athlete must learn while healthy to differentiate performance pain from injury pain and when injured to discriminate between benign pain and harmful pain. The athlete also must deal with the distraction of minor aches and pains, the extreme pain of acute injury at its occurrence, the recurring pain of overuse injury, and the persistent pain of unresolved injury.

Remarkable feats of pain tolerance by athletes have long been noted in the pain literature (Melzack, 1961). Stock car racer Neil Bonnett (personal communication, March 11, 1990) described how he sorted out pain and emotion during a wreck in which he suffered a fractured sternum:

> When I wrecked I knew I was hurt. . . . If that would have been the first wreck that I had ever had in a car I would have been jumping up and down scared to death and going crazy. . . . When the crew got to the car I said "Just take it easy" . . . [then] they were joking with me. I got to the hospital and they told me my heart rate was normal.

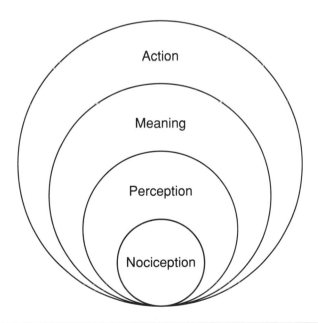

Figure 4.2   A conceptual model of pain.

In whatever form, pain presents a challenge. The athlete may quite effectively deal with the acute pain associated with injury but may have difficulty with more enduring pain. An example is Mike, a former competitive hockey player and recreational distance runner who suffered a severe work-related injury that would have been fatal had he not had the presence of mind to direct his rescuers in proper first aid. He underwent a lengthy series of surgeries, which he managed with remarkable effectiveness, and then established a regular rehabilitation regimen of swimming. However, his inability to tolerate chronic pain during daily activity and the loss of function that his injury brought eventually caused problems in his personal life.

The longer pain lasts the more likely it is to lead to pervasive emotional disruption, including depression and performance anxiety, and the greater the likelihood it will interfere with rehabilitation. The challenge of pain to the athlete is all the more noteworthy because of the implicit assumption that athletes cope effectively with pain. In sport, much remains to be done to improve the abilities of the athlete, coach, and health providers to understand, communicate about, and manage pain.

Cognitive Response to Injury

Emotional distress is typically accompanied by *thoughts* of distress, which reflect the specific circumstances of the precipitating events as well as the psychological makeup of each individual. Emotional distress gives rise to distortions in thinking that reflect inaccurate interpretations of the situation at hand. Similarly injury can also give rise to cognitive distortions (T.W. Smith, Aberger, Follick, & Ahern, 1986; T.W. Smith, Follick, Ahern, & Adams, 1986) as individuals seek to understand its meaning. When injury is complicated by significant enduring emotional distress, cognitive distortion is further exaggerated.

Beck and his associates (Beck & Emery, 1985; Beck, Rush, Shaw, & Emery, 1979) identified five categories of cognitive distortion that represent prevailing tendencies toward flawed interpretations of events. In relation to injury these are characterized as follows:

1. Catastrophizing—exaggerating the severity of injury
2. Overgeneralization—incorrectly extending the expected impact of injury to aspects of playing ability or daily behavior that are not likely to be affected
3. Personalization—taking undue personal responsibility for injury or giving it some exaggerated special meaning in relation to oneself
4. Selective abstraction—attending to specific aspects of injury that have little meaning in the overall context
5. Absolutistic/dichotomous thinking—simplistically reducing complex experiences to all-or-none categories

These distortions in thinking are particularly well suited to cognitive behavioral interventions (Turk, Meichenbaum, & Genest, 1983); for detailed examples of cognitive distortion, see Table 4.2.

Thoughts that at first appear distorted will in some instances be accurate. Consequently, it is important that the treatment provider listen carefully to an athlete's concerns. This begins with a clarification of the athlete's thoughts on injury and an analysis of their accuracy based on objective assessment of the situation. Once the treatment provider understands the athlete's concerns, they can be dealt with more effectively.

Absolutistic/dichotomous thinking is of special concern relative to pain and unfortunately is a type of thinking to which athletes, coaches, and to an extent health professionals are prone in the assessment of pain. This reflects a failure to appreciate the diversity of the pain experience and its emotional and cognitive concomitants. In many cases, there

---

Table 4.2
Cognitive Distortions

Catastrophizing

At the time of injury: "I'll never be able to play again."
Following a pain flare-up: "I'll never get over this pain."

Overgeneralization

Following a shoulder injury: "I'll probably lose my running speed, too."
"At the rate I'm going with my rehabilitation I'll probably screw up my grades, too."

Personalization

"Why am I the one who always gets injured?"
Upon observing the athletic trainer to be in an unpleasant mood: "My trainer must think I'm not trying hard enough."

Selective abstraction

"The last player with a knee injury didn't recover and neither will I."
"If the coach had let me train in my own way this would have never happened."

Absolutistic/dichotomous thinking

"My pain is either physical or it's in my head."
"Because I'm injured I'm worthless to the team."

is a tendency to identify pain as mental or physical, or alternately, as real or imagined. But pain resists such simple classification. Efforts to simplify pain are potentially damaging to the athlete and tend to undermine treatment relationships. One of the more common and erroneous assumptions is that all pain behaves like acute pain. Acute pain and chronic pain behave in distinctly different ways. Acute pain is characterized by accelerated heart rate, pallor, sweating, and other sympathetic autonomic signs. In chronic pain, autonomic signs are typically absent, although muscular guarding and other body language indicators may be prominent (Keefe & Block, 1982). As chronic pain persists, it becomes increasingly linked to cognitive and environmental factors. Displays of pain come to reflect the physical and emotional suffering that are consequences of injury (Fordyce, 1988).

A Cognitive Schema of Injury

In problematic injury situations, athletes show increased tendencies toward absolutistic/dichotomous thinking and other cognitive distortions. Such examples of faulty thinking are typically based on deeply rooted thought processes or schema that reflect fundamental personal assumptions about cause and effect in the world. A *cognitive schema* may be defined as a unifying construct integrating diverse sets of information and thereby enhancing the meaning of a particular situation. A cognitive schema of injury is now proposed that includes three elements: impairment, ability, and pain (Heil & Russell, 1987) (see Figure 4.3). Impairment is an objective medical assessment of physical status as demonstrated in physical exam and diagnostic testing. Ability is simply what a person is able to do and may vary relative to a given level of impairment across individuals or within a particular individual across time. Pain is a complexly determined subjective perception linked to sensory input and personal interpretation. Although pain is related to impairment and disability, it may vary independently of these two factors. The primary goal of medical treatment, such as surgery, is to resolve impairment; the purpose of rehabilitation is to enhance ability. Both are intended to decrease pain in the long run, although their short-term effects may be to increase pain.

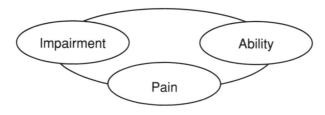

Figure 4.3   Cognitive schema of pain and injury.

Impairment, ability, and pain are on a continuum of relatively increasing subjectivity and complexity of assessment. For all of the subtleties of impairment and ability, the private nature of pain renders it most difficult to effectively assess. Pain is readily obvious to the athlete and may be much more compelling in its manifestation relative to impairment or ability. Impairment and ability, in turn, are most apparent to treatment providers. In routine rehabilitation, resolution of impairment and pain and enhancement of ability are typically simultaneous, resulting in readiness to play; however, this is not always the case. When simultaneous resolution and enhancement do not occur, problems are in the making.

Each athlete, coach, and health professional has a schema of injury that reflects personal knowledge and experience. The most frequent flaw in a schema of injury is an overemphasis on the interdependence of impairment, disability, and pain and a related failure to appreciate their potential independence. For example, people often assume that greater impairment implies greater pain, which is not always the case.

When the athlete feels unready to return to play (in contrast to the recommendations of treatment providers), one of two concerns is likely operating: The athlete either feels that his or her sport skills are not up to par or doubts that the injury is healed. The first concern, that skills are inadequate, results in a diminished sense of self-efficacy. In many cases, this is best viewed as a normal performance anxiety that will resolve with return to play. The coach's input will help the treatment provider clarify the accuracy of this concern.

A second and potentially more problematic concern is doubt about recovery from injury. This is typically evoked when impairment resolves and ability improves, as objectively assessed, but pain remains. As a result the athlete confuses benign pain (a safe pain that is associated with recovery from injury) with harmful pain. In this situation, the presence of pain elicits concerns regarding impairment and ability as well as fear of reinjury. More broadly speaking, what occurs is a discrepancy between the athlete's cognitive schema of injury and that of the treatment providers. When such a discrepancy occurs, it is important to proceed cautiously. The treatment providers should reassure the athlete of the benign status of the pain, clarify the bases of objective medical opinion, and emphasize the complex nature of the pain experience. (For more information on measuring and managing pain, see chapters 8, 11, and 13.)

Concluding Comments

The impact of injury on the athlete's psyche is potentially great. A comprehensive perspective of injury should encompass emotional and cognitive factors as well as pain. This chapter has described the response to injury as a grief process and emphasized its dynamic and cyclical nature. The stress of injury may disrupt cognitive function and lead to faulty interpretations of the meaning of pain and injury. The links between emotions, cognitions, and pain are complex, and this chapter proposes a cognitive schema of pain and injury as a way of conceptualizing their interrelationships. Ultimately, it is most important that treatment providers understand the meaning of pain and injury to the athlete.

II
PART

Behavioral Risk Factors for Sport Injury

A broad array of factors interact to influence injury risk. To a certain degree, risk is a consequence of the rules of the game and how they are routinely applied in a given setting. The nature and quality of personal equipment and sports facilities are also significant. Perhaps less apparent, but equally important, are the roles of behavioral factors such as training intensity, risk taking, attitudes toward pain and injury, life stress, drug and alcohol use, and coping skills. Concerns regarding behavioral factors have crystalized into two areas of investigation: psychological (especially psychosocial) risk factors and overtraining syndrome. The following two chapters are devoted to these topics and are characterized by an interactional multifactor approach to risk assessment and management.

In "Psychological Risk Factors and Injury Prevention," Mark Andersen and Jean Williams introduce a comprehensive model of stress and athletic injury. In describing the relationship of stress and injury, Andersen and Williams present the biological substrates as well as the attentional and cognitive concomitants of the stress response within the larger context of psychosocial behavior. They also describe an innovative approach to the assessment of the psychological and attentional elements of the stress response and offer recommendations on how to identify high-risk athletes.

In the chapter entitled "Overtraining Syndrome," Juergen Froehlich presents a pragmatic clinical perspective on diagnosis, treatment, and prevention. The author presents theoretical bases of the concept of overtraining, emphasizing the complex physiological dynamics but also highlighting the influence of psychological factors. The chapter provides insightful speculation on the relationship of overtraining to injury and describes the roles of the physician, sport psychologist, coach, and athlete in the identification and management of overtraining syndrome.

5
CHAPTER

Psychological Risk Factors and Injury Prevention

Mark B. Andersen and Jean M. Williams

Early work on the relationship between psychological factors and athletic injury risk was often a product of coaching or clinical experience (Ogilvie & Tutko, 1966). Recently, more scientific advances have been made in ferreting out the psychological factors and potential mechanisms involved in injury risk. Those advances will be the focus of this chapter.

We have postulated that the mechanism behind the life events–injury relationship lies in an individual's stress responsivity (Andersen & Williams, 1988). For example, in cardiac medicine, individuals who react to stress tests with large and prolonged stress responses are at greater risk for later cardiac problems. A similar relationship exists between life events, stress responsivity, and injury.

A Model of Stress and Athletic Injury

The proposed model of the psychological factors involved in athletic injury (Andersen & Williams, 1988) provides a framework for assessing injury risk and suggests interventions for reducing the likelihood of injury for the high-risk athlete (see Figure 5.1). This model owes much to earlier stress research (Allen, 1983; R.E. Smith, 1979) and was developed from a synthesis of the stress-illness, stress-injury, and stress-accident literatures.

Central to the model is the stress response with its mutually influencing cognitive and physiological/attentional elements. In any athletic situation,

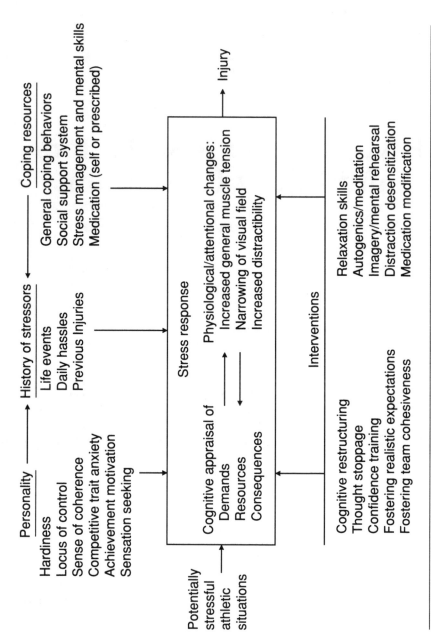

Figure 5.1 A model of stress and athletic injury.

participants will experience different cognitive responses; for example, competition may produce positive feelings of challenge, excitement, and joy (eustress) or negative feelings of dread, anxiety, and discomfort (distress). The type of affective response an athlete experiences can easily influence injury risk. Distress may be more likely than eustress to lead to injury. Physiological/attentional responses are rooted in endocrinological changes (e.g., elevated adrenocorticotropic hormone [ACTH] and catecholamine levels, release of glucocorticoids) and autonomic nervous system changes (e.g., activation of the sympathetic nervous system). Observable changes in sympathetic nervous system arousal may include an increase in respiration, pupillary dilation, increased sweating, piloerection, generalized muscle tension, tremor, increased distractibility, and emotional lability. Less observable, but often experienced by the individual, are changes such as vasoconstriction in the viscera ("butterflies"), nausea, tunnel vision, and "adrenaline rush." From these physiological events, attentional changes may follow.

Stress-injury relationship research has been conducted largely within the realm of athletics. In football alone, several studies have shown a relationship between life events, stress, and injury, with high-stress athletes having a greater likelihood of injury than low-stress athletes (e.g., Bramwell, Masuda, Wagner, & Holmes, 1975; Cryan & Alles, 1983; Passer & Seese, 1983). High levels of stress also contribute to a greater likelihood of accidents in the general population (Selzer & Vinokur, 1974; Stuart & Brown, 1981).

Life events stress research was our starting point for examining the relationship between stress and injury. As is often the case, there are few simple relationships, and subsequently we investigated other factors. Besides "history of stressors" (including life events, daily hassles, and previous injuries) there are two other broad categories of factors that may influence stress responsivity either directly or indirectly. Personality factors (intrapersonal) and coping resources (behavioral and social) can have substantial effects on potential injury and are thus included in the model.

The Stress Response

The way in which the cognitive and physiological elements of the stress response interacts, especially in stress-inducing athletic situations, influences the likelihood of injury. Those changes that we believe are involved in increased injury risk are discussed next.

Physiological/Attentional Changes. The changes during stress that may be the major culprits in stress-injury relationships are generalized muscle tension, narrowing of the visual field, and increased distractibility. Unwanted simultaneous contraction of agonistic and antagonistic muscle groups in generalized muscle tension (often called guarding or bracing) reduces flexibility, motor coordination, and muscle efficiency, which can easily set the athlete up for a variety of injuries such as strains, sprains, and fractures. If the athlete's muscles are "fighting" themselves, he or she may not be able to quickly generate the motor patterns necessary for moving out of harm's way in a dangerous situation (e.g., a baseball or racquetball approaching the head).

Narrowing of peripheral vision during stress is often reported anecdotally. For example, a quarterback might report that he experienced tunnel vision during a crucial point in the game and was not able to "see" secondary receivers who were not being guarded. Research by Weltman and Egstrom (1966) demonstrated that novice divers, when placed in a stressful situation (open ocean rather than a pool), showed greater peripheral narrowing than experienced divers. Substantial peripheral-vision narrowing during stress has been demonstrated in a laboratory setting, with individuals who score high on life stress experiencing greater narrowing than individuals who score low on life stress (Andersen & Williams, 1989; J.M. Williams, Tonymon, & Andersen, 1990, 1991). This narrowing of vision could prevent the athlete from picking up cues in the periphery that might otherwise enable her or him to avoid an injurious situation (e.g., in football, an unexpected block or tackle from the side).

The cause of peripheral narrowing under stress is not clear. It may be that when the demands of a situation exceed the athlete's resources (e.g., behavioral, attentional, perceptual), available resources are allocated to more central tasks, leaving the periphery with fewer resources for processing information. (See Kahneman, 1973, for a more thorough description of allocation of resources during stress.) A recent peripheral vision and stress study suggested that in a dangerous situation a person also fails to respond as quickly as would be possible in a less stressful situation (Andersen & Williams, 1989). This delay or hesitation could set up the individual for injury. The slowed-reaction-time interpretation of peripheral narrowing is not firmly established but offers another avenue for research into this interesting phenomenon.

Attentional distractibility also may predispose the athlete to injury if attention to irrelevant cues pulls him or her off task. For example, at a gymnastics meet several events take place simultaneously. If a gymnast is highly stressed and something happens in another part of the arena that results in wild applause, the gymnast's attention may be drawn off the task at hand. This shift of attentional focus may lead to slips, falls, and poor landings.

Cognitive Appraisals.   Logically connected to the physiological/attentional aspects of the stress response are the cognitive appraisals of the athlete. For example, an athlete's attitudes about competition may influence the likelihood of injury. If the athlete views competition as challenging, exciting, and fun, this sort of "good" stress (eustress) may help the athlete remain on task, stay focused, and "flow" with the competition. Injury risk in this situation would probably be lower than when the athlete feels "bad" stress (distress), for example, if the athlete views competition as anxiety producing, or as potentially embarrassing, or as a tribulation.

If confidence is down, the athlete may feel that he or she does not have the resources to meet the demands of the situation. The feeling that "I'm going to blow it" or "this person is going to cream me" can easily contribute to an acute stress response and the accompanying physiological/attentional changes that set up the athlete for injury. Also of great importance is what the athlete thinks are the consequences of performance. Thoughts such as "if I don't do well I'll be cut" can lead to exaggerated stress responses.

The cognitive appraisals of an athletic situation and the physiological and attentional responses to stress constantly modify and remodify each other. For example, a relaxed body can help calm the mind just as anxious thoughts can activate the sympathetic nervous system. Individual differences in stress responsivity may either inoculate the athlete against injury or exacerbate his or her risk.

Psychosocial Factors and Stress

The question of interest is, What psychological factors influence the stress response? The three major contributors are the personal history of stressful experiences, personality traits, and resources that help in coping with stress (social and behavioral). The model also suggests that personality variables and coping resources act either directly on the stress response or as moderator variables for the effects of stress history. In doing so, they may act independently or in combination.

History of Stressors.   This includes life events and daily hassles. The previous injury history may be important to consider as well, in that an athlete may return to play before he or she is fully recovered physically. Also, the athlete may be physically but not psychologically prepared to return to sport competition.

Life Events.   The study of the influence of past stressful events on health began with studies on the relationship of major life events to illness outcome. In the now-classic study of T.H. Holmes and Rahe (1967), the researchers demonstrated a connection between the number of major life changes a person experiences (e.g., divorce, relocation) and the person's likelihood of becoming ill. The original scale, developed to measure life events (Social Readjustment Rating Scale; SRRS), listed 40 major events ranging from death of a spouse to minor violations of the law. Within a few years the life-events approach to health research was applied to athletic injury, when T.H. Holmes (1970) found a positive correlation between major life events and injury in football players.

Since Holmes conducted the football investigation, there have been over 20 studies of stress and athletic injury risk, with 18 of the 20 finding some type of positive relationship between life stress and injury. The best evidence for high-life-stress athletes being more injury vulnerable still involves football. This documentation encompasses six studies, from T.H. Holmes's study in 1970 to Blackwell and McCullagh's in 1990. Similar findings have occurred across 14 other sports as diverse as Alpine skiing, race walking, figure skating, gymnastics, soccer, and track and field (see J.M. Williams & Roepke, 1992, for a more thorough review).

Generally, research has shown that the risk of being injured increases in direct proportion to the level of life-event stress. The strength of the life stress–injury relationship, however, varies considerably across studies. Athletes with high life-event stress are two to five times more likely to be injured than athletes with low life-event stress. The largely positive findings across sports and competitive levels is compelling considering the diversity in measures of life stress and definitions of injury. Eight questionnaires have been used to assess life stress with most including both general and athletic stressors and distinguishing between positive and negative stressors. The criteria for injury have varied from the athlete's seeing an athletic trainer but not modifying activity or reducing practice time (e.g., Blackwell & McCullagh, 1990) to the athlete's missing more than a week of practice (e.g., Coddington & Troxell, 1980). Because of these different operational definitions, it is impossible to determine relative injury risk either across sports and competitive levels or for positive versus negative stressors.

Daily Hassles.   Chronic daily hassles are the everyday stresses and strains of living that may or may not be connected to major life events (e.g., job dissatisfaction, loneliness). These hassles have been shown to be predictors of health outcome (Kanner, Coyne, Schaefer, & Lazarus, 1981), psychological distress (Monroe, 1983), and stress responsivity (J.M. Williams et al., 1990, 1991) but not injury vulnerability (Blackwell & McCullagh, 1990; R.E. Smith, Smoll, & Ptacek, 1990a). They are included here as potential contributors to injury outcome because both injury vulnerability studies had methodological limitations. An assessment of both life events and daily hassles may still give us a better overall picture of athletes' stress and their potential injury risks.

Personality.   The general health literature has demonstrated that personality variables such as hardiness (Kobasa, 1979), locus of control (Rotter, 1966), and sense of coherence (Antonovosky, 1985) are related to health outcomes. Except for locus of control, research into the relationship between these variables and athletic injury is lacking.

Competition anxiety (Martens, 1977), sensation seeking (Zuckerman, Kolin, Price, & Zoob, 1964), and achievement motivation are included in the model because of their direct relevance to sport. High competitive trait-anxious athletes, when placed in stressful situations, exhibit strong stress responses and thus are more likely to incur injury. The roles of sensation seeking and achievement motivation in injury are at present speculative. Perhaps sensation seekers may actually be at greater risk of injury because of their willingness to take chances. Alternately, they may be at lower risk because they are less likely to cognitively appraise extremely demanding situations as stressful. High achievement motivation may place an athlete at risk in certain situations. For example, when the athlete feels a strong need to excel but has inadequate skills, frustration and stress may result. A high achiever also may experience relatively greater stress when confronted with a superior opponent.

Many of the personality measures currently in use are "generic" and do not reflect the personality in a sport situation. For example, someone who scores high on sensation seeking in general may be a very cautious and controlled competitor. Only when researchers have used sport-specific anxiety (Blackwell & McCullagh, 1990; Passer & Seese, 1983) and locus of control (Dalhauser & Thomas, 1979) measures have differences been detected in injury vulnerability. Athletes with an internal locus of control were less likely to be injured, and athletes with lower competitive trait anxiety were less likely to experience a severe injury. Research using interactional models and sport-specific measures is needed to illuminate the role of personality in injury.

Coping Resources. There is evidence that an athlete's coping resources influence injury outcome both directly and indirectly. J.M. Williams, Tonymon, and Wadsworth (1986) found that the strongest predictor of injury among volleyball players was a low level of coping resources. These authors used the Miller and Smith Vulnerability to Stress Questionnaire (1982), which measures general coping resources (e.g., eating, sleeping, and exercise habits) and social support resources (e.g., social activities and friendships). R.E. Smith, Smoll, and Ptacek (1990a) found that male and female high school varsity athletes low in both social support and psychological coping skills (e.g., ability to concentrate, stay positive, and regulate arousal) exhibited the greatest injury risk. A major methodological advance of this study was the finding that social support and coping skills interact to predict vulnerability or resistance to injury. Other studies found a similar relationship between social support and athletic injury (Hardy, Prentice, Kirsanoff, Richman, & Rosenfeld, 1987; Petrie, in press).

Assessing Injury Risk

The proposed model of stress and athletic injury suggests that in a potentially stressful situation, individuals with high life stress, many daily hassles, certain personality factors, and few coping resources will exhibit greater peripheral vision narrowing, more attentional distractions, and higher levels of generalized muscle tension. How the athlete's peripheral vision, muscle tension, and related motor-skill performance change from baseline to stress conditions during athletic performance is an important practical question. When this question is evaluated in conjunction with the assessment of key psychological variables, a clear picture of injury risk may emerge. This multimodal approach to assessment has proven fruitful in medical research. For example, in assessing risk of cardiac disease, researchers measure Type A behavior, administer stress tests, and monitor patients physiologically.

A variety of options are available for injury risk assessment depending upon the availability of time, equipment, funding, and staff. To extend the predictive power of injury risk assessment, we propose a two-step evaluation that incorporates physiological and attentional factors. (This type of testing can be incorporated into the preparticipation screening that many sport organizations require.) The first step is to obtain some combination of measures of personality, history of stressors, and coping resources that are pertinent to the athletes being assessed. Sport-specific measures should be used whenever possible. The second step is physiological and attentional factors assessment, which is described in detail subsequently.

We recommend a protocol for assessing generalized muscle tension that includes measurement (by electromyography, i.e., EMG) of a noninvolved muscle (e.g., frontalis) while the athlete performs a complex visual motor task (e.g., rotary pursuit) under baseline and stress conditions. Stress conditions might include some combination of environmental conditions, crowd noise, or other factors relevant to the athlete's sport situation. An increase in muscle activity in a noninvolved muscle group during stress indicates an overall pattern of excess muscle tension. Deterioration in performance of the visual-motor task during stress indicates a disruption of motor skills. These changes predict increasing injury risk and diminished performance.

Changes in peripheral vision from baseline to stress conditions can be measured with a relatively inexpensive color perimeter device modified for this purpose (for a detailed description see J.M. Williams, Tonymon, & Andersen, 1990). Substantial decreases in peripheral vision during stress suggest greater risk of injury and a related impact on performance.

Procedures such as those reviewed here are in preliminary stages of development. Their greatest value at this time is as applied research models that can generate a better understanding of sport injury. Methods should not be used to label an athlete as "injury prone" or to exclude an athlete from sport, because such actions can result in a self-fulfilling prophecy. The information gained by such assessment should be used to identify high-risk individuals whose health and performance can be improved by psychological intervention.

Interventions

The model of stress and athletic injury offers a two-pronged attack on the major psychophysiological culprit behind injury, the stress response. Practitioners may moderate the stress response by addressing the cognitive appraisals, the physiological/attentional aspects, or both. A variety of approaches can accomplish this, as shown in Figure 5.1. In an archival review of injury data, Davis (1991) found that progressive relaxation and imagery training reduced swimming injuries by 52% and football injuries by 33%. These and related mental training techniques have been covered by many authors (e.g., Harris & Williams, in press; Schmid & Peper, in press) and will not be reviewed in more detail here. (See chapter 11 regarding the use of related procedures in injury management.) Continued preventive intervention in conjunction with program evaluations will give us a better handle on which techniques and approaches are the most feasible, cost-effective, and beneficial.

Concluding Comments

Recent comprehensive interactional models of psychosocial risk factors, along with methodological advances, offer promising avenues of research into injury vulnerability and practical applications for injury reduction. Self-reports of life events, daily hassles, personality, social support, and other coping resources, coupled with measures of muscle action and perceptual change, can identify the high-risk individual. From this assessment, potential intervention strategies for reducing risk can follow.

6

CHAPTER

Overtraining Syndrome

Juergen Froehlich

Physical exercise induces physiological reactions that result in adaptive changes of the organism. For hours or for a few days those changes may parallel transitory symptoms of fatigue and decreased performance until a higher level of adaptation is established. According to Selye's (1956) theory of adaptation, each athlete has a capacity to achieve a higher level of adaptation in the face of combined physical and mental stresses from training, environment, profession, and other life circumstances. But if the balance between load and coping capacity is disturbed, an athlete is in danger of developing overtraining syndrome.

A Definition of Overtraining

Participants of a 1983 round-table discussion uniformly agreed that an accurate and universally acceptable definition of overtraining is not available (Ryan, Brown, Frederick, Falsetti, & Burke, 1983), and this is still true. Accordingly, terms such as *burnout, overreaching, overwork, overtraining, staleness*, and *overtraining syndrome* often are not uniformly used. Following are working definitions of these terms.

When heavy training work loads are applied for a long time, the athlete is in danger of moving beyond a critical point resulting in a prolonged period of decreased performance and a profound feeling of fatigue. This, in conjunction with a complex set of other subjective symptoms and objective signs (which will be discussed at length later in the chapter), indicates *overtraining syndrome* (Kuipers & Keizer, 1988). The training process resulting in this syndrome will be called *overtraining*. *Staleness* is used either to describe the initial reaction to overtraining (Silva, 1990) or to define a prolonged state of overtraining syndrome, lasting several weeks (Kuipers & Keizer, 1988; Ryan et al., 1983). An overtraining syndrome of lengthy duration can lead to the state of physical and emotional exhaustion and frustration that characterizes *burnout* (Fender, 1989; Henschen, 1986; R.E. Smith, 1986).

In contrast, *overreaching* or *overwork* means a short period of heavy training that deliberately exceeds the athlete's coping capacity. This is often practiced in training camps that assign a heavy workload for a short period of time (Ryan et al., 1983). This intentional training overload is used as a stimulus (Harre, 1979) to speed processes of physiological adaptation that usually occur more slowly during periods of normal training. There is a general empirical consensus that "overreached" athletes can recover within 2 or 3 weeks (Kuipers & Keizer, 1988; Ryan et al., 1983).

In recent years, research in overtraining has increased, yet there is still a lack of controlled studies in specific sports. The pathophysiological and pathopsychological mechanisms of the overtraining syndrome remain unclear; however, no investigation has identified overtraining syndrome as a manifestation of a primary organic disease process.

Symptoms and Signs of Overtraining Syndrome

A variety of psychological and physiological features characterize a colorful mosaic of clinical and laboratory findings about overtraining syndrome. These findings suggest that overtraining syndrome is characterized by disturbed regulation of the central nervous system, the autonomic nervous system, and the neuroendocrine system, with resultant physical symptoms and behavioral changes. The leading symptoms are decreased performance and rapid onset of fatigue during exercise. The athlete experiences a "run down" feeling, a general loss of motivation, and diminished concentration. Additional diagnostic signs either may indicate general systematic disturbances (cardiovascular, digestive, or nervous system) or, in contrast, may reflect single organ dysfunction. Because the same symptomatology might alternately indicate organic disease as well as a psychophysiological disorder, careful clinical investigation of symptoms including laboratory testing is necessary.

Clinical Findings

Based on clinical findings, European sport physicians and exercise physiologists (e.g., Israel, 1976) differentiate between two types of overtraining syndrome: sympathetic and parasympathetic. The sympathetic type shows symptoms similar to those of hyperthyroidism and is characterized by increased activity of the sympathetic nervous system. The sympathetic type affects the state of health enormously and is clearly reflected in both objective signs and self-reports (i.e., the athlete feels sick). Athletes involved in nonendurance sports, beginner athletes, teenagers, and females are most susceptible to this syndrome. In contrast, the parasympathetic type may show only nondescript signs and consequently is difficult to recognize and often diagnosis is delayed. Clinical observation (Israel, 1976) shows that parasympathetic overtraining syndrome is preceded by a short period of increased activity of the sympathetic nervous system, although parasympathetic activity subsequently dominates. Highly trained endurance and elderly athletes are most affected by this type of overtraining syndrome. Characteristic clinical findings that identify the leading common and "type-specific" symptoms are presented in Table 6.1.

Table 6.1
Overtraining Syndrome:
Characteristic Clinical Findings

Common symptoms

Decreased performance
Rapid onset of fatigue
Generalized pervasive fatigue
Loss of motivation
Emotional instability
Reduced concentration
Increased incidence of injuries
Increased susceptibility to infections

Sympathetic	"Type-specific" symptoms	Parasympathetic
Increased	Resting heart rate	Not altered
Retarded	Heart rate recovery following exercise	Quick
Decreased	Body weight	Not altered
Decreased	Percent body fat	Not altered
Decreased	Appetite	Normal
Disturbed	Digestion	Normal
Present	Insomnia	Absent
Absent	Increased sleep duration	Present
Present	Irritability, restlessness	Absent
Present	Heart palpitations	Absent
Absent	Apathy, disinterest	Present
Present	Depression	Absent

An important clinical feature of overtraining syndrome is increased susceptibility to infections with corresponding symptoms, suggesting some kind of impaired immune response. According to Ryan et al. (1983), chronic muscle soreness may be also a symptom of the overtraining syndrome, as may headaches or exaggeration in postural hypotension. Some cases of chronic fatigue syndrome in athletes appear to be related to overtraining (Eichner, 1989). Costill (1986) suggested that many athletes lose competitive drive and enthusiasm for training, developing aversions to the whole training program, training facilities, or athletes they regularly train with. In contrast, a strong desire to compensate for decreased performance with higher training work loads may actually mask early signs of overtraining. Decreased self-confidence is often evident and thus a consequence of the repeated experiences of weakness and failing. Psychological features such as mood disturbance appear to be sensitive indicators of the onset of overtraining (Druckman & Bjork, 1991; Silva, 1990). Israel (1976) suggested that disturbed coordination of excitatory and inhibitory mechanisms in the cortex may lead to dysphoria and may provoke conflicts in the social environment. Many authors agree that the overtrained athlete may finally experience a typical clinical depression, signaling burnout (Israel, 1976; Kindermann, 1986; Kuipers & Keizer, 1988; Ryan et al., 1983).

Morgan, Brown, Raglin, O'Conner, and Ellickson (1987) and Murphy, Fleck, Dudley, and Callister (1990) used standardized psychological assessment instruments to monitor the psychological impact of heavy training loads. In a series of studies, Morgan et al. (1987) administered the Profile of Mood States (POMS) to swimmers and wrestlers and found that mood disturbances increased with greater training loads. In a study of elite judo athletes, Murphy and his colleagues (1990) used a series of psychological measures, including the POMS, and found increases in fatigue, anger, and anxiety with high-volume training loads. However, the results varied somewhat in relation to the type of training (conditioning vs. sport-specific training). Although these psychological studies demonstrated certain changes related to increased training load, they were not designed to assess the presence or absence of a concurrent overtraining syndrome, as determined by comprehensive physiological and psychological assessment.

Laboratory Findings

In spite of the wide spectrum of clinical findings about overtraining, little is known about underlying physiological changes. The research presently available reports the following changes in overtrained athletes: Reductions in maximum work capacity and maximum plasma lactate during exercise tests (Kindermann, 1986; Lehmann et al., 1990). Also reported have been lowering of hemoglobin, hematocrit, and red blood cell count (Lehmann et al., 1990; Ryan et al., 1983) and changes in blood chemistry levels such as urea (Kindermann, 1986), creatinine phosphokinase (Kindermann, 1986; Lehmann et al., 1990; Ryan et al., 1983), glucose (Lehmann et al., 1990), and others. The hormonal system has shown changes in basic levels of testosterone, free testosterone (i.e., ratio of testosterone to sex-hormone-binding globulin), and the ratio of free testosterone to cortisol (Kindermann, 1988). Researchers have also observed altered response of plasma catecholamine levels during exercise (Kindermann, 1986, 1988; Lehmann et al., 1990) and decreased response of adrenocorticotropic hormone, cortisol, human growth hormone, and prolactin to insulin-induced hypoglycemia (Barron, Noakes, Levy, Smith, & Millar, 1985) as well as change in basic levels of these measures (Neisler et al., 1989). Six studies found lowered immune globulin levels and changes of other immune parameters (Israel, 1976; Kindermann, 1988; Kuipers & Keizer, 1988; Lehmann et al., 1990; Neisler et al., 1989; Tharp & Barnes, 1989). Changes in neurophysiological functions have been indicated by increased excitatory states of various muscles assessed by nervous stimulation of muscles at rest (Mies, 1957); increased fusion frequency on intermittent stroboscopic light stimuli; increased latency of motor responses to visual stimuli (Derevenco, Florea, Derevenco, Anghel, & Simu, 1967); and reduction in stereosynchronization in electroencephalogram (EEG) recordings (Sologub, 1982). Kindermann (1986) found that reduced maximum work capacity appears to be related to disturbances in sympathetic adrenal regulation that result in impaired anaerobic energy supply.

Research on overtraining syndrome has not yet established normal ranges of function. Furthermore, athletes in general are likely to show not only differences from the general population but also broad ranges of individual differences. To present generally normal values may be misleading. The key is to evaluate the athlete individually, monitoring him or her regularly and comparing the obtained data longitudinally.

Contributing Factors

Due to the limited research and the lack of well-documented case studies, we must rely on clinical experience to identify contributing factors. Workload intensity seems to play the major role in overtraining (Israel, 1976; Ryan et al., 1983), in particular frequent intensive, anaerobic workouts without adequate regenerative training or rest (Kindermann, 1986). Ryan et al. (1983) emphasized that incomplete recovery occurs most frequently when athletes participate in too many events and rest too little between competitions. (For example, this occurs in tennis and in road racing when athletes are paid for tournaments or races.) On the other hand, training cycles that last too long without intermittent competitions may result in monotony. In general, any kind of monotony during training may affect the athlete's capacity for compensation.

Experience shows that the sympathetic type of overtraining syndrome is caused when athletes undertake high-intensity anaerobic workouts without sufficient aerobic base (which has to be built up before intensity of training can be increased). Increasing the frequency of high-intensity workouts in endurance training typically triggers the parasympathetic type of overtraining syndrome (Israel, 1976; Kindermann, 1986).

Athletes may get stuck on the idea that they must push themselves hard to catch up with their training partners. Costill (1986) identified fear of failure, excessive expectations from the coach or the public, and demands of competition as additional causative factors. In team sports and during intensive training camps, changes in the moods of athletes are contagious (Ryan et al., 1983). Ryan et al. (1983) suggested that highly motivated athletes and particularly women seem to be at high risk for overtraining syndrome.

Demands of training and competition are not the only factors in the development of overtraining syndrome. A complex set of psychological factors is involved, including personality structure, social environment, relations with family and friends, and educational, professional, and work-related factors. Intolerable emotional stress sometimes plays the major role. Any kind of infection has to be considered, in particular when training is resumed too quickly after illness, preventing sufficient convalescence (Israel, 1976; Kindermann, 1986). Inadequate nutrition or caloric deficiency (Kindermann, 1986; Ryan et al., 1983) may also be important and should be monitored carefully in sports in which extreme weight-loss measures and eating disorders have been observed (e.g., wrestling, women's distance running, and dance).

Injury Risk and Overtraining Syndrome

Injury risk is clearly increased in overtraining syndrome. Two different patterns appear to be involved: injury and overtraining occurring in parallel as separate consequences of the same underlying mechanisms, or injury occurring as a secondary effect of overtraining symptoms.

When injury and overtraining occur in parallel, all the factors contributing to overtraining syndrome may simultaneously affect the musculoskeletal system and result in overuse injuries. This is reflected in the predisposition of overtraining athletes to stress fractures (Stanish, 1984) and other musculoskeletal problems. There is also an increased risk of chronic connective tissue overuse and inflammation such as tendinitis. Israel (1976) pointed out that compensated latent traumata will become manifest under prolonged overload.

Injury risk may also be directly related to excessive training or may be caused by a reduction in the body's capacity to recover and repair tissue. According to Ryan et al. (1983), hormonal changes may be involved in this reduced recovery process. The authors also indicated that stress fractures can occur as reduced appetite and food intake result in substantially lowered blood levels of calcium. This is apparently quite common in female ballet dancers and amenorrheic athletes across a broad range of sports (Lloyd et al., 1986; United States Olympic Committee, 1987).

When injury occurs as a consequence of overtraining syndrome itself, chronic muscle soreness in conjunction with mental and emotional instability may affect nervous coordination of working muscles and the perception of movement and fatigue. Therefore, the athlete may not identify risky situations arising during training or competition adequately or quickly enough to avoid impending acute injury. This may happen especially during intensive exercise and in sports that involve high speed or direct body contact.

Diagnosis and Differential Diagnosis

In many cases of overtraining syndrome, the athlete in combination with the coach or sport psychologist will be able to recognize and manage the situation. In cases of doubtful etiology, a sport physician must be consulted. Depending upon the clinical presentation of symptoms, differing series of diagnostic tests might be necessary. However, there is great variability between individuals in most of those measures, and furthermore these tests can be complicated, expensive, and inconvenient to the athlete. Consequently, diagnosis is primarily based on medical history and the empirically identified physical and psychological characteristics of the syndrome (Kuipers & Keizer, 1988).

The most affordable, simple, and effective diagnostic method is to monitor the athlete regularly for signs of overtraining syndrome (see Figure 6.1). The athlete, coach, and sport psychologist need to keep long-term data of the monitored variables, which ideally are supplemented by regular examinations by a sports physician every 4 to 8 weeks in combination with body fat measurements (a decrease in percent body fat may indicate sympathetic overtraining syndrome) and blood tests (e.g., an increase in red cell sedimentation rate, lowering of red and white blood cell counts and hemoglobin, urea, and creatinine phosphokinase levels). If these data fail to demonstrate specific or remarkable changes, performance tests, which include lactate measurements (e.g., decreases in maximal working capacity and in maximal plasma lactate levels), hormonal assays (e.g., decreases in the levels of testosterone and free testosterone, and the free-testosterone-to-cortisol ratio), or immunological measurements may be necessary (Kindermann, 1986, 1988). Due to the long-term effects and individual changes involved in overtraining syndrome, the athlete must be compared to herself or himself and not to group values (Kindermann, 1988; Ryan et al., 1983).

The sports physician must rule out the presence of any disease, psychophysiological disorder, or other problem whose symptoms mimic those of overtraining syndrome. The physician must search for chronic illness or injuries that may show only few symptoms and therefore be difficult to recognize. Kuipers and Keizer (1988) investigated athletes who were considered to be suffering from overtraining syndrome but found that some had myocarditis, mononucleosis, or a tropical disease. Focal infections (e.g., of paranasal sinuses, teeth, or skin) or allergies (which demonstrate disturbance in the immune system) need to be taken into consideration. Chronic fatigue syndrome shares many of the symptoms of overtraining (Eichner, 1989). The physician must also consider affective and anxiety disorders as well as substance use and eating disorders as a primary cause. With the wide range of diseases that must be taken into consideration, consultation with other specialists may be necessary.

Daily record

Resting heart rate at awakening
(count for 60 s)   _____

Morning weight   _____

Time to bed   _____

Hours slept   _____

Feelings of muscle soreness   _____

Evening fluid intake   _____

General health and mood
self-estimation   _____

Perception of training load
(sense of exhaustion after
single workout)   _____

Periodic record (4 to 8 week intervals)

Body fat   _____

Performance tests   _____

Figure 6.1 Overtraining syndrome diagnostic monitor: athlete checklist.

Effective Therapy for Overtraining Syndrome

Early detection of overtraining syndrome is the key for treatment. The syndrome sometimes can be reversed within a few weeks, but it may last several months, depending on the severity of the individual case, the timeliness of diagnosis, and the effectiveness of treatment. The athlete should be well informed about his or her condition including projected time (weeks or months) until complete recovery. He or she should know that recovery happens stepwise and that setbacks may occur (Israel, 1976). The athlete, coach, psychologist or sport psychologist, and sport physician must communicate regularly to coordinate their efforts.

For short-term overtraining and overreaching, Costill (1986) recommended interruption of training for 3 to 5 days and resumption with lower total volume but maintained intensity. In general, overtraining syndrome requires a drastic cutback of training, and all competitions should be dropped until recovery. In order to allow necessary rest, the athlete should alternate each training session with a day off (Kuipers & Keizer, 1988). In severe cases, coaches should suspend sport-specific training and substitute it with other forms of nonspecific exercise (Israel, 1976). Sometimes it may be useful for the athlete to omit a complete competitive cycle and orient training to the next competitive season. The athlete who has sympathetic overtraining syndrome needs to build up a sufficient aerobic base, beginning with low-intensity endurance training and proceeding with slowly increasing work loads. Parasympathetic overtraining syndrome requires a cutback of high- and low-intensity endurance training and more emphasis on a few strictly limited, intensive, anaerobic work loads (Israel, 1976). Monotony of training and frequent repetition of single workouts must be avoided. Motivation is enhanced by the introduction of variety and novelty into training regimens.

Stanish (1984) emphasized that it is foolish to assume that enforced rest is a panacea. Complete cessation of training may induce an acute exercise-abstinence syndrome. This syndrome typically occurs days or weeks after abrupt discontinuation of athletic training and shows clinical features such as cardiac complaints (e.g., heart palpitations, irregular heartbeat, chest pain), disturbed digestion and appetite, sleep disorders, increased sweating, depression, and emotional instability (Baekeland, 1970; Israel, 1967). Exercise-abstinence syndrome has similarities to overtraining syndrome and may even exacerbate the athlete's symptoms.

Treatment must consider both psychosocial and biological factors. Israel (1976) and Kindermann (1986) recommended sufficient rest, sleep, and relaxation and proper nutrition. Any illness or injury needs immediate diagnosis and consequent treatment by a sport physician, if necessary in coordination with other specialists. To cope with emotional conflicts or psychological demands, the athlete should consult a sport psychologist. Ongoing monitoring through repeat testing of mood (e.g., by the POMS or other psychological measures) facilitates evaluation of overtraining syndrome. The essential element in a successful sport psychology intervention is the reestablishment of appropriate performance goals (Henschen, 1986). Self-regulation procedures (autogenic training, mental imagery, relaxation training, visualization, and yoga) seem to be very effective. In case of a profound depression or neurotic adaptation, Israel (1976) recommended treatment via autonomic nervous system regulation. This includes deliberately awakening the athlete in order to maintain an appropriate sleep schedule in the case of hypersomnia or short-term administration of sedatives in the case of insomnia.

Regularly performed laboratory and psychological tests will help the physician determine if therapy is progressing effectively. Demonstrable progress gives athletes and coaches confidence and motivation to continue to apply the therapeutic measures. No progress indicates either ineffective treatment or a prolonged course of recovery.

In general, overtraining syndrome is reversible if treated adequately. Burnout resulting in dropout from sport is mostly related to an improper evaluation of the situation or to a treatment that is too short or otherwise inadequate.

Prevention

Due to the complexity of overtraining syndrome, preventive measures require a multimethod approach. The importance of ongoing monitoring by coach and athlete and timely medical and psychological evaluation has already been noted. One of the most important factors is a well-balanced training program, which gradually increases work loads in a logical progression (Kuipers & Keizer, 1988; Ryan et al., 1983). Because most of the cardiovascular adaptations seem to occur in 3-week cycles, the athlete can normally adapt to a certain percentage increase in work load within 3 weeks (Ryan et al., 1983). The risk of overtraining will be reduced if training follows the natural biological response of adaptation (a wavelike design), with each cycle having a different main focus of intended adaptive change. Such periodization represents an essential tool for prevention of overtraining syndrome.

The coach and athlete need to evaluate regularly the relationship between training load and performance. Too often recovery, an essential component of athletic training, is overlooked. It is not surprising that athletes sometimes perform better after a forced rest period that was caused by a mild illness or slight injury. Most athletes should be discouraged from doing additional workouts simply because they feel particularly good during training. My personal experience is that athletes' perceptions of great shape in combination with their inabilities to critically evaluate their own mental states may be a sign of increased sympathetic activity and may indicate impending overtraining syndrome (of either type). Intensive workouts should be alternated with training sessions consisting mainly of relatively low-intensity endurance activities. Before starting interval or intensive workout periods, the athlete must establish a good endurance or aerobic base.

Ryan et al. (1983) recommended that coaches keep records of workouts, set goals, and stick to them. Good communication between athlete and coach is a basic preventive principle as is involvement with a sport psychologist. Coaches and sport psychologists should regularly discuss self-monitored data (as presented in Figure 6.1) with the athlete, frequently evaluate the athlete's mental outlook, and be informed of important changes in the athlete's family and social environments. Chronic negative changes in self-monitored data (e.g., decrease in weight, insufficient evening fluid intake, chronic muscle soreness, increase in resting heart rate of 5 to 10 beats per min) may signal the beginning of overtraining syndrome.

Standardized laboratory tests performed every 4 to 8 weeks inform the sport physician, coach, and athlete about positive or negative training adaptations and indicate whether and how training load can be increased. Results indicating decreased performance may be the first objective signs of overtraining syndrome. Drop in body fat (which is simply measured) is diagnostic of sympathetic overtraining syndrome. Blood tests (e.g., hemoglobin, hematocrit, red blood cell count, creatine phosphokinase, urea, and hormonal levels) sometimes help detect early signals of overtraining syndrome (Kindermann, 1986, 1988; Kuipers & Keizer, 1988).

Training must be adjusted if any kind of physical or emotional stress has already affected the athlete's performance. If the athlete develops an infectious disease, intensity or volume of training should be drastically reduced or training should even be suspended. Any infection lasting more than 2 or 3 days should be carefully diagnosed and adequately treated, especially when fever is present or the lymphatic system is involved. During the athlete's convalescence, the coach must pay close attention to the appropriate gradual increase in intensity and duration of training and should not assign the athlete too much work too soon. In a double-blind study of 20 swimmers, preventive application of intramuscular-injected gamma globulins every 4 weeks shortened the duration of banal infections and improved athletes' perceptions of physical fitness (Froehlich, Simon, Schmidt, Hitschhold, & Bierther, 1987).

Athletes should take care of disturbed relations in their family and social environments. Younger athletes need support from their parents (Hellstedt, 1988). Enough rest and sleep are obligatory, and a well-balanced sports-adjusted nutrition program is also a preventive measure. Substrates of energy metabolism, in particular glycogen, and fluid and minerals lost through perspiration require immediate repletion. Coach, sport psychologist, and sport physician must watch for first signs of anorexia, especially in female athletes.

Concluding Comments

Because of the increasing time athletes spend training, overtraining syndrome is becoming more common, resulting in unexpectedly poor performances and high risks of injury. Not enough is known about the psychophysiological mechanisms underlying adaptation to training and overtraining syndrome. The best and most affordable preventive measure still remains monitoring of the athlete, which should be done by coach, sport psychologist, and sport physician. But athletes also must learn to monitor and critically evaluate their own physical and mental states and to communicate with their coaches. Coaches should have "the confidence to let athletes do less rather than make them do more at times" (Ryan et al., 1983). The possible links between overtraining syndrome, increased injury risk, burnout, and premature career termination merit further investigation.

III
PART

Injury Assessment

Effective diagnostic assessment is the cornerstone of successful treatment. The psychological assessment of sport injury should be timely, efficient, and sensitive to elements of context as well as to the injured athlete's personal concerns. The overarching goal of assessment is to determine the cost of injury and the strength of the athlete's coping resources—and their relative balance. Understanding the role of sport in the athlete's life is essential. Knowledge of the sport milieu and of how injury is likely to be viewed by others who share this world with the athlete is also important. A timely and sensitive approach to diagnosis can uncover the source of adjustment problems and pave the way for prompt and precisely focused treatment.

Part III contains three chapters. Chapter 7, "A Framework for Psychological Assessment," is broad in scope, reviewing the wide range of issues that are relevant to assessment. The chapter identifies and discusses factors associated with injury, as well as those that precede and follow injury, and reviews controversial concepts including secondary gain and the injury-prone athlete.

Chapter 8, "Diagnostic Methods and Measures," surveys the techniques with which diagnostic assessment is implemented. The chapter emphasizes the benefits of a carefully conceived and conducted diagnostic interview and reviews psychological tests and measures that are particularly suited to the assessment of athletic injury. This chapter also provides recommendations for selection, administration, and feedback of these tests and highlights the value of including supplemental sources (such as coaching and sports medicine staff) in obtaining a truly comprehensive assessment. This chapter also provides a detailed treatment of multimodal pain assessment.

Chapter 9, "Conducting Assessment and Intervention," presents practical recommendations about conducting timely, efficient, and appropriate assessment. The chapter emphasizes the importance of a programmatic approach and proposes a general intervention strategy that varies according to injury severity, psychological adaptation, developmental issues, and sport and lifestyle issues that influence the meaning of injury to the athlete. The chapter provides specific protocols for consultation-liaison assessment and for the evaluation of acute and chronic injury and includes a Sports Medicine Injury Checklist to help the health professional identify psychological adjustment problems.

7
CHAPTER

A Framework for Psychological Assessment

John Heil

In the life of the athlete, injury is perhaps the ultimate stressor. Injury occurs frequently and can severely disrupt the athlete's ability to pursue athletic goals. A thorough psychological diagnostic assessment goes beyond the objective evaluation of injury to identify the personal meaning of injury to the athlete. We assume that all injury carries some degree of psychological cost. The fundamental strategy of psychological diagnostic assessment is to identify the subjective cost of injury to the athlete as well as his or her coping resources. This involves attention to a broad array of physical, psychological, and social factors related to the athlete's unique needs and to the role that sport plays in his or her life.

In contrast to the nonathlete, the athlete is both uniquely challenged by injury and particularly well prepared to cope with it. An athlete's advantages typically include a goal orientation, proclivity for physical training, strong motivation to return to optimal function, and good pain tolerance. The athlete likely has more experience than the nonathlete in coping with injury. But there are disadvantages for the athlete as well. Return to normal daily function is simply not good enough for the athlete, who obviously needs a longer recovery in order to meet the performance demands of sport (although the athlete often expects quick recovery). Due to the great investment of time, energy, and emotion (and perhaps money) in sport, the athlete experiences a greater loss with injury and a potentially greater threat to self-esteem than does the nonathlete. The relative balance of the positive and negative factors

Positive	Negative
Motivation	Sense of loss
Pain tolerance	Threat to self-image
Goal orientation	Sport performance demands
Physical training habits	Expectations of quick recovery

Figure 7.1 Psychological factors in rehabilitation of athletes.

associated with injury will determine the speed and effectiveness of rehabilitation (see Figure 7.1).

Diagnostic Overview

A comprehensive framework for thorough diagnostic assessment includes factors associated with injury as well as those preceding and following injury. These are summarized in Table 7.1.

Factors Preceding Injury

Personal attitudes and behaviors as well as events in the recent and remote past reflect on an athlete's coping ability and his or her readiness to face the challenge of injury. Factors such as medical and psychological history and evidence of somatization provide insight into the strength of the foundation on which coping ability is based. Awareness of stress and significant changes in sport and in the athlete's life is quite informative. These events, which put an athlete at risk for injury "before the fact" (see chapter 5), also put the athlete at risk for problems after injury. The psychologist (or other member of the sports medicine team) should also consider the potential role of overtraining syndrome, the approach of major competitions, the effects of marginal player status, and other sport-related health risk factors (e.g., drug use or eating disorders).

Medical History. It is useful to know if the athlete has any preexisting medical conditions or a problematic medical history (e.g., repeated injury, multiple surgeries, lengthy hospitalization), particularly if they were marked by difficulty in coping. A recurring injury that has posed significant difficulty in the past is particularly noteworthy. An athlete's first serious injury may be extremely disruptive with subsequent injury less

Table 7.1
Diagnostic Overview

Factors preceding injury

Medical history
Psychological history
Somatization
Life stress and change
Sport stress and change
Approach of major competition
Marginal player status
Overtraining
Sport-related health risk factors

Factors associated with injury

Emotional distress
Injury site
Pain
Timeliness
Unexpectedness

Factors following injury

Culpability
Compliance with treatment
Perceived effectiveness
Treatment complications
Pain
Medication use
Psychological status
Social support
Personality conflicts
Fans and the media
Litigation

so as the athlete learns coping methods. However, the repeated stress and strain of injury over a career may, at some point, undermine the recovery process. The National Hockey League Physicians Society has expressed concern about the cumulative effects of injury on athletes' psychological and physical well-being (Kizilos, 1989).

Psychological History.   Repeated or recent problems with psychological adjustment are cause for concern, because there may evolve a reciprocally reinforcing relationship between injury and psychological difficulties. Evidence of poor adjustment is reflected by prior psychological disorder, a history of drug problems, or difficulty in psychosocial adjustment including trouble in school and with the law. The psychologist's knowledge of remote history becomes increasingly important as the athlete demonstrates problems in adjusting to injury. In some cases the athlete may feel that such a thorough history-taking effort is intrusive, which can undermine the treatment relationship. However, information is often available indirectly through medical records.

It is also important to determine the relative balance of needs met through sport involvement and those met by other aspects of the athlete's life. When an athlete's sense of self-efficacy and self-esteem largely depends upon athletic prowess, injury is especially threatening.

Somatization. Somatization is characterized by the inability to differentiate somatic sensations arising from physical illness and those that typically accompany emotional distress (C.J. Taylor, 1984). The somatic component of emotion is well conveyed in the body metaphors we use in speech (e.g., "butterflies in the stomach," "pain in the neck," "uptight," "choking"). From this perspective, somatization may be viewed as an information-processing deficit whereby a person overinterprets and mislabels somatic sensations. Virtually everyone makes occasional somatization-type information-processing errors, especially under duress. Limiting such processing errors is a component in learning to differentiate benign pain from injury.

A small segment of the general population is prone to psychophysiological disorders and difficulty in coping with injury and illness (Ford, 1983; Fordyce, 1976). Although manifested in varying degrees, in its extreme form somatization is characterized by a long history of pain and varied somatic complaints, frequent use of medications, and a high rate of use of medical services for vaguely defined conditions. Following injury, the person who is prone to somatization tends to focus on pain and somatic complaints while generally denying emotional distress. To the observer, the physical complaints may appear overstated and emotional distress underreported. In diagnostic interview, the patient's conversational style is vague and discursive and typically directed away from discussion of psychological factors and toward complaints of pain.

Somatization is most common among young athletes and among others whose sport participation is not truly elective. This includes situations such as required physical education programs or prescribed rehabilitation programs. An interesting but unanswered question is whether a natural selection process operates in sport that eliminates those prone to somatization as athletes move up the hierarchy of achievement in competitive sport.

Life Stress and Change.   There is growing evidence that life stress, in the form of either major life changes or chronic daily hassles, is predictive of injury. Risk that life stress will lead to injury is greatest in the segment of the athletic population characterized by limited psychosocial support and poor coping ability (R.E. Smith, Smoll, & Ptacek, 1990a). It appears appropriate to pay careful attention to the athlete when major negative life changes coincide with injury because the demands of one problem may undermine the athlete's ability to cope with other problems. Instruments like the Social Readjustment Rating Scale (Holmes & Rahe, 1967) and the Adolescent Perceived Events Scale (Compas, Davis, Forsythe, & Wagner, 1987) may serve as useful checklists for adults and adolescents, respectively. A detailed treatment of life change stress is provided in chapter 5.

Sport Stress and Change.   There are few settings in which the potential for sudden and dramatic change is as ever-present as in sport. All athletes must cope with the fact that one day they can be winners and the next day losers. In this context change means challenge, whether it is following up on an outstanding performance or bouncing back from a poor one. As a consequence, even positive changes can be stressful. Recent sport change events constitute important markers. Inventories such as the Social and Athletic Readjustment Rating Scale (Bramwell, Masuda, Wagner, & Holmes, 1975) and the Athletic Life Experiences Survey (Passer & Seese, 1983) provide useful guides to review the athlete's current status.

The psychologist can also obtain important information indirectly through consultation with the coaching staff. Change in team status, steady improvement or decline in performance, and remarkably good or bad play in a critical situation can be easily identified, and change in playing conditions or positions is also noteworthy. Where interpersonal problems exist among players and staff prior to an athlete's injury, return to play may be more complicated.

Natural transitions in sport such as a change in level of competition from high school to college can bring new and greater challenges (Pearson & Petitpas, 1990). Movement to a higher competitive level brings increased mental and physical demands, and in addition the athlete often must adjust to a new social or geographic environment.

Approach of Major Competition.   Investigators have observed increases in injury and illness as major competitions approach (Kerr & Minden, 1988; Nideffer, 1983). This is likely due to the combined effects of the heavy training load that often precedes major competitions and the psychological stress of the competition itself. Long-distance travel, which may influence sleep and diet, may also play a role. Because of the potentially recurrent nature of this problem, it is useful to identify factors that lead an athlete to be at risk before a major competition; factors can include attentional deficits, increasing anxiety, and a tendency to increase training load. Once identified, these factors can be addressed preventatively to help the athletes prepare for the approach of subsequent major competitions.

Marginal Player Status.   Highly motivated marginal players may be prone to take risks in order to enhance their status and opportunities. They may be particularly concerned about losing opportunities as a consequence of injury and may attempt to hide injury. They may also hide injury if they are sensitive to being labeled as "not tough" (Rotella & Heyman, 1986).

Research has raised but failed to answer the troubling question of whether marginal players are at increased risk of injury because they may be expected and directed to engage in more dangerous behavior or may be issued lower quality equipment (e.g., Pargman, 1986). Of equal concern is the plight of those who play low-status sports, those who may have inadequate medical care, or, those who have inferior sports equipment.

Overtraining.   Overtraining is manifested as increased fatigue and decreased performance in conjunction with a potentially broad array of related symptoms that include emotional instability, increased susceptibility to infection, and sleep disturbance. Overtraining occurs when training load exceeds the athlete's physiological coping capacity. Overtraining syndrome is difficult to diagnose because of the broad variability of symptoms and the absence of a definitive diagnostic procedure. Overtraining syndrome is related to staleness and burnout, which will also complicate recovery (see chapter 6 for a detailed treatment).

Sport-Related Health Risk Factors.   Athletes have been identified as a population at risk for substance abuse and eating disorders as well as problems related to competitive stress. Recreational and ergogenic drug use is widely noted (Tricker & Cook, 1990; Wadler & Hainline, 1989). Drug use has a broad variety of potential psychological and medical effects. Substances that may result in anxiety include nicotine, caffeine, alcohol, cocaine, ginseng, antihistamines, and cold preparations containing ephedrine or pseudoephedrine. Anxiety may also arise in withdrawal from opiates, sedatives, alcohol, nicotine, and tranquilizers. Depression may be influenced by tranquilizers and antihypertensives such as beta blockers (Stout, 1988).

The use of steroids and related agents in sports that place a premium on size and strength is well recognized as are a variety of health-related risks (American College of Sports Medicine, 1987b). The most immediately relevant of these is increased likelihood of soft tissue injury. Adverse psychological reactions including mood inflation, imperturbability, poor judgment, and aggressiveness (Gregg & Rejeski, 1990; Lubell, 1989b) are being increasingly observed. Psychotic reactions may also be precipitated by steroid use (Stout, 1988).

In "weight class" sports (e.g., wrestling) there is a concern regarding the health impact of extreme weight loss measures including the use of diuretics and laxatives, fluid deprivation, and other means of intentional dehydration (American College of Sports Medicine, 1976). These practices are also common in sports that subjectively evaluate physical form (e.g., women's gymnastics or dance); participants in these sports appear to be at greater risk for bulimia or anorexia with consequent medical and psychological problems. Where extreme weight loss or heavy training result in amenorrhea there is evidence of increased risk for stress fracture (Lloyd et al., 1986).

Factors Associated With Injury

The greater the overall impact of the injury at the moment of its occurrence, the greater the emotional challenge the athlete faces during rehabilitation. The factors to be considered include emotional distress, the site of injury, and the immediate experience of pain, as well as the timeliness, culpability, and unexpectedness of injury.

Emotional Distress. The greater the psychological trauma, the greater the likelihood of treatment complications. Significant psychological impact is indicated by any of the following:

1. Extreme fear, anxiety, agitation, or hopelessness observed or reported at the time of injury
2. Catastrophizing thoughts occurring at the time of injury (especially those that persist in spite of reassuring evidence to the contrary)
3. A sense of derealization or depersonalization
4. Incomplete memory of circumstances of the injury
5. Retrograde or posttraumatic amnesia (of even brief duration)

The more extreme the emotional response relative to injury severity and the more limited the athlete's coping resources, the greater the cause for concern. Reinjury especially following a difficult rehabilitation course can be disproportionately disturbing if it calls to mind prior trauma or triggers persistent catastrophizing thoughts. Relatively mild emotional response to a threatening situation may be explained by an athlete's strong sense of social support, native coping ability, and prior experience with injury. Timely medical care that engenders trust and confidence at the time of injury enhances coping (Jacobs, 1991). The adaptive use of denial as a defense mechanism may also play a role. The factors discussed subsequently also contribute to the degree of psychological trauma.

Injury Site. Injury to a part of the body that is highly prized or for which there is a special fear has greater psychological impact than other injuries (Eldridge, 1983). Injuries to the face, the genitalia, and the hand tend to be most problematic (Chambers, 1963; Ford, 1983; Grunert, Devine, Matloub, Sanger, & Yousif, 1988), and injuries that cause significant disfigurement are also problematic. Traditionally, women are more sensitive to injuries that cause loss of physical attractiveness, whereas men are more sensitive to loss of functional ability (Ford, 1983).

There is cause for special concern when injury occurs to a paired organ (e.g., eye, kidney, testicle) for which one of the set is already absent or dysfunctional.

Pain.   Pain as an immediate response to injury reflects not only the severity of tissue damage but also anxiety and expectations regarding the impact of injury on performance. Loeser (1991) offers an anecdotal case report to illustrate this. A collegiate quarterback who had returned to play following a severe knee injury stayed down after a tackle, apparently in severe pain. He was briefly examined on the field and reassured that the knee was still intact. His pain seemed to diminish quickly, and he was able to walk with assistance off the field. On the sidelines, this now-reduced pain continued as he tried with difficulty to "walk it off." He eventually reached down to feel his lower leg and found a bone was fractured and pushing out through the skin. At this instant the pain once again became severe.

Pain that appears out of proportion to the magnitude of injury may signify a breakdown of coping mechanisms. Pain response that appears mild relative to extent of tissue damage has often been noted and is attributed to a positive mind-set (e.g., Beecher, 1956).

Timeliness.   Even relatively minor injury at a key point in an athlete's competitive season or career can be of tremendous consequence. Season-ending injuries can create a sense of incompleteness that lingers into the next competitive cycle. There is evidence that injuries become more likely near the end of a natural cycle of activity—and that these injuries lead to more problems psychologically (Braverman, 1977).

Individuals may hold superstitions regarding timing of injury, or groups may share such expectations. For example, there is a long-standing belief among soldiers that death or injury is most likely on the last mission before rotation off combat duty (Ford, 1983). There is also evidence to suggest that injury or illness is more likely on the anniversary of a significant prior trauma (Dlin, 1985).

Unexpectedness.   In low- and moderate-risk activities, a highly proficient athlete may have a more troubled reaction to serious injury than one who is less skilled or experienced. Braverman (1977) noted this in ski and work-related injuries. In contrast, when athletes understand and accept high risks, distress may be less. Beecher (1946, 1956) observed dramatically greater pain tolerance and less need for medication in soldiers wounded in combat compared to general medical patients with injuries of comparable severity.

For the athlete who eludes the dangers inherent in sport it may be particularly distressing to lose playing time to an accident outside of sport or to illness. For example, it can be tremendously frustrating for a competitive downhill skier to slip on the ice while walking or for an auto racer to be injured in a motor vehicle accident while out for a drive with friends.

Factors Following Injury

The greater the chronicity of injury whether due to severity or to rehabilitation complications, the greater the likelihood of psychological adjustment problems. Progress in rehabilitation, psychological status, and response of significant others to injury are key factors, which psychologists may assess by monitoring compliance with treatment, the perceived effectiveness of rehabilitation, treatment complications, pain, medication use, psychological status, social support, personality conflicts, responses of fans and the media, and litigation.

Culpability.   Where there is a preoccupation with culpability for injury, whether attributed to oneself or another, adjustment problems are more frequent. If the one injured assumes responsibility for the occurrence of injury or interprets injury as a failure, feelings of guilt are likely. In team sports, injured athletes may also feel they have let their team down. Significant others who have an investment in the athlete's competitive success (coaches, teammates, parents, family) may react in a way that enhances guilt. Some sports (e.g., tennis, gymnastics) can require a substantial financial sacrifice by families of children who show competitive promise, and some families evidence dissatisfaction following an injury.

Anger may result if the athlete blames someone else for an injury (Ogilvie & Tutko, 1966), such as a coach for putting the athlete at unneccesary risk or a health professional for providing inadequate care. Such anger may create problems in interpersonal relations between the athlete and the one being blamed.

The athlete is more likely to be disturbed by injury that occurs as a consequence of an intentional, calculated action to do harm than by injury that occurs during routine play (Ford, 1983). This can be all the more disturbing because of the tendency for such destructive behavior to go relatively unpunished. For example, Daniel was an elite team sport athlete who suffered head and neck injuries in a brawl in which he was not an aggressor. He was hit with a blind-sided attack against which he was unable to defend himself. His sport career was ended and he was unable to work. Through a long and complicated course of rehabilitation, he tolerated his injuries stoically. There was always great poignancy as he described the other athlete's clear intent to do harm and the subtle encouragement of such behavior provided by the opposing team. Daniel stated that he could accept being hurt in the course of the game but to be injured intentionally made him feel that the other player took his career away.

Compliance With Treatment.   The importance of compliance with treatment in ultimate recovery is readily evident. From a diagnostic point of view the advantage of this behavior is that it is typically easily observed. Compliance is not a unidimensional function of patient personality but rather the consequence of a variety of factors including the nature of treatment, competing environmental demands, the patient–health care provider relationship, and individual patient characteristics (Meichenbaum & Turk, 1987). Failure to comply is a problem in its own right and is predictive of other issues as diverse as rehabilitation scheduling difficulties and overall motivation (Duda, Smart, & Tappe, 1989; Fisher, Domm, & Wuest, 1988). If there are compliance problems, it is useful for the psychologist to assess the logistics of rehabilitation, considering factors such as scheduling convenience and comfort of the training room environment. Alternatively, poor compliance may be a function of the factors subsequently discussed.

Perceived Effectiveness.   The athlete's willingness to report a positive motivational set and satisfaction with treatment progress are positive prognostic indicators (Duda, Smart, & Tappe, 1989; Fisher, Domm, & Wuest, 1988). When treatment is perceived to be progressing effectively, mood is generally good (McDonald & Hardy, 1990). Where health care providers and the athlete share favorable impressions of treatment effectiveness, treatment appears to be on course.

In the early stage of severe injury, denial (regarding injury severity and recovery) is often an appropriate way to diminish the immediate impact of the trauma. However, prolonged reliance on this defense mechanism, as evidenced by failure to accept realistic goals, is problematic.

Treatment Complications.   Treatment setbacks as well as unsuccessful attempts to return to play are of concern not only because they delay rehabilitation but also because of their psychological impact. Setbacks tend to enhance a sense of failure and vulnerability and raise fears of reinjury, and they can lead the athlete to question the quality of care. In complicated injury situations iatrogenic problems may have a similar effect on the athlete. Lengthy treatment plateaus even when anticipated by treatment providers can be a source of distress as well.

Pain.   The tolerance of pain in one form or another is a routine aspect of sport performance for most athletes. However, pain is typically well controlled, usually ceasing significantly following activity and in some instances giving way to enhanced mood (Morgan & O'Conner, 1988). Injury-related pain is less under individual control and poses a somewhat different self-management problem. Even for athletes who show remarkably good tolerance for performance pain, the pain of injury can be quite distressing.

Toleration of pain and the broad scope of its impact on functioning are related not only to severity of pain but also to the individual's interpretation of the meaning of pain. Consider an athlete undergoing resistance training in the rehabilitation of injury. If the athlete interprets pain as related to building muscle strength, he or she will probably be willing to continue activity. If the athlete fears that pain means exacerbation of injury or reinjury, he or she obviously will be less willing to continue training. Interpretation of pain as a danger signal may lead to protective bracing or guarding, hesitancy in approaching particular situations, or outright avoidance. Detailed recommendations regarding pain assessment are presented in chapter 8.

Medication Use.   Monitoring for correct use of medication as well as for potential side effects is prudent. Medication is often not taken according to instructions. For about two thirds of the 750 million new prescriptions written each year, there is partial or complete noncompliance (Meichenbaum & Turk, 1987). Specific instructions provided by the physician regarding what to do if symptoms increase or decrease or if side effects occur can be reinforced by both the psychologist and the sports medicine specialist. There is an estimated 2 to 3% incidence of psychological symptoms with the use of medications commonly prescribed for injury and illness (Hall, Gruzenski, & Popkin, 1979). Persistent medication seeking by the athlete signals problems with pain tolerance, which may in turn reflect problems in psychological adjustment; that is, the athlete may use psychoactive medicines as a coping tool.

Psychological Status.   Pervasive dysphoric mood with signs of depression, anxiety, anger, and guilt is relatively easily recognized. Although some depression or anxiety following severe injury is understandable and certainly not abnormal, persistent symptoms that do not respond to informal support and encouragement should evoke concern. Often psychological difficulties following injury may remain masked and may be discerned only with careful observation. When anxiety or fearfulness is situation specific (e.g., fear of reinjury only in circumstances that resemble those in which injury occurred), it is less apparent. Diminished concentration and memory may also become obvious only in performance situations. Distractibility and forgetfulness during rehabilitation and failure to understand the nature of injury and treatment following adequate explanation suggest problems.

Dysphoria may also be indirectly represented in behavior. Disturbed sleep, gastrointestinal distress, and non-injury-related pain (e.g., headaches) merit prompt attention because of the added stress they create for the athlete and the impact they may have on the speediness of rehabilitation. Communication among treatment providers and coaching staff regarding the athlete's psychological status facilitates accurate assessment.

Social Support.   The positive role of social support in the management of injury is widely recognized in sport psychology (Duda et al., 1989; Fisher et al., 1988; Rosenfeld, Richman, & Hardy, 1989). Social support provides reassurance, a safe environment for the expression of emotions, and encouragement in the use of problem-solving skills. It reduces anxiety and increases one's sense of self-efficacy (Sarason, Sarason, & Pierce, 1990). Support from coaches, teammates, friends, and parents, as well as from sports medicine professionals, is valuable.

Although positive support is typically the norm, there can be negative responses from teammates, coaches, and others. In a survey of over 500 collegiate volleyball players, subjects reported negative responses such as pressure to return to play from coaches (24%) and teammates (6%) (Hankins, Gipson, Foster, Yaffe, & O'Carroll, 1989).

Personality Conflicts.   Athletes and treatment providers share the same goal—safe, speedy return to play. However, they hold much different perspectives on the rehabilitation process. The treatment provider's focus is on objective signs of healing and progress in rehabilitation, which he or she evaluates according to a "norm" of recovery for athletes with similar injuries. In contrast, the athlete's perspective is subjective, reflecting personal hopes and desires. A compelling desire to return to play can lead the athlete to feel impatience and frustration with treatment providers who are perceived as not getting the athlete healthier fast enough.

Conflicts may also arise with family, friends, coaches, or teammates. These may be due to frustration and irritability that reflect the athlete's difficulty in adjusting to injury. Alternately, conflicts may evolve out of inappropriate responses by significant others.

Fans and the Media.   The reactions of fans and the media to an athlete can have a significant effect—good or bad. Geoff Petrie (see chapter 2) comments on the potentially devastating role that this reaction can have on athletes. The media have a tremendously influential role not only in reporting events but also in shaping opinion.

However, the potential for support is just as strong. Stock car racer Neil Bonnett (personal communication, March 11, 1990) reported needing an extra hospital room to accommodate the flowers and cards he received from fans following a serious injury. He commented, "When I was really down and out I lay here on the couch and read those things day after day. It really meant a lot." He was especially struck by those who identified themselves as fans of another driver who were nonetheless concerned about him, having appreciated his achievement as a driver.

Although nothing compares with the visibility of professional and major college athletics, sports at all levels receive newspaper coverage. Even though the audience for high school sports and minor collegiate programs is small and the scope of the media that serve them is modest, the media impact within the local community can be significant. For the treatment provider, knowing when and how the injured athlete is presented in the media is important.

Litigation.   Following a neck injury that left him a quadriplegic, Citadel football player Marc Buoniconti filed suit against his physician, trainer, and school. Although his doctor was eventually exonerated from a $22-million lawsuit, Buoniconti was awarded an $800,000 independent settlement from the school and the athletic trainer. This is but one of many lawsuits filed each year at all levels of sport.

There is a growing trend toward litigation in both sport and medicine. Civil suits for liability in athletic injury have been directed to medical personnel (for negligent treatment or diagnosis), coaches and teachers (for negligent supervision or instruction), and to those responsible for equipment and facilities (Lybbert & Laycock, 1987). More extreme examples of violent behavior resulting in injury have been subject to criminal proceedings (Reed, 1976).

Although a person's desire for justice when wronged can be great and justice can be much deserved, it can be costly as well. Even for the injured party, litigation can be prolonged, expensive, and stressful. It tends to reinforce a focus on the worst elements of the past event at the expense of a more positive and adaptive future focus. Health providers who specialize in the treatment of chronic injury widely believe that ongoing litigation can inhibit recovery.

Diagnostic Controversies

This chapter has described important situational and personal factors in injury risk, but additional items merit mention because of their complex and controversial nature. Two concepts that often arise in conjunction with injury management problems are those of the injury-prone athlete and of secondary gain. Unfortunately, both concepts are often misunderstood and at times may be invoked to the disadvantage or misfortune of the athlete. These concepts may function as diagnostic shortcuts that fail to address the diversity and complexity of the underlying dynamics that contribute to problems with injury.

The Injury-Prone Athlete

It is generally much easier to identify an injury-causing activity (e.g., football or mountain climbing vs. soccer or hiking) than an injury-prone athlete. When one is considering an individual athlete, it is probably of greater utility to identify injury-prone attitudes (e.g., playing with injury) or behaviors (e.g., steroid use). This approach goes beyond simply labeling a problem and provides some direction toward a solution.

It has been suggested that the concept of injury proneness may, in many cases, draw attention away from dangers inherent in certain environments and undermine the adoption of needed safety practices (Sass & Crook, 1981). This calls attention to the important role to be played by sport governing bodies in monitoring injury, making rules, and setting equipment standards.

Epidemiological research has identified children, the elderly, and those engaging in substance use to be at relatively increased risk for sport injury. The mechanism appears to be deficits in attention and motor skills (Sass & Crook, 1981). Concerns about injury proneness also apply to "special" populations including people who are psychologically and physically disabled. This is especially significant in light of the growing involvement of these groups in sport activities. Careful identification of appropriate medical limits for sport participation, such as those addressed in preparticipation medical screenings, is an important component in the management of this dimension of injury risk (American Academy of Pediatrics, 1988; Hudson, 1988).

Secondary Gain

Injury is a negative event in that it bars the athlete from a highly prized activity—sport. In our sympathetic society, however, the injured person gains some favorable consequences, such as increased attention from significant others, sympathy and social support, release from day-to-day responsibilities, escape from stressful situations, and medication use. These favorable consequences, which occur in conjunction with the generally undesirable injury, are termed *secondary gains*. The losses of injury and the benefits of secondary gain constitute a complex set of interacting forces that reshape the athlete's world while he or she is injured. Secondary gains are subtle in their influence and generally operate outside the athlete's conscious awareness.

Secondary gain is positive in that social support, sympathy, attention, advice, and concern can boost the athlete's morale and make her or him feel less alone in the uphill battle to regain health. However, secondary gain can be a mixed blessing when it reinforces and maintains the "sick" role, thereby interfering with and delaying rehabilitation. Luckily, this seldom happens with a highly motivated athlete who had good preinjury functioning.

Where the benefits of the sick role outweigh those of recovery, rehabilitation will proceed more slowly than is medically prognosticated. The sports medicine professional must, at this time, examine the total situation with a particular look at the athlete's attitude toward sport and the secondary gain she or he receives from remaining injured. In general, situations of slowed rehabilitation with entrenched secondary gain represent an uncomfortable compromise between a desired ideal outcome (return to play at an equal or improved level) and the fear of a worst-case scenario (return to play with performance failure or reinjury). Secondary gain is rarely a solitary factor of slowed recovery but is usually only one element of a set of contributing factors. Others may include traumatic conditioning, fear of reinjury, pain problems, and personality style, which typically interact in a complex fashion.

When injury is a convenient way out of an otherwise unrewarding athletic situation, secondary gain may play a compelling role in nonrecovery. In such a case the treatment provider may wish to facilitate a more direct and appropriate transition out of sport for this person.

When the sick role persists in young athletes and secondary gain seems to be delaying rehabilitation, the situation is possibly a parent-child relationship problem. The parents may be pressuring the child to participate when he or she does not wish to do so, or they may be making unrealistic demands for success. Where further assessment reinforces the initial impression that parental pressure is having a disruptive impact on the attitude of the athlete, the psychologist should counsel the parents directly.

Concluding Comments

Psychological assessment requires attention to factors that occur in conjunction with injury and during the process of rehabilitation as well as those that precede injury. Injury should be considered not just an event but a force setting up a chain of events that include disruption of sport and daily activities, the athlete's personal reaction to the disrupting impact of injury, and the response of persons significant to the athlete. These multiple effects are interactive, collectively influencing an athlete's state of mind. A comprehensive assessment strategy facilitates early identification and intervention in problem situations and improves the quality of care that can be provided.

8
CHAPTER

Diagnostic Methods and Measures

John Heil

Diagnostic assessment paints the overall picture of injury and its impact on the athlete. The many and varied diagnostic methods and measures are the tools that psychologists use in making assessments. The nature of the picture, in turn, reflects the tools themselves as well as the skill with which they are used.

The heart of assessment is personal interview. It may vary from highly structured interview to open and free-form discussion, and it elicits information from both self-report and nonverbal behavior. But diagnosis is not simply a series of questions; it is a process, the goal of which is not only to collect information but also to establish a treatment relationship. In general, establishing confidence and trust is more important than collecting information. The process of evaluation can be intrusive, and the psychologist should try to minimize intrusion. The approach to evaluation should balance the receptivity of the athlete, the severity of the psychological impact, and the degree of time urgency.

The psychologist can supplement the personal interview with varied forms of assessment devices ranging from the simple and straightforward (such as a rating of pain) to the lengthy and complex (such as the Minnesota Multiphasic Personality Inventory, or MMPI). Sport-specific assessment instruments are available as well as those for use with the general population. The use of psychological testing has a controversial history in sport. The psychologist should carefully consider which measures to use and where in the assessment process to introduce them.

Supplemental sources of information are of great value in the psychological assessment of athletic injury. Of particular significance is the objective evaluation of injury provided by the physician or sports medicine specialist. The psychologist (or other member of the sports medicine team) should routinely check this objective evaluation against the athlete's perception of injury. The coach is also a source of useful information ranging from the impact of injury on the athlete's team status to the athlete's general ability to cope with stressful situations. Parental input is critical with young athletes, and media reaction is important to athletes in high-visibility sports. When interviewing those providing supplemental information, the psychologist should determine the degree to which they support the athlete and understand his or her situation, because this plays a tremendously important role in the athlete's ability to cope with injury.

Assessment should identify personal cost and coping resources—and their relative balance in the life of the athlete. The specific diagnostic factors presented in the preceding chapter are the pieces that we use to assemble the picture of injury. They not only contribute to the overall picture but gain added meaning in relation to it. Personal cost is reflected by the severity of injury, the likelihood of enduring performance deficits, the length of downtime, the timeliness of injury, and the influence these have collectively on the athlete's future performance.

Of greatest concern from a psychological perspective are the athlete's level of distress and how well she or he has mobilized coping resources in response. These factors can vary greatly across athletes with similar injuries. It is useful to think of distress as a summative measure of emotion and pain, spoken and displayed. The extent of emotion and pain is often rooted in the personal meaning attached to injury, for which Lipowski (1969) offered a range of possibilities including the following:

1. A challenge to overcome
2. An enemy that threatens to destroy
3. Punishment for past transgressions
4. Evidence of inherent weakness
5. Relief from demands and responsibilities
6. An irreparable loss
7. A tool for manipulating one's environment to meet personal or financial needs

Establishing a Treatment Relationship

Assessment begins with establishment of the parameters of treatment. Because the athlete's first impression of the psychologist will be lasting, the psychologist should approach the athlete in a way that recognizes her or his specific concerns and is sensitive to issues relevant to sport participation. Competitive sport discourages the athlete from displaying vulnerability and encourages self-reliance; injury is an inherent challenge to this attitudinal set. Due to this, and to the anxiety inherent in any new interaction with a psychologist, it is understandable that the athlete may be reluctant.

Treatment should be viewed as a collaborative interaction. Although the psychologist should establish a sense of authority as a professional, she or he should regard the patient-athlete as the leading authority on himself or herself. Typically the athlete knows much more about the particular sport than does the psychologist. Collaborative treatment is especially appropriate when treatment focuses on performance enhancement as opposed to the management of psychological disorder.

The psychologist should emphasize the performance-enhancing aspects of treatment and identify speedy rehabilitation and mental readiness for return to play as the general goals (unless otherwise indicated). The psychologist can describe the purpose of intervention as helping the athlete use personal coping skills to his or her best advantage. This can be followed by a description of the techniques that can be used such as goal setting, pain control, mental preparation for competition, stress management, and sleep management.

It is important that the psychologist clarify what is confidential and what is not and describe how he or she interacts with other members of the sports medicine team. (More on confidentiality is provided in chapter 16.) It is often useful for the athlete to know about the psychologist's background and professional orientation.

Assessment is a two-way process. The athlete assesses the psychologist according to professional presentation, personality, ability to establish rapport, and knowledge of both psychology and sport. That treatment will follow from assessment should not be a foregone conclusion. The psychologist who can gain the athlete's respect and confidence will be most likely to establish an enduring and effective treatment relationship.

Initial Interview

Ideally, the initial interview serves as an implicit statement of the athlete's importance to the athletic program as well as a supportive intervention expressing concern about the athlete's well-being at a time when he or she is not able to perform. The interview not only serves to identify key issues but also to mobilize the athlete's use of coping skills (Crossman & Jamieson, 1985). The latter most likely occurs where the interview prompts subsequent self-evaluation and action. The psychologist should conduct the diagnostic interview in a way that demonstrates professionalism, sincerity, and sensitivity to the patient's status as an athlete. These factors are conveyed through good eye contact, careful listening, attention to nonverbal cues, and willingness to address the athlete's questions in detail.

From a purely diagnostic point of view, the more information gathered the better. However, interviewing can be intrusive. Information gathered at the expense of a good treatment relationship is usually of relatively little practical value. Whenever questions appear to cause the athlete discomfort, the psychologist must balance the acquisition of information with the establishment of a good treatment relationship. Ravizza (1988) recommended a simple approach whereby psychologist and athlete agree that the psychologist will ask questions freely and that the athlete will say "not now" when he or she does not wish to answer. Once a trusting treatment relationship is established, the athlete will eventually answer many questions that are initially met with reluctance. Other questions do not need to be answered; simply asking them can be enough to raise awareness or initiate a coping response. The athlete may refuse—to her or his detriment—to answer some questions that may very well need to be answered; the psychologist must accept this as well as the fact that some athletes will refuse intervention altogether.

The patient who clearly needs psychological treatment but who actively or passively refuses intervention can be a source of great frustration for the psychologist and for other members of the treatment team. This is illustrated in the personal case report that follows. Tom, who had been a golf teaching pro for many years, was hospitalized for evaluation of long-standing mouth and jaw pain. Psychological evaluation of depression was requested as part of his overall workup. The interview revealed a series of tooth extractions for alleviation of pain. Pain continued after the initial extractions and, in turn, prompted further extractions. As the scope of his problem had grown he had given up his work as a golf pro and had stopped playing golf altogether, choosing instead to sit in his hospital bed toothless and evidently depressed. To understand the depth of his loss of interest in golf I asked Tom what he would do if a friend came to his house, drove him to a golf course, and suggested that they play a round. He said he would refuse. I recommended treatment for depression to Tom, but he responded with little enthusiasm. Soon after, he was discharged. A follow-up phone call and then a letter encouraging treatment met with no response from him or his family. Although frustrated, I felt I had done all I could at the time. Sometimes patients like Tom will later decide they are ready for treatment. Showing respect for the limitations patients set can be the first step in a person's eventually seeking treatment, though it may be weeks or months later.

The central goal of assessment in injury is to determine the athlete's level of distress. This "distress quotient" is a measure that is the sum of emotion and pain either stated directly or demonstrated in behavior. Because the interrelationships of pain, emotion, and injury are complex, systematic assessment of pain is of special importance.

Evaluating Pain

The diversity and complexity of pain are recognized in the International Association for the Study of Pain (1986) definition, which describes pain as a "sensory and emotional" experience characterized by "actual or anticipated" injury. The multidimensionality of the pain response is reflected in the hard wiring of the biological system that propagates its transmission. There appear to be two primary lines of pain transmission, one carrying sensory information and the other conveying a more cognitive-emotional component. This latter system functions as an alarm mobilizing the organism into a vigilant and ready state. It conveys a sense of danger, mobilizes cognitive problem-solving mechanisms, and elicits a search for the "meaning" of the pain.

Pain demands a multimethod approach to assessment (Chapman et al., 1985). The diagnostic interview, which is the central element in the overall process, should provide information regarding quantitative and qualitative aspects of pain, the meaning that the athlete attaches to pain, and the extent to which pain influences the athlete's sense of control and serves as a guide to subsequent behavior. The initial questions regarding the quantity and quality of pain provide insight into the "meaning" dimension of pain.

The simplest approach to the quantitative assessment of pain is the use of a self-report such as the one shown in Figure 8.1. The numbers 0 to 10 represent "no pain" to "worst possible pain." This method simplifies assessment of pain across a variety of situations. For example, the psychologist should obtain measures of average daily pain, pain at its worst, and pain at its least. In conjunction with the report of pain severity, identification of specific factors or situations that increase or decrease pain is useful. This line of questioning provides insight into the challenges posed by sport, rehabilitation, and daily life activities. It also offers a perspective on the scope of the athlete's natural coping methods and their perceived effectiveness. The athlete whose least pain and average daily pain ratings are equivalent likely has poor pain management skills, as seen in the athlete's inability to lower pain levels.

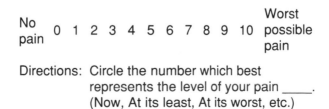

Directions: Circle the number which best
         represents the level of your pain _____.
         (Now, At its least, At its worst, etc.)

Figure 8.1   A quantitative self-report pain measure using a numerical scale.

The psychologist can further refine quantitative assessment by having the athlete rate pain separately for both intensity and "bothersomeness," a distinction some patients will have difficulty appreciating. The psychologist can illustrate the distinction by pointing out that in the moment an individual is, for example, laughing at a joke or intently absorbed in some activity, the impact of pain on thoughts and feelings is diminished although pain intensity remains unchanged. This shows the patient that even as pain remains constant, one's sense of distress can vary.

The visual analog scale shown in Figure 8.2 is a written self-report method of pain rating that may be used as an alternative to the 0-to-10 scale. In using the visual analog scale, the athlete places an X at a point on a continuous 100-mm line anchored by the terms *no pain* and *worst possible pain*. The psychologist subsequently scores the mark in number of millimeters (from 0 to 100). Because the scale offers 101 data points, it is more useful psychometrically than a 10-point scale. Also, because no numbers appear on the scale, it is assumed that the athlete's memory of prior ratings interferes less with subsequent ratings of pain.

An open-ended request for a description of pain is the simplest approach to qualitative assessment. This provides important psychological as well as medical diagnostic information. Descriptions of pain that are vivid and detailed as well as those characterized by catastrophizing ("muscles tearing apart" vs. "tightness") and personalization ("like being stabbed with a knife" vs. "stabbing pain") are signs that pain is particularly severe or otherwise distressing.

Observation

We are all familiar with the maxim that actions speak louder than words. Although attention to body language should be a routine aspect of diagnostic assessment, it is especially important where pain and injury are involved. Demonstrations of pain or pain behaviors indicate severity of pain and associated distress. Pain behaviors are observable across a variety of categories including vocal (e.g., sighing), facial (e.g., grimacing), gestural (e.g., rubbing), and postural (Keefe & Block, 1982). Postural cues

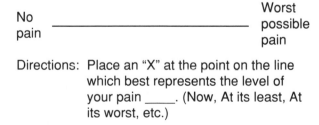

Figure 8.2 A quantitative self-report pain measure using a visual analog scale.

include excessive stiffness and other protective or compensatory positioning typically referred to as bracing or guarding. The psychologist should evaluate variations in pain behavior during an interview relative to interview content; pain behaviors often increase with discussion of issues that concern the athlete. Observations of pain behaviors across a variety of settings (e.g., rehabilitation, sport activities) reflect the athlete's overall level of distress and the circumstances that are precipitating factors.

Bracing and guarding can lead to chronic muscle tension. If maintained following return to play, this tension can interfere with the biomechanics of skill execution and if persistent can even lead to the development of myofascial pain syndrome. This is illustrated by the case report that follows. Sandy was a late-middle-aged golfer whose game was steadily on the rise relative to her circle of golfing companions—until a low-grade chronic shoulder pain problem evolved. There was no precipitating trauma, and no pain interfered with day-to-day activities other than golf. Medical evaluation and treatment and variations in style of play had virtually no impact on the problem. As she discussed this situation, her distress grew more evident as did the severity of her guarding behavior. When this observation was pointed out to Sandy she was quite surprised. Although initially puzzled and somewhat defensive, she seized on this observation as an opportunity for improvement and wanted to hear more. In the discussion that followed, other fears and concerns associated with performance and injury, of which Sandy had been previously unaware, became apparent. This, in turn, opened the way for further problem solving.

Psychological Testing

The purpose of psychological testing in injury is to help the psychologist elicit information about the athlete's personality style and coping skills and determine how these have been affected by injury or other circumstances. Psychological testing offers a relatively concise, time efficient, and objective measure of athlete functioning. In a sense, it provides a second opinion that is more objective than the diagnostic interview. The disadvantages of testing are that the patient may perceive it as impersonal, unnecessarily time-consuming, or threatening. Those unfamiliar with psychological testing will often attribute greater power or meaning to test results than is appropriate. When test results are shared with the athlete, used as a framework to provide feedback, and presented as hypotheses about behavior (rather than statements of fact), the disadvantages are greatly minimized.

A great variety of psychological tests and measures are available to the practitioner. As a general rule, sport-specific instruments are preferable to those designed for the general population; however, most sport-specific tests are in developmental stages. Reviews of the tests most frequently used with athletes (Anshel, 1987; Ostrow, 1990) are available to guide the psychologist in the selection and interpretation of test results.

Use in Sport

Both the research and applied uses of testing in sport have been controversial. Personality research in sport has been criticized on conceptual, methodological, and interpretive grounds (LeUnes & Nation, 1989). Efforts to differentiate athletes in various sports or at positions within sports on the basis of personality measures have been generally unsuccessful. However, researchers are increasingly observing the tendency of highly successful athletes to be in good psychological health relative to less successful peers (LeUnes, Hayward, & Daiss, 1988).

The applied use of testing in sport in the 1970s met with a great deal of resistance. This can be largely attributed to a misunderstanding by athletes and coaches of the nature, purposes, and limits of psychological testing. Unfortunately, this misunderstanding extended to some psychologists who failed to effectively incorporate testing as part of overall intervention. Controversy was fueled by the frequent use of tests for selection purposes and by athletes' natural reluctance to be evaluated in this way. The problems inherent in psychological testing are more pronounced when it is used for one-time screening for selection purposes than when it is used in ongoing consultation. This controversy led the National Football League (NFL) Players' Association to rule against the use of psychological testing in the NFL, a significant setback for the field of sport psychology. Nideffer (1981) suggested that this controversy could largely have been avoided had psychological testing been used in ways that respected the underlying concerns of those being tested.

The psychologist should be aware that strong preconceptions about psychological testing may already be in place in a given setting. This not only may limit the effectiveness of testing but also may influence the credibility of the praciticner. However, new developments in testing and a better understanding of how to use tests in applied situations have fostered their continued use in sport.

Assessment Devices

A number of factors influence the decision about which assessment device to use in a given situation. These include the athlete's psychological status and current life circumstance, the research and applied goals of the intervention, and the personal preference of the practitioner. Next is a brief review of a number of psychological assessment devices including the POMS, the MMPI, pain drawing, and others.

POMS.   The Profile of Mood States (McNair, Lorr, & Droppleman, 1971) assesses transient mood states across six dimensions: tension-anxiety, depression-dejection, anger-hostility, vigor-activity, fatigue-inertia, and confusion-bewilderment. The advantages of the POMS include its speed and ease of administration as well as its face validity (Eichman, 1978). It is available in shortened formats—37 items (Schacham, 1983) and 5 items (Dean, Whelan, & Meyers, 1990)—which facilitate its use in applied performance settings. However, there are no controls for response set, and therefore it is of limited use where denial is prominent.

The POMS has been used widely with athletes. In initial work by Morgan and Pollock (1977) with Olympic athletes, a distinctive healthy profile emerged, which was marked by elevation of vigor-activity above the mean with all other measures below the mean. Referred to as the "iceberg profile," it is predictive of athletic success (see Figure 8.3). Subsequent research with a variety of athlete groups supports these initial findings (LeUnes et al., 1988).

The POMS also appears to be a sensitive measure of change over time in athletes' emotional responses to injury. Perceived effectiveness of rehabilitation and self-report of mood on the POMS are highly correlated (McDonald & Hardy, 1990). Two additional POMS profiles are presented in Figure 8.4 and 8.5. The first profile (Figure 8.4) is of a university basketball player seen soon after a successful surgery that would allow him to participate in sport following rehabilitation. However, because injury occurred in his senior year it marked the end of his collegiate career, and he had no opportunity for a professional career. His response is most notable for diminished energy level and increased anger. In interview, he was cooperative and expressed a level of distress that was consistent with both his current circumstances and self-report on the POMS.

The second profile (Figure 8.5) is of a university track-and-field athlete seen following surgery. He was expected to be able to return to competition but only following a long rehabilitation. In initial interview, the athlete indicated significant psychological distress. Two days later he presented a remarkably positive outlook on both his current emotional state and his expectations for return to competition. His new outlook was clearly exaggerated and out of keeping with both the severity of his injury and his earlier indication of distress. His POMS results resembled the iceberg profile except for modest elevations of tension and fatigue. Because there is no control for a social desirability response set, it is quite easy to "fake good" (which the athlete is assumed to have done on this profile). However, when the psychologist carefully considers test results in light of overall evaluation, their effectiveness is optimized. In this case test results helped confirm the impression of strong denial and predicted subsequent problems in rehabilitation because of unrealistic expectations.

MMPI.   The Minnesota Multiphasic Personality Inventory, initially developed in 1942 by Hathaway and McKinley, is the most widely used

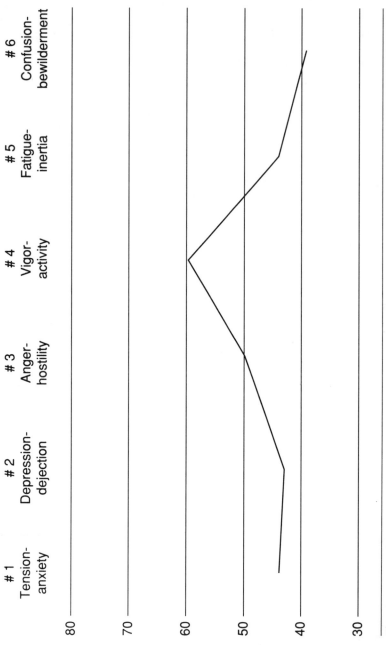

Figure 8.3 Profile of Mood States: "iceberg" profile.

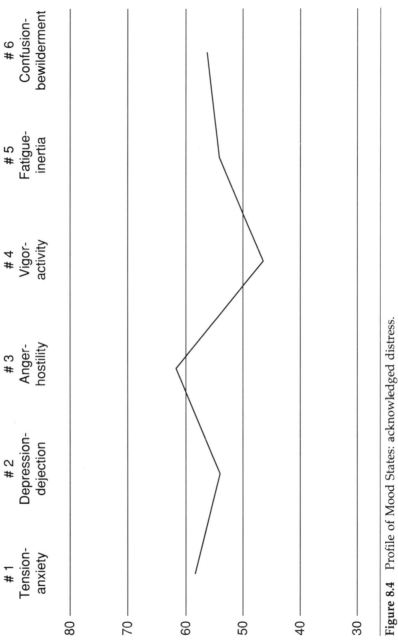

Figure 8.4 Profile of Mood States: acknowledged distress.

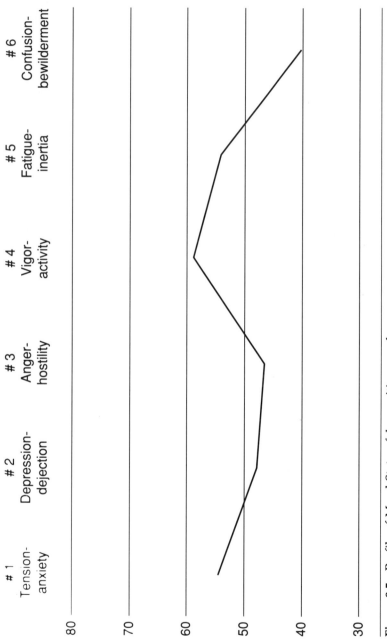

Figure 8.5 Profile of Mood States: false positive mood.

test of enduring personality traits. It has been used in thousands of research studies with diverse psychiatric, medical, and healthy populations. Research using the MMPI with sport populations has generally found a positive correlation between psychological health and performance (LeUnes & Nation, 1989).

Its basic form is composed of 8 clinical scales (1—hypochondriasis, 2—depression, 3—hysteria, 4—psychopathic deviance, 6—paranoia, 7— psychasthenia, 8—schizophrenia, 9—mania) and 2 general measures (5—masculinity/femininity, 0—social introversion) for a total of 10 scales. The scales are typically indicated by number rather than name, because they carry a broader meaning than is implied by their name. There are also three validity scales (L, F, K) that assess response style (for more information, see the subsequent section in this chapter on response style). Dozens of additional scales have been subsequently devised. The recently revised instrument, MMPI-2, addresses many criticisms initially directed against the original instrument and renders it more suitable for contemporary use (Hathaway & McKinley, 1989). There are a number of interpretive guides for the MMPI and MMPI-2, many of which are readily available through computerized scoring systems.

The MMPI is especially useful in the evaluation of psychological complications that occur in conjunction with medical problems (Fordyce, 1979). Two distinctive patterns, designated in this text as the somatization profile and the acknowledged distress profile, have been noted among individuals who fail to rehabilitate from injury. The somatization profile (often referred to as the conversion V profile) is characterized by the elevation of Scales 1 and 3 with a relatively low Scale 2. People who respond in this manner tend to complain about pain and discomfort across a wide variety of situations, to experience magnification of symptoms in times of distress, to use these complaints in the place of more adaptive coping mechanisms, to deny the impact of psychological distress, and to resist psychological treatment. For example, the profile presented in Figure 8.6 is of an athlete with an interest in a variety of sports. He had failed to rehabilitate effectively from a complicated leg injury, was minimally compliant with rehabilitation goals, used pain medication excessively, and was hostile to treatment providers and family. His behavior in the diagnostic interview was consistent with that predicted by the MMPI. He subsequently refused an intensive rehabilitation approach to treatment.

The acknowledged distress profile, in contrast, is characterized by candid recognition of psychological distress. There may be mixed symptoms of anxiety with or without phobic reaction, depression, and disruption in thought processes. This is indicated by elevation, singly or in combination, of Scales 2, 7, and 8. The profile presented in Figure 8.7 is of a recreational athlete severely injured in a near-fatal on-the-job accident. One year later, after a long series of surgeries, she was referred for psychological treatment because of emotional difficulties related to physical

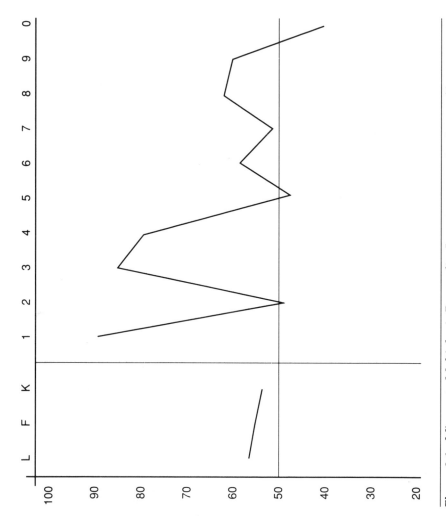

Figure 8.6 Minnesota Multiphasic Personality Inventory: somatization profile.

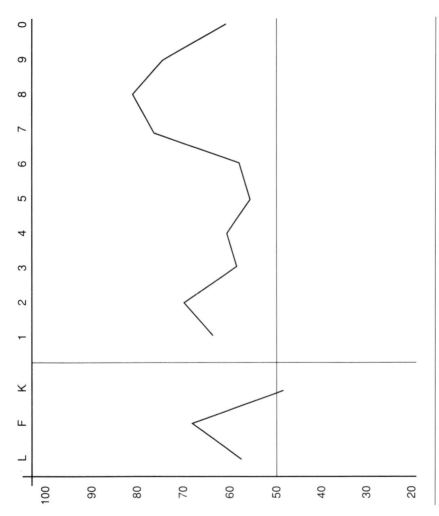

Figure 8.7 Minnesota Multiphasic Personality Inventory: acknowledged distress profile.

limitations, pain, and disfigurement. She was quite candid in her acknowledgment of significant emotional distress, as reflected in her MMPI profile.
At the time of evaluation she was engaged in an aerobic conditioning
program, which included biking and swimming and from which she
reported significant benefit. Her initial approach to treatment was quite
positive and led to notable gains.

The MMPI is also useful in the prediction and early identification of
problems in response to injury. It has been used prior to surgery to
effectively predict difficulties in postsurgery rehabilitation (Spengler &
Freeman, 1979; Wise, Jackson, & Rocchio, 1979). It is relatively well-known
to physicians and is often requested in difficult rehabilitation situations.
Although criticism has been leveled at the MMPI for its failure to predict
organic pathology in low-back pain (Hendler, Mollett, Talo, & Levin,
1988), these criticisms are based on a misunderstanding of the MMPI
(which is not intended as an alternative to medical exam) and to a poorly
contrived diagnostic strategy (by which psychological profiles are used
to predict organic pathology). Psychological function and physical function are independent dimensions that need to be separately assessed and
that, in turn, collectively provide a comprehensive picture of adjustment
to injury.

Pain Drawing.   Pain drawing is a relatively simple diagnostic tool that
allows pain sufferers to graphically portray their pain. Although used in
a variety of formats, it typically includes an outline (front and back view)
of a human figure with accompanying instructions for using symbols to
identify type and site of pain. Pain drawing is easy and provides information not readily evident in other forms of self-report. It is especially useful
for its clear portrayal of pain distribution through the body. This face
valid diagnostic tool is a useful adjunct to the evaluation of back pain in
conjunction with both medical examination and psychological evaluation
(Ransford, Cairns, & Mooney, 1976).

Three general elements of pain drawing serve as the basis for prediction
of difficulty in adapting to injury. These include relatively large quantitative estimates of pain, unusual or atypical qualitative presentation of pain,
and an unusual or clearly inappropriate response to instructions. To obtain
a quantitative measure, the psychologist can use specially designed tem-
plates to calculate the number of pain sites or the overall percentage of
the body described as painful. The larger the pain relative to that typical
for a given injury, the greater the likelihood of difficulty in adaptation to
injury. Unusual distributions of pain or the presence of whole-body pain
often indicate the development of secondary pain syndromes.

Qualitative responses can be evaluated according to typical patterns of
pain distribution for a given injury. In the case of back injury, known
patterns of nervous enervation (myotomal and dermatomal distributions)

serve as a standard against which self-report is compared. Unusual responses such as representation of pain outside body boundaries or embellishment of the drawing with added comments or symbols are again predictive of difficulties in rehabilitation. Pain drawing can predict rehabilitation problems and can indicate successful rehabilitation (Fordyce et al., 1986). The drawing in Figure 8.8 represents a normal or typical response to serious back injury. In contrast, the drawing in Figure 8.9 suggests somatization and problems in rehabilitation. As can be seen, the impression created by pain drawing can be quite compelling.

Other Measures.   A variety of other sport-specific and general psychological measures are useful in the evaluation and treatment of the injured athlete. For example, the Social and Athletic Readjustment Rating Scale (Bramwell et al., 1975) and other measures of life stress and change offer concise summaries of athletes' life situations (see chapter 5 for information on measures of life stress and change). Because these are easily administered and readily understandable to those without psychological training, they are useful instruments in the hands of the physician or sports medicine specialist.

Although a growing number of sport-specific tests are available, they are limited in that they do not directly address the specific issues relevant to the injured athlete. However, instruments such as the Competitive State Anxiety Inventory-II (CSAI-II) (Martens, Burton, Vealey, Bump, & Smith, 1982), the Sport Competition Anxiety Test (SCAT) (Martens, 1977), and the Psychological Skills Inventory for Sports (PSIS) (Mahoney, Gabriel, & Perkins, 1987) may be used to assess the athlete's readiness for return to play following injury. Nideffer's (1976, 1990) Test of Attentional and Interpersonal Style (TAIS) is the most useful of the sport-specific measures because of the broad base of attentional and interpersonal elements it assesses. Individuals whose TAIS responses are characterized as overloaded by internal stimuli (OIT), reduced attentional focus (RED), obsessiveness (OBS), and lacking in behavior control (BCON) are most likely at risk for rehabilitation complications.

Borg's (Borg & Ottoson, 1986) Rating of Perceived Exertion Scale, which was initially designed as a measure of effort for use with aerobic activity, is suitable for monitoring effort expended on a wide range of physical tasks. For the injured athlete who tends to overdo activity (and experience repeated reinjury), the psychologist can use the Rating of Perceived Exertion Scale to assess effort and to help set appropriate limits during rehabilitation.

The Millon Behavioral Health Inventory (MBHI) (Millon, Green, & Meagher, 1982) is specifically designed for use with ill or injured people. It is composed of eight scales that identify basic coping styles, six psychogenic attitude scales that identify factors that may precipitate or complicate physical illness, and an additional six scales to assess the extent

Using the symbols, indicate the areas on your body where
you feel the described sensations. Include all affected areas.

Aching	Numbness	Pins and needles	Burning	Stabbing	Other
▲▲▲▲	= = = =	ooooo	XXXX	/ / / / /	• • • • •

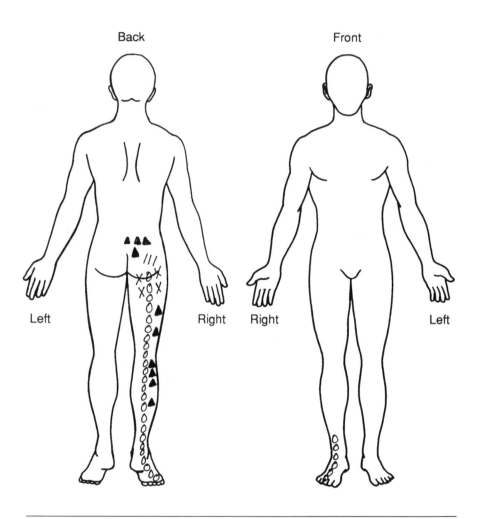

Figure 8.8   Pain Drawing: typical response.

Using the symbols, indicate the areas on your body where you feel the described sensations. Include all affected areas.

Aching	Numbness	Pins and needles	Burning	Stabbing	Other
▲▲▲▲	= = = =	ooooo	XXXX	/ / / / /	• • • • •

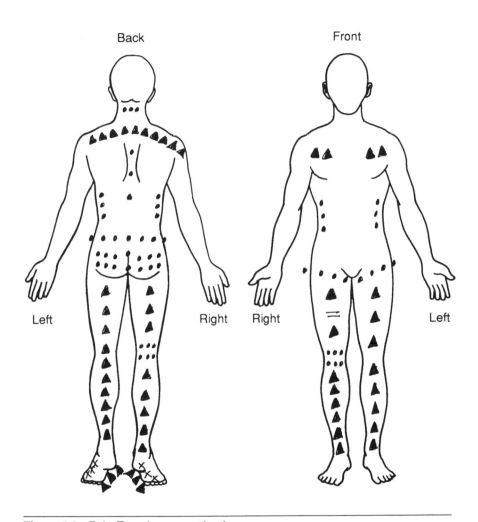

Figure 8.9   Pain Drawing: somatization.

to which emotional factors are likely to complicate response to specific medical problems. This instrument is unique in that it makes specific predictions about the ways in which patients are likely to relate to health personnel and various treatment regimens. High levels of somatic anxiety indicated on the MBHI have been found to correlate with poor compliance in injured athletes (Wittig, 1986).

When injury fails to respond to routine management strategies, the athlete's thorough understanding of the severity and variability of pain across a broad range of situations takes on increasing importance. The athlete can gain such an understanding with the use of a pain-activity diary. Relatively simple to design, this diary includes a listing of the athlete's scheduled activities (including sedentary periods and sleep) with a rating of pain level (e.g., on a scale of 0 to 10) during each activity. Ratings may be tabulated and summarized by day and by activity. The pain-activity diary raises the athlete's awareness about pain and factors related to its occurrence and provides practitioners with a better understanding of the relationship of pain and life activities.

The Pain Rating Index of the McGill Pain Questionnaire is a series of 78 terms commonly used to describe pain (Chapman et al., 1985; Melzack, 1975). These are organized into 20 subsets of similar terms that are categorized as either sensory (e.g., *sharp, burning, aching*) or affective-evaluative (e.g., *exhaustive, fearful, agonizing*). The Pain Rating Index facilitates the qualitative description of pain. Responses may also be tabulated to provide a quantitative measure. The ease of administration and face validity of the instrument give it much practical value.

Administration and Feedback

A number of fundamental considerations guide the use of psychological tests. Foremost, the individual should be informed of the reasons for testing. Athletes have the right to know to whom test results will be provided, and they should be informed themselves of the results of their testing. In informing athletes of test results, psychologists should not simply provide a report but should present feedback in a way that the athlete finds meaningful.

Nideffer (1981) offered the following series of recommendations about the feedback process. The psychologist should

1. preface feedback with an explanation of the limitations inherent in testing;
2. be concise, emphasizing a few key points;
3. provide clear and unambiguous feedback, avoiding the use of psychological jargon;
4. balance the positive and negative aspects of feedback;

5. place feedback in a situational context, for example, in the form of a prediction about behavior in a given situation; and
6. provide the athlete with an opportunity to ask follow-up questions at a later date.

The two brief feedback scenarios presented next are based on psychological testing and observed behavior. They reflect an underlying assumption that traits are behavioral tendencies with potential advantages and disadvantages. The first scenario is of an individual whom testing shows to be withdrawn and mildly depressed. He is also detached from team members following injury and is progressing slowly through rehabilitation, occasionally missing treatment sessions. The sample feedback statetment follows:

> You seem to be good at drawing inward as a way of gaining strength, which has probably helped you through some tough situations. But, of course, a person can overdo this. Withdrawal may lead you to be out of touch with people who are important to you and may cause you to feel lonely and isolated. When you get out of touch with others in this way it can make it difficult for you to remain motivated in your rehabilitation.

The second scenario involves an athlete who appears in psychological testing to be impulsive and energetic. She shows a history of quick return to play following injury but with subsequent reinjury. A sample of how feedback might be provided in this case follows:

> You have a go-for-it attitude, and your willingness to take risks has let you succeed in situations where others didn't. But now that you are injured you are having a difficult time holding back and setting safe limits for yourself. Your go-for-it attitude tends to cause you to push too hard too soon and interferes with your recovery.

Interpretation of test results should incorporate as much relevant information as is available including reasons for referral, results of diagnostic interview, and information from supplemental sources.

Response Style. Response style is a reflection of the attitude with which the athlete approaches the test. Often, but not always, response is honest and straightforward, and in such a case, interpretation is similarly straightforward. However, less candid response renders interpretation more difficult. Three such response styles have been observed: fake good, fake bad, and conservative (Nideffer, 1981).

In the fake good response, the athlete exaggerates strengths and places himself or herself in the most favorable light possible. This is more common among those with a simplistic understanding of psychology, and it may also reflect the strong emphasis on a positive attitude in sport.

Psychologists are more likely to see the fake good response where testing is conducted for team selection purposes rather than as part of an ongoing consulting relationship. In distinct contrast to this is the fake bad style. Although this response is not uncommon in clinical situations, it is relatively rare for athletes to present themselves in an unfavorable light. When this response is observed, the psychologist should assume it to be a statement of significant distress that demands prompt response until proven otherwise. Alternately, the fake bad response may reflect the athlete's hostility or rejection of the test situation. The psychologist will find this differentiation (significant distress vs. hostility/rejection) is relatively easy to make with appropriate follow-up. The conservative response style reflects a play-it-safe attitude. The athlete is reluctant to state either strengths or weaknesses strongly or definitively. Difficult to detect, this response often reflects a lack of trust by the athlete.

Test instruments vary in the degree to which they are able to identify the influence of these deviant response styles. The psychologist needs to be vigilant to the potential for such bias in response and adjust interpretation accordingly.

Inconsistent Pain Response. Athletes will sometimes demonstrate inconsistency in pain report and behavior, appearing either to overreport or underreport pain severity. Complaints of pain that appear extreme relative to typical response for similar injuries (based on objective medical opinion) or which appear inconsistent across different situations may raise questions regarding the athlete's credibility. The psychologist should interpret these inconsistencies in light of the situation-specific nature of pain; the more severe and chronic the pain the more likely it is to become contingent upon environmental factors. Variations in attention, expectation, muscle tension, and autonomic arousal mediate changes in the perception of pain both somatically via modulation of the nociceptive system and cognitively in the interpretation of the "bothersomeness" of pain. These mediating factors may be triggered by circumstances that elicit fear, anxiety, or uncertainty, causing behavior to vary in a way that appears inconsistent.

The emphasis in sport on having a positive attitude, being tough-minded, and playing with pain subtly encourages athletes to underreport pain and injury. Athletes may further be encouraged to hide pain from treatment providers if they fear that they may be withheld from play. This has been noted in dancers and musicians as well (Clanin, Davison, & Plastino, 1986; Rozek, 1985). With these considerations in mind, treatment providers should regard inconsistency in behavior or report initially as diagnostic of a potential problem that needs to be carefully assessed and treated appropriately.

Supplemental Sources of Assessment Information

Valuable information about the athlete may be available directly from the physician, sports medicine specialist, coach, and parent. Information may also be available indirectly from medical records, sport performance data, and, in some cases, the media. The more complex and problematic the injury situation, the more important it becomes for the psychologist to incorporate these supplemental sources into the overall psychological evaluation. All who are involved closely with the athlete have an important perspective on the athlete's mood and coping ability. The psychologist who interacts with the athlete outside the office environment will likely gain a greater appreciation of the athlete's situation-specific response to injury and will find information from the medical staff and coach much more accessible. This practice also improves relations among treatment team members.

A thorough evaluation of the injured athlete is not complete without an understanding of the type and severity of injury and the anticipated course of rehabilitation. In some cases the athlete's perspective on injury and recovery differs from the perspectives of health care providers. A significant gap in understanding may signal a communication problem or may be a sign of an athlete's denial.

It is important that the psychologist know the athlete's preinjury ability level. Fortunately, few areas of human endeavor are as thoroughly and systematically evaluated as sport. The coach, although limited by his or her understanding of injury, is the definitive source of information about the athlete's ability. Differences between the athlete's and the coach's appraisals of sport performance are cause for concern. In treating an athlete from a high-visibility sport with regular media coverage, the psychologist must know how the athlete's injury situation has been presented by the media. Positive or derogatory media comments, whether accurate or inaccurate, can have a noteworthy impact on the athlete.

As a general rule in evaluation, information from various sources should converge toward one conclusion. When the psychologist notes divergent perspectives on injury or performance, problems are likely.

Concluding Comments

Diagnostic methods and measures are gateways to effective treatment. The psychologist's selection and use of methods and measures should respect prevailing practices and attitudes in specific sports and should be individualized to reflect the unique situation of each athlete. Wherever possible, the psychologist should use sport-specific tests. Their use will appear more logical to the athlete, aiding the psychologist in explaining test results and applying them to sport performance. The psychologist should observe and interact with the athlete in multiple settings (e.g., the office, the training room, and the playing field or arena). This enhances rapport with the athlete and provides opportunity to assess the opinions of coaches and other members of the sports medicine team regarding the athlete's adjustment to injury. Effective assessment is ongoing, utilizes multiple sources of input, and moves through a convergence of information to a central set of hypotheses about the athlete's adjustments to injury.

9
CHAPTER

Conducting Assessment and Intervention

John Heil

This chapter summarizes the issues discussed in prior chapters and presents a plan for comprehensive assessment of the injured athlete's psychological status. This assessment becomes the basis for a rational intervention strategy, which is introduced here and developed in subsequent chapters.

The factors that the psychologist should take into account can be summarized as follows:

1. Severity of the injury
2. Premorbid psychological status
3. Psychological adjustment to injury
4. Physical and psychosocial development factors
5. Level of achievement and commitment to sport
6. Choice of sport
7. Gender
8. Racial and other cultural considerations
9. Health status

The two most critical elements are severity of injury and the athlete's psychological adjustment to injury. Severity of injury affects the level of pain and discomfort, the length of downtime, and the rigors of rehabilitation, factors that determine the challenge of rehabilitation. Psychological adjustment, in turn, determines the athlete's response to injury and affects coping ability: Will he or she respond with feelings of hopelessness and depression or with optimism and a willingness to strive for excellence during rehabilitation? The developmental stage of the athlete (i.e., the level of physical and psychosocial maturity) provides an orienting framework within which psychologists may assess sport and lifestyle issues relevant to each athlete.

A comprehensive assessment-intervention strategy and a brief overview of related interventions open this chapter. These are followed by sections that present a life-span developmental perspective and review sport and lifestyle factors that influence the meaning of injury and its psychological impact on the athlete. The chapter concludes with a series of assessment-intervention protocols designed to guide the initial interview.

A Comprehensive Assessment-Intervention Strategy

Because of the great variability in injury scenarios, a comprehensive strategy to guide assessment and subsequent intervention is essential. This strategy is outlined in the flowchart in Figure 9.1 (Heil, 1988), which presents a programmatic approach to injury management that emphasizes timely and efficient delivery of services as well as coordination of care. Based on the assumption that psychological management is an important, ongoing aspect of treatment, this strategy incorporates a sport psychology of performance and a clinical psychology of behavioral disorders. There is a strong foundation in clinical practice and research for this approach and for the specific recommendations provided regarding intervention. In a sense, this plan defines what the sport psychology of injury can be at its best. A comprehensive program such as this is most practical with highly competitive athletes, for whom commitment to sport, cost of injury, and emphasis on expedient return to play create a great sense of urgency. However, this plan is more broadly applicable, because all athletes are affected by severity of injury, difficulty in psychological adaptation, and developmental issues.

Interventions are cued initially to severity of injury and subsequently to degree of difficulty in psychological adaptation. Five categories of injury severity are defined:

1. Mild—an injury requiring treatment without interruption of training
2. Moderate—a relatively more severe injury that interferes with ongoing training and limits participation
3. Major—an injury requiring a long duration of downtime, often with surgery or hospitalization
4. Sport disabling—an injury which, because of severity or timing, prevents the athlete from returning to prior levels of competitive performance
5. Catastrophic—an injury that causes permanent functional disability

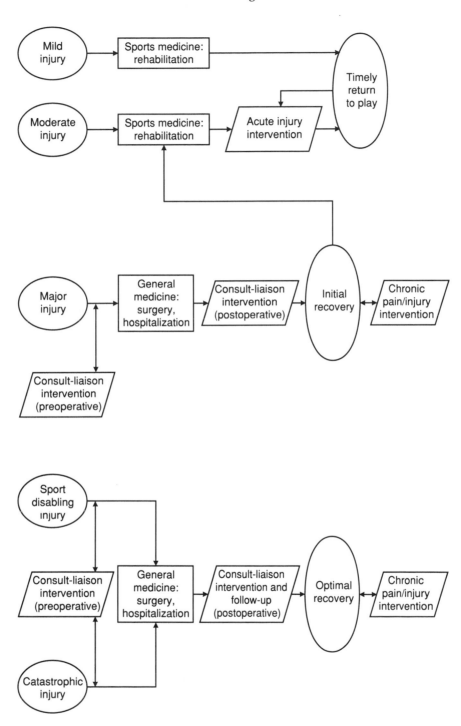

Figure 9.1   Injury treatment flowchart.

More detailed information about when and how to conduct assessment is provided in the sections that follow.

Assessment-Intervention Overview

Figure 9.1 presents an overview of the recommended treatment program. The speed and intensity with which psychological intervention proceeds are determined by the degree of psychological and physical distress and the intensity of the athlete's commitment to speedy return to play.

For mild injury, the intervention strategy is to enhance stress management and pain management skills and to help the athlete deal with other difficulties concomitant with injury such as stiffness, sleep disruption, or worrisome thinking. This is most easily accomplished when the athlete has already developed mental training skills and has a working relationship with a sport psychologist. Where there is not a working relationship with a sport psychologist, intervention in the case of a mild injury is not typically necessary. This is because athletes are generally resilient enough to deal with minor injury and because a diagnostic interview with an unknown person can be intrusive. Where timely return to play is not forthcoming or special concerns are identified (e.g., repeated overuse injury, apparent fear of reinjury), an acute injury assessment can be conducted.

The approach to moderate injury similarly focuses on stress management and pain management. An additional concern, however, is the impact of downtime on the athlete and its potential effect on mental readiness. The athlete can use mental training to help maintain mental performance skills and deal with the stress of injury. This intervention can be conducted proactively on a routine basis to speed recovery and prevent potential problems. It may also be initiated reactively in response to specific concerns raised by the athlete or the sports medicine professional.

Because of the trauma of major injury, the focus of intervention is primarily on the athlete's current level of psychological adaptation and secondarily on more long-term treatment goals. With major injury, the athlete is taken out of the more familiar sport rehabilitation environment and thrust into a general medical environment to undergo treatments that may include hospitalization and surgery. A preoperative consultation-liaison intervention that provides training and guidance in psychological preparation techniques may help the athlete deal with anxiety regarding surgery (or other medical procedures). Intervention may also be helpful when the athlete or physician is concerned about the overall benefits of surgery. The goal of intervention in this case is to clearly identify and assess the pros and cons of treatment approaches.

A routine postoperative consultation-liaison intervention is useful. Of brief duration, it provides the athlete support and reassurance during hospitalization and can be used to identify any potential rehabilitation problems. Thus, problems that do occur can be treated on a timely basis. As recovery progresses, the athlete typically shifts from the general medical environment to the more familiar sports medicine setting. Psychological interventions may conclude at this time or be modified to suit the new setting. For any problems that occur in the late stage of rehabilitation, intervention should follow the acute injury model. If recovery is not forthcoming, the psychologist should consider a more comprehensive chronic pain and injury intervention.

In sport-disabling injury (as in major injury), the primary focus is on the psychological status of the athlete and his or her adaptation to the trauma of injury and treatment. The issue of career termination adds complexity and challenge to this situation. Postoperative intervention is recommended routinely (with preoperative intervention conducted as needed). Follow-up treatment focused on career termination and lifestyle reorientation is also recommended. When persistent problems interfere with recovery, a chronic pain and injury assessment is indicated.

In catastrophic injury, intervention is focused on the psychological impact of the trauma and on the mobilization of coping resources during the initial phases of medical treatment. Preoperative or preprocedural consultation-liaison intervention may be indicated as part of a comprehensive psychological treatment program. In cases of brain or spinal cord injury, a thorough evaluation of physical, cognitive, and emotional factors is necessary. Once treatment providers have addressed the immediate issues, attention should be turned toward long-term goals regarding medical management and independent living. The patient can deal with issues of loss regarding both athletic career and functional ability most effectively as part of an ongoing treatment process. Significant problems with recovery relative to predicted treatment course indicate the need for a chronic pain and injury intervention.

Just as advances in sports medicine have accelerated the speed of injury recovery, this vigorous and proactive approach to intervention keyed to injury severity and psychological adaptation is designed to accelerate psychological recovery and readiness for return to play.

A Developmental Perspective
on Assessment and Intervention

The processes of physical and psychosocial development that characterize change through the life span are most coherently represented in a biopsychosocial developmental model. This broadly based perspective helps place in context the diverse physical, psychological, and social elements that bear on injury. Early work on physical assessment of injury by the Institute of Sportsmedicine and Athletic Trauma (Nicholas, 1976) identified relationships between physical maturation and change, and sport injury. From this, Nicholas (1976) identified a distinct sequence of developmental stages. Upon this physically derived developmental model I have superimposed a psychosocial perspective based on work in developmental and sport psychology. From this integrated perspective the psychologist can conceptualize decisions regarding injury risk and treatment in relation to the changing role of sport through the athlete's life. Thus, for similar injuries experienced by a Little League athlete and a major league player, different diagnostic and treatment considerations are brought to bear.

This biopsychosocial model provides an orienting perspective from which the psychologist can draw into focus other idiosyncrasies of each athlete's situation. This developmental model is detailed by stages in the following sections. Sport and lifestyle issues that influence assessment and intervention are presented subsequently.

Childhood

For children up to 6 or 7 years old, play is the major source of physical activity. Safety is an essential concern because injury causes more deaths in this age group than the next six causes of death combined (Christopherson, 1989). However, the risks associated with accidental death decrease with increasing age and motor ability (Langley, 1984).

From age 6 or 7 to the end of adolescence, the child has more opportunities to participate in formal sport activities than at any other stage. The rapid development of the musculoskeletal system during this period leads to strength and endurance imbalances. This makes the athlete more vulnerable to injury (Nicholas, 1976). In addition to being at risk for the overuse injuries typically seen in adults, children and adolescents are at risk for injury to areas of active growth. These include the growth plates or physes and articular cartilage (Clain & Hershman, 1989).

However, musculoskeletal injury is not the only risk; competitive stress can lead to psychophysiological disorders in young athletes. Dermatologic and gastrointestinal problems have been noted in particular (American Academy of Pediatrics Committee on Sports medicine, 1983). Parental pressures and unrealistic expectations of coaches contribute to a disturbing incidence of psychological and psychophysiological disorders among child athletes, especially elite performers (Nash, 1987).

Injury and psychological pressure both contribute to sport attrition (Gould, 1987). Injury is likely to threaten the sense of mastery of the youthful athlete for whom sport has provided an important early achievement experience. Alternately, injury or illness may provide a way out of an intolerable sport situation for the athlete who fails to meet performance goals of parents or coaches. Because of the child's dependency on parents at this stage, parents play an important role in the management of injury and need to be included in the treatment process. Psychologists should consider and address as necessary parents' potential role in the etiology of problems. (See chapter 16 for more information on the role of parents in injury management.)

Adolescence

Through puberty and adolescence (approximately to age 20), rapid physical growth and development continue. Athletic activities are the leading cause of nonfatal injuries among American youth ("Teens' health," 1990), and many factors contribute to this injury risk. Gains in physical prowess occur in tandem with more demanding training regimens and increasing pressure to play in spite of pain. The required level of excellence in performance increases, and athletes perceive growing pressure for competitive success. Related injury- and health-risk behaviors such as drug use (Anderson & McKeag, 1985, 1989) and extreme weight loss measures appear. Finally, many adolescents develop a more calculated approach to risk taking, and more dangerous sport activities become accessible.

These factors collectively contribute to the risk of physical injury as well as to problems in psychological adjustment. The profound and potentially devastating effects of competitive pressure on the athlete aspiring to elite status have long been noted (McDermott, 1982; Michener, 1976). High school–aged elite athletes (in sports such as tennis, gymnastics, and skiing) may enter specialized training programs away from home and parents, exacerbating the potential impact of competitive pressure.

Natural selection leads to a weeding out of those less physically and mentally fit, and injury appears to be an important factor in this process. However, injury is threatening to the adolescent struggling with issues of dependence and independence, not only because of the loss of valued activity but also because medical care implies increased dependence. During this stage the individual either moves up the ladder of achievement in the pursuit of competitive excellence or relegates sport to a recreational role. Through adolescence parents continue to play an important but diminishing role in injury management. In working with the adolescent athlete, the psychologist must strike a particularly delicate balance between confidentiality, the athlete's responsibility for decision making, and parental participation (Rotella & Heil, 1991).

Early Adulthood

In early adulthood (ages 20 to 40) athletes reach a peak of physical ability and achievement in sport. To the individual for whom competitive sport is a vocation, the question of the short-term gain of continued play in spite of injury versus long-term health cost is particularly compelling. The greater the degree of professionalization, the more complicated the resolution of this question becomes.

During early adulthood, many athletes will retire from competitive sport at the end of collegiate careers; most professional athletes also will conclude their careers by the end of this period. Postcompetitive physical screening in conjunction with recommendations for maintenance of fitness in light of injury history is of great value. To many athletes, sport will have served as an important component of personal identity. This loss may be sorely felt, especially by those who have failed to achieve outside the realm of athletics.

By the conclusion of this period, athletic pursuits are generally relegated to leisure and must be balanced against career and family responsibilities. With age the "weekend athlete" becomes increasingly injury prone, due to insufficient training and to overexertion in competition. An interesting anomaly, the addicted athlete, is seen among adult groups. Usually this is a recreational athlete whose drive to participate in sport is so compelling that physical, emotional, or social well-being may be compromised. (See chapter 13 for more information.)

When physical activity is well suited to social and physical constraints and becomes established as a life-long behavior, it will significantly enhance health and well-being (Pelletier, 1979). Alternately, inactivity leads to an early decline of physical fitness and functional ability, and injury may well tip the scale in this direction.

Middle Adulthood

During the years of middle adulthood (ages 40 to 60), a person's children leave home and occupational activities stabilize, often providing an increase in leisure time. However, physical ability decreases, and the person must adjust activity accordingly. At this age individuals become particularly prone to overuse injuries, and the need for setting appropriate limits becomes increasingly important, especially given that recovery from injury slows with age. Individuals who initiate and energetically pursue sport activities at this stage of life may experience enhanced vigor and vitality and a strong sense of achievement. Others may find it necessary to initiate exercise programs for weight control or other health reasons. For this group, compliance is a critical issue. In remaining active, these people help stave off the specter of age-related physical decline.

Few athletes continue careers in professional sports at this age, but the growing availability of Masters-level competition provides an appropriate competitive outlet. For example, Tom resumed running in middle adulthood following a mediocre college career. In less than 5 years he rose to a top national Masters ranking. The rapid and gratifying sense of personal development he gained was in marked contrast to the relatively slow, measured career progress he made as a nationally known research scientist.

The extent to which midlife crisis may be played out (for good or ill) in the pursuit of sport during this stage of life is an interesting but unanswered question (Astle, 1986; Little, 1969).

Late Adulthood

The later stages of adulthood (age 60 and older) are marked by loss of physical expertise and fitness as well as by increasing prevalence of chronic medical conditions. However, there is also increased leisure time and greater opportunity for participation in physical activity. Sport and fitness programs may meet a wide variety of social, emotional, cognitive, and medical needs (Van Camp & Boyer, 1989). Those for whom exercise has been a lifelong activity may show remarkable vitality. Walter Stack began running at age 58 as a complement to his long-standing involvement with swimming. By age 70 he had run 34,000 mi and 70 marathons (Bishop, 1978). Age-group events provide an appropriate competitive outlet for those less stout of heart.

With advancing age, medical problems occur with increasing frequency, and the risk of injury increases. Poorly contrived physical fitness programs can have a tremendously deleterious impact on health. In contrast, it is becoming increasingly clear that well-designed activity programs are useful in the management of a variety of chronic diseases (Ward, Taylor, & Rippe, 1991).

Sport and Lifestyle Issues Affecting Assessment and Intervention

The biopsychosocial developmental model provides a perspective from which the psychologist can bring into focus other sport and lifestyle issues. These include the athlete's

1. level of achievement and commitment to sport,
2. choice of sport,
3. gender,
4. racial and other cultural considerations, and
5. health status.

An athlete's level of achievement and commitment to sport provide important insight into the nature of his or her sport experience. The athlete who embarks on the quest for competitive excellence enters a survival-of-the-fittest scenario, in which fewer and fewer athletes successfully reach levels of performance culminating in bona fide professionalism. This has been described by Kroll (1970) in his Personality-Performance Pyramid.

For those so committed, sport offers its own life cycle of sorts. Important sport-related tasks and transitions may interact with events unfolding in the context of the broader development cycle of everyday life. Transitions in sports such as moving to a higher level of competitive excellence (or alternately failing to do so) and retirement are of critical significance (Pearson & Petitpas, 1990).

For youthful, aspiring athletes who seek to move up the ladder of success, commitment and achievement generally increase with age. However, there are many exceptions to this rule. In some sports (e.g., gymnastics), athletes may peak at very young ages. Olympic champions Olga Korbut (in 1972) and Nadia Comaneci (in 1976) led a trend to predominance of gymnastics by prepubescent females. The delayed puberty that is now common among competitive female gymnasts has important psychosocial consequences (Iversen, 1990). Other athletes may first approach sports seriously in adult life and so experience a personal peak of excellence in Masters-level competition. There are also competitive athletes whose achievements are quite modest but who nonetheless are intensely committed; these athletes clearly should receive treatment of comparable intensity to that provided to the more successful elite athlete.

Choice of sport is noteworthy as well. Each sport is like a subculture, with participation guided by special rules, demands, and expectations. Knowing the sport helps the psychologist to know the mind-set toward which the athlete tends to gravitate. It also provides valuable information in regard to health risk factors such as extreme weight loss measures, eating disorders, and drug abuse. Choice of sport also tends to reflect the availability of medical services (e.g., Division I collegiate football vs. competitive running). The psychologist is encouraged to include the performing artist among those athletes who can benefit from his or her services. It is essential to be sensitive to the distinct perspective that characterizes artistic pursuits.

Gender, race, and other cultural factors are compelling social issues in contemporary sport with far-reaching implications. These same factors are of practical significance in terms of assessment and intervention. For more information see the special issue of *The Sport Psychologist* entitled "Working With Various Populations" (G. Roberts, 1991) and the special issue of *Sports Illustrated* entitled "The Black Athlete" ("The black athlete," 1991). For additional information on women's issues see Haycock (1986) and Puhl, Brown, and Voy (1988).

The physical and mental limitations of special populations and the distinct perspective of the special athlete on sport participation merit attention. Karl Ellingson (1981), who lost an arm in a motor vehicle accident at 13 years of age, described his motivation for making solo walks of the Appalachian and Pacific Coast trails in adult life.

I made the decision not to wear my artificial arm. . . . Working one-handed was frustrating, slow, awkward and clumsy at times—such as pitching a tent in a gale using teeth, knees, shoulder, and head besides my good left hand—but it could be done. The discipline required to get up and go rain or shine with numb fingers folding a frosted tent and pulling on wet cold boots meant I was really free—free to do what I wanted. (pp. 1, 2, 31)

(The special issue of *The Sport Psychologist*, "Working With Various Populations" [G. Roberts, 1991], also contains information on intervention with special populations.)

Careful assessment of the role of sport and lifestyle factors guides and refines the psychologist's approach to assessment and intervention so that it meets the unique needs of each athlete.

Injury Assessment and Intervention Protocols

Effective intervention requires an accurate and thorough assessment of the athlete's situation. Ideally, in conducting the assessment the psychologist should emphasize the athlete's importance in the sport program and express concern for her or his welfare. These contacts with the psychologist should identify existing or potential problems, prompt subsequent self-assessment, and enlist the athlete's coping abilities. For intervention to be successful it must be individualized; thus factors that must be assessed include injury severity, the degree of related psychological distress, developmental status, and other sport and lifestyle factors.

Assessment protocols are presented next with practical recommendations regarding their use. These are the acute injury assessment, the consultation-liaison assessment, the chronic pain and injury assessment, and the Sportsmedicine Injury Checklist.

Acute Injury Assessment

The acute injury assessment (Heil, 1988; see Figure 9.2) is optimally designed for use in moderate injury, although it is appropriate in cases of minor injury in which the coach or sports medicine professional expresses concern about the athlete. It is also useful for an athlete who is recovering from severe injury and is making the transition from a general medical to a more sports medicine-based approach to treatment. Focused on current factors that are relatively easily reported or observed, this is the most proactive and preventive of the injury assessment approaches. In its comprehensive form it is designed with attention to three goals: early identification of rehabilitation problems; identification of concurrent problems, which either preceded or arose from injury; and clarification of the coping resources available to the athlete. The breadth, depth, and formality of this assessment should be adjusted to suit the presenting context of injury.

There are five sections to the acute injury assessment: rehabilitation process, pain, psychological status, life circumstances, and coping resources. Of these, the initial three are most essential and can be used as a short form of this assessment interview.

Regarding rehabilitation process, there are several key questions. Does the athlete attend treatment sessions and demonstrate good effort? Does

Acute Injury Assessment

Rehabilitation process

- Compliance
        Attendance
        Effort
- Knowledge
        Nature of injury and treatment
        Specific rehabilitation goals
- Perceived effectiveness

Pain

- Rehabilitation
- Day-to-day activity
- Sport performance

Psychological status

- Mood (in general)
- Fear/anxiety (in specific situations)
- Psychophysiological problems

Life circumstances

- Sport-related stress/change
- General life stress/change
- Overtraining prior to injury

Coping resources

- Personal
        Positive, optimistic attitude
        Stress management
- Social support
        Sport
        Family and friends

Figure 9.2   Acute injury risk assessment outline.

he or she understand the nature of injury and treatment and specific rehabilitation goals? Does the athlete perceive rehabilitation as effective? Discrepancies between the perceptions of the athlete and the treatment providers concerning effort or effectiveness are noteworthy. Thus, the treatment provider should tactfully ask the athlete how he or she perceives his or her own effort.

Although pain is a routine aspect of rehabilitation, how the athlete manages pain is of great importance. The key question here is how well the athlete tolerates pain during rehabilitation and in daily activities. With return to play, poor performance or increased complaints of pain may signal either fear of reinjury or concern that treatment has been inadequate. In this situation, it is important to determine if the athlete can differentiate benign pain from harmful pain.

Obvious emotional distress, either reported or observed, is cause for concern. Athletes may be particularly reluctant to directly admit psychological distress, but the psychologist can observe signs of distress indirectly. Signs include hesitancy or outright anxiety in specific rehabilitation or performance situations, as well as complaints of fatigue, sleep problems, headaches, gastrointestinal distress, or other psychophysiological problems. Differences between self-reported and observed psychological status are particularly noteworthy.

In reviewing the athlete's situation, the psychologist should look for what may complicate rehabilitation or be complicated by injury, such as stressful events in sport and in daily life. The possibility of overtraining should be considered.

Also important are the athlete's coping resources, in terms of availability and the effectiveness with which they are used. A good social support system may be available, but the athlete who withdraws in times of distress is deprived of its benefits. The athlete who has formal training in sport performance-enhancement methods should be encouraged to use these during rehabilitation.

The sports medicine specialist, physician, and coach are important secondary sources of information. The physician and sports medicine specialist can provide useful input regarding rehabilitation compliance and progress as well as impressions of psychological status. The coach can provide input on the athlete's psychological functioning as well as insight into recent sport situation changes, signs of overtraining prior to injury, and the readiness for return to play.

As discussed in chapter 8, psychological testing should be used with discretion. It is most appropriate where significant problems are identified and more information is needed. The POMS is particularly useful because of its brevity and ease of administration. Sport-specific measures such as the CSAI-II (Martens et al., 1982) may help determine readiness for return to play. Brief questionnaires regarding the rehabilitation process such as those used by Fisher et al. (1988) are also useful.

If in the absence of other problems the athlete experiences difficulty in returning to play, the role of pain in performance should be examined. Specifically, it is important to determine how pain triggers the athlete's action, either directly in behavior or cognitively in the form of attention shifts. The psychologist should look carefully for protective bracing or guarding, hesitancy in approaching performance situations, or outright avoidance and should check with the coach and sports medicine staff to determine if increased pain is due to failure to adhere to physical limitations.

The psychologist should individualize the acute injury intervention based on the athlete's development, sport, and lifestyle. Examples of issues of concern for some sport and life situations follow.

There is the possibility of emotional distress if otherwise minor injury is perceived as resulting in disfigurement or decreased attractiveness. In highly competitive athletes, the timing of even minor injury may undermine hopes for competitive success. For the early or middle adult suffering injury soon after embarking on a new exercise program, the psychologist should devote extra attention to facilitating resumption of the program. Chapters 11 and 13 provide additional information on identification of and intervention with pain problems.

Consultation-Liaison Assessment

The goals of consultation-liaison assessment are to provide a concise impression of psychological function, practical recommendations for the medical team regarding patient management, and brief timely psychological treatment as needed. Specialized services may be provided in conjunction with surgery preoperatively and postoperatively and with ongoing hospitalization.

A worksheet for the consultation-liaison assessment is provided in Figure 9.3 (Heil, 1986). It identifies four areas of inquiry: medical status, psychological status, adjustment to injury and treatment, and psychological history. The POMS is well suited for use in consultation-liaison assessment.

The psychologist must understand the athlete's medical status in order to assess the appropriateness of the athlete's emotional response to injury and to assess how realistic expectations are regarding recovery. Much of this information is available from medical records, which the psychologist may review prior to meeting with the athlete. However, it is also important to consult with the physician and to note treatment complications.

The initial meeting should begin with a brief assessment of psychological status and of the athlete's receptivity to the interview at that moment. These factors help determine the tone, timing, and intensity of intervention. It may be best to conduct a minimal assessment informally and plan

Consultation-Liaison Assessment

Name: _____ Date: _____ Age: _____

Sport: _____ Team status: _____

Diagnostic review

Medical status

Injury/illness _____

Related medical history _____

Treatment _____ Complications? _____

Rehab plan _____ Time loss _____ Function loss _____

Psychological status

Mood _____ Distress level appropriate? _____

Pain _____ Sleep _____

Adjustment to injury and treatment

Treatment hassles _____

Psychological reaction to injury _____

Rehabilitation goals _____

Future orientation _____

Loss/grief _____

Psychological history

Recent life/sport stress _____

Prior adjustment problems _____

Social support system _____

Impression

Adjustment to injury and treatment _____

Prognosis for rehabilitation _____

Recommendation

Figure 9.3   Consultation-liaison assessment worksheet.

to return later. Alternately, the athlete may be in distress and may want to express his or her concerns at length and in detail.

The psychologist should promptly identify the athlete's special worries or concerns about hospitalization and treatment and should review the circumstances of injury. The psychologist should also identify the athlete's expectations regarding the course of rehabilitation, anticipated downtime, and impact of injury on playing ability and should evaluate the athlete's sense of loss or grief. Evidence of traumatic conditioning with injury or denial regarding the impact of injury on performance should be observed and noted. Life and sport stress at the time of injury should be identified, and the quality and availability of social support should be evaluated as well. The psychologist should conduct a more detailed review of psychological history as appropriate.

Postoperative assessment should enable the psychologist to predict whether the athlete is on course for effective rehabilitation or is at significant risk for problems. If the athlete is at risk, additional psychological intervention should be recommended. If the athlete is in psychological crisis, intensive treatment should begin immediately.

Preoperative assessment may guide athletes in psychological preparation for surgery, assist them in the decision-making regarding surgery itself, or identify those at risk for psychological complications following surgery. Pre- and postoperative treatment approaches are described in detail in chapter 12.

The psychologist may fine-tune the consultation-liaison assessment in accord with developmental, sport, and lifestyle issues. Some special concerns for specific sport and life situations are as follows. Be aware that children may underreport severity of pain in order to avoid injections or other medical procedures. Where surgery or other intensive treatment is considered on an elective basis with the successful adolescent (or child) athlete, the psychologist should differentiate the athlete's wishes from those of the parents; where these are in conflict, they should be a focus of intervention. When surgery is planned for the late adolescent or early adult who is likely nearing the end of a competitive career (e.g., nearing graduation from high school or college), the relative costs and benefits of return to play for a short period should be assessed in comparison to the impact of reinjury on lifelong recreational sport activity.

Chronic Pain and Injury Assessment

When treatment is unsuccessful and the athlete has problems adapting to injury, then chronic pain and injury syndromes develop. Complaints of pain contrasting with minimal objective medical findings are usually the case in these syndromes. As pain turns chronic, critical physiological and psychological changes take place. Often, sensitization occurs whereby the same level of pain-inducing stimuli at the periphery leads to increasing levels of pain registered in the brain. (For more on this complex biological process see chapter 17.) As pain endures, related behavior changes (e.g., sleep disturbance and chronic muscle tension) further exacerbate pain and contribute to a sense of loss of control. This can lead to irritability, diminished motivation, and depression.

Relative to the acute injury and consultation-liaison assessments, the chronic pain and injury assessment is more comprehensive and in-depth. It should include a review of the broad range of diagnostic risk factors that precede, follow, and occur in conjunction with injury. (See chapter 7 for a complete review of these.) Among the factors preceding injury, problematic medical history, history of difficulties in psychological adjustment, and a tendency for somatization are prognostic indicators of poor adaptation. Evidence of significant trauma in conjunction with injury is also noteworthy.

Figure 9.4 is an extensive guide to the assessment of chronic pain and injury. (See chapter 8 for more information regarding the specific methods and measures listed.) The assessment guide may be used in whole or in part at the discretion of the psychologist. The guidelines for pain assessment in diagnostic interview are most important and should be used in their entirety. Questions should address mood as well as the variability of pain across situations and its impact on performance. The use of psychometric measures is less critical but still quite valuable. The input of significant others as part of assessment is also quite important.

Fordyce (1976) described complaints of pain as a form of social communication, the meaning of which for a particular patient remains to be determined. At times patients' ratings of pain may appear to bear little relationship to medical findings, functional ability, or observed behavior. Pain behaviors may fluctuate across different situations and may be magnified in times of stress. This may lead treatment providers to suspect malingering (although this is rare). If these suspicions are conveyed to the athlete, the relationship between athlete and treatment provider can become strained, contributing a crisis of trust to an already difficult situation. Consequently, athletes may be cautious or even suspicious in diagnostic assessment as to whether or not the physician is giving their complaints serious attention. Establishing trust during the initial interviews is important, and it begins with acceptance of the athlete's complaints of pain as true and honest.

Chronic pain and injury assessment should incorporate two perspectives of the athlete's psychology: the behavioral and the dynamic. The general objective of a behavioral analysis is to identify the antecedents and consequences of pain. To what extent are pain behaviors followed directly by reinforcing consequences? To what extent does pain allow avoidance of unpleasant situations? When the person hurts, what positive events take place that otherwise wouldn't, and what negative things do not happen that otherwise would (Fordyce, 1976)? Direct positive

Chronic Pain and Injury Assessment

Diagnostic interview

- Self-report

    Quantitative (1 to 10 scale or visual analog scale)

      Severity

      Bothersomeness

    Qualitative (open-ended description)

    Environmental contingencies

      Things that increase pain

      Things that decrease pain

Observation

- Pain behaviors (type and frequency)

- Variability during interview

Psychometric assessment

- Psychological testing

    Minnesota Multiphasic Personality Inventory

    Millon Behavioral Health Inventory

- Other measures

    Pain-activity diary

    Pain drawing

Alternate sources

- Sports medicine professional

- Coach

- Parent

Figure 9.4   Chronic pain and injury assessment outline.

reinforcers for pain typically include increased attention and medication use. The indirect negative reinforcers include avoidance of aversive tasks and time out from ongoing life responsibilities. The various antecedent factors that elicit pain cause pain response to vary from situation to situation. Identifying these factors allows the psychologist to identify situations that present the greatest challenge during rehabilitation.

To assess the dynamic perspective, the psychologist must understand the personal meaning of injury to the athlete. Does the injury threaten his or her lifestyle or generate a sense of loss? The dynamic analysis offers a subjective perspective to complement the more objective behavioral analysis. For more information on this diagnostic process see Fordyce (1976), Ford (1983), and Brena and Chapman (1982).

In conducting the chronic pain and injury assessment, the psychologist should consider specific developmental, sport, and lifestyle factors. Some situations that the psychologist should be alert for are listed as follows. With special populations (i.e., people who are mentally and physically handicapped), the psychologist must differentiate issues related to recent injury from those related to disability. When working with racial and ethnic minorities, the psychologist should explore the possibility that conflicts between treatment providers and the athlete may grow out of subtle cultural differences. When injury leads the late-aged adult to withdraw from sport as well as from other social contacts, that person may be experiencing age-related cognitive difficulties; because of the cognitive benefits of regular exercise, this group should be encouraged to return to sport following injury.

The Sports Medicine Injury Checklist

The psychological status of the injured athlete is of concern to all treatment providers. The sport physician and the sports medicine rehabilitation specialist are in unique positions to monitor the athlete's psychological well-being, and their input contributes significantly to the comprehensiveness of psychological evaluation. The importance of identification and triage of psychological problems is widely recognized among sports medicine rehabilitation specialists (Furney & Patton, 1985). Physicians implicitly recognize these same concerns as an aspect of overall patient care.

The sports medicine specialist typically spends a significant amount of direct contact time with the injured athlete. In addition, this practitioner often interacts with the athlete during periods of health—especially where the sports medicine specialist is directly affiliated with the team (as in the collegiate setting). As a consequence, the sports medicine specialist is able to use his or her understanding of what is typical behavior for the athlete to provide useful insights into the impact of injury on that person. The physician is best able to assess the appropriateness of the athlete's pain in response to injury.

Because chronicity of injury and psychological complications are mutually reinforcing, the benefit of early identification is great. Bridges (1987) developed a checklist to enhance the early identification chronic pain syndrome. The Sports Medicine Injury Checklist (Heil, 1988) (Figure 9.5) extends the work of Bridges (1987) by identifying factors of particular relevance to athletes. The checklist is divided into a relatively brief "acute phase" section and a more lengthy, detailed "chronic phase" section. There is no formal weighting of items. The checklist is best considered simply as a guide to inquiry and evaluation, which when followed ensures a comprehensive diagnostic approach.

The differentiation between acute and chronic adaptation to injury is ultimately subject to clinical interpretation. Traditionally, injury-related symptoms that persist beyond 6 months have been regarded as chronic. However, there is increasing evidence that chronic syndromes can be identified as early as 6 weeks following injury (E.W. Johnson, 1987).

The acute phase section of the checklist allows the user to unobtrusively identify potential difficulties in the immediate postinjury period. Most of the items can be assessed through direct observation and during treatment. An athlete's failure to comply with the rehabilitation regimen and persistent difficulties in pain management are the most reliable early indicators of rehabilitation problems. Obvious emotional distress is also a significant indicator, although it is much less frequently seen. Persistent fatigue and sleep problems may signal adjustment difficulties, and signs of anxiety demonstrated only in conjunction with specific performance situations suggest fear of reinjury. When either physical or psychological difficulties become evident, the psychologist should seek the athlete's input on how well rehabilitation is progressing. The athlete's perception of recovery influences the degree of emotional distress being experienced (McDonald & Hardy, 1990). When the athlete's perspective on injury differs substantially from objective medical opinion, problems are in the making.

Prolonged or repeated difficulties with rehabilitation and pain inevitably lead to the development of psychological sequelae. When problems persist in spite of continued appropriate medical treatment, a more detailed review of the athlete's psychological status is necessary. The chronic phase section of the checklist is designed for this purpose. It is composed of two parts: a rather lengthy section on current factors and a more brief listing of elements of personal and family history. The assessment of current factors relies significantly on observation of the athlete's behavior. Although the sports medicine professional can observe many of these behaviors, it may be necessary to consult with coaching staff on factors such as performance problems and interpersonal relationships. Other items—for example, the ability to identify realistic goals for recovery—require careful discussion with the athlete. It is essential to determine if

Sports Medicine Injury Checklist

<u>Acute phase</u>

_____ Failure of pain to respond to routine management strategies

_____ Failure of athlete to comply with recommended rehabilitation program

_____ Rehabilitation setbacks

_____ Emotional distress (depression, irritability, confusion, guilt, withdrawal)

_____ Irrational fear or anxiety in specific situations in the otherwise well-adjusted athlete (may be seen as avoidance of feared situation)

_____ Overly optimistic attitude toward injury and recovery

_____ Persistent fatigue

_____ Sleep problems

_____ Gross overestimate or underestimate of rehabilitation progress by athlete

<u>Chronic phase</u>

Current factors

_____ Persistence of pain beyond natural healing

_____ "Odd" descriptions of pain

_____ Inconsistency in "painful" behavior or reports of pain

_____ Failed attempt(s) at return to play

_____ Performance problems following return to play

_____ Inability to identify realistic goals for recovery

_____ Recent stressful changes in sport situation

_____ Stressful life circumstances (within the last year)

_____ Depression (including changes in sleep, appetite, energy, and libido)

_____ Strained relationships with coaches, teammates, or friends

_____ Personality conflicts between treatment providers and athlete

_____ Poor compliance with scheduled visits and medication use

_____ Additional medical treatment sought by athlete without consulting current treatment providers (including emergency room visits)

_____ Iatrogenic problems

_____ Repeated requests for pain (especially psychoactive) medication

_____ Evidence of illicit drug use (recreational or ergogenic)

History

_____ Multiple surgeries at pain site

_____ Chronic pain in the same or another physiological system (may be resolved)

_____ Family members with chronic pain

_____ Problematic psychosocial history (behavior problems in school; vocational, marital, or legal problems; history of physical or sexual abuse)

_____ Problematic psychological history (repeated or prolonged psychological adjustment problems; alcohol/drug problems; eating disorders)

Figure 9.5   Sports medicine injury checklist.

the athlete is able to distinguish benign pain that occurs routinely during rehabilitation and harmful pain that signals reinjury.

Problems in emotional adjustment may be more noticeable under careful scrutiny. However, the athlete may tend to deny these and may reflect them indirectly as a worrisome obsessive focus on pain or alternately as performance problems. Emotional difficulties may show themselves in increasing irritability, which results in strained relations with coaches, teammates, friends, and treatment providers.

Knowledge of the athlete's personal history helps treatment providers place other observations in perspective. As a general rule, a history of difficulty in adapting to psychological stressors is predictive of present difficulties. The assessment of history often requires probing questions; however, much of this information is available in medical records. Because of their intrusive nature, questions regarding history should be presented with sensitivity to the athlete's privacy. How probing one should be is a matter of clinical judgment. Treatment providers should also be vigilant to signs of drug use and eating disorders especially when the athlete has a known history of these behaviors. (See chapter 15 for more information.)

The physician and the sports medicine rehabilitation specialist provide the first line of psychological intervention with injured athletes. The psychologist and the physician and the sports medicine specialist are encouraged to work cooperatively to develop strategies for identification, management, and referral of athletes with difficulty in adjustment to injury. The Sports Medicine Injury Checklist is designed with this in mind. Pain drawing (see chapter 8) is a useful complement to this checklist in the hands of the medical professional. A more detailed treatment of the role of the physician and sports medicine rehabilitation specialist in the psychological management of the injured athlete is provided in Part V.

Concluding Comments

This chapter has presented a comprehensive strategy for assessment and intervention that also guides the practitioner in developing a programmatic approach to the psychological management of athletic injury. It is proactive and is congruent with the performance-enhancement philosophy that characterizes sport psychology and the speedy return to play that is emphasized in sports medicine. The individualized approach to assessment and intervention presented rests on four key elements: severity of injury, psychological adjustment to injury, developmental status, and sport and lifestyle issues. Four psychological assessment protocols are presented as practical guides to assessment. These are the acute injury assessment, the consultation-liaison assessment, the chronic pain and injury assessment, and the Sports Medicine Injury Checklist. The last of these protocols addresses the important role that the sports medicine professional plays in psychological assessment.

IV
PART

The Treatment of Injury

The heart of any applied health discipline is its approach to intervention and treatment. Given the diversity of sport injury in relation to severity, psychological adjustment, developmental concerns, and other sport and lifestyle issues, there is a wide range of potential psychological interventions for athletic injury. The treatment approaches presented in Part IV combine a health-oriented psychology of performance and a clinical psychology of behavior disorder. They span a continuum ranging from uncomplicated injury to subclinical syndromes to diagnosable disorders.

Chapter 10, "A Comprehensive Approach to Injury Management," focuses on routine approaches to the management of the injured athlete. It identifies education, goal setting, social support, and mental training as the pillars upon which injury intervention programs are built. The first three of the four elements of treatment—education, goal setting, and social support—are presented in detail in this chapter.

Chapter 11, "Mental Training in Injury Management," focuses on the fourth of the key elements, because the great richness and complexity of mental training warrant an in-depth review. The topics presented include continued performance-enhancement training, rehabilitation rehearsal, healing imagery, biofeedback, pain management, and fear of injury. Fear is intimately connected to injury both as a potential antecedent and as a consequence. How well fear of injury is managed influences injury risk before injury and rehabilitation effectiveness following injury. Because of the ubiquity of pain in sport, its potential deleterious impact, and a generally poor understanding of the psychobiology of pain, this topic is thoroughly reviewed.

The two subsequent chapters present treatment approaches for rehabilitation that is complicated by either severity of injury or problems in psychological adjustment. Chapter 12, "Specialized Treatment Approaches: Severe Injury," provides guidelines for management of injuries that require hospitalization and surgery as well as sport-disabling, catastrophic, and fatal injuries. The role of sensation seeking in sport and its relationship to injury are critically reviewed.

Chapter 13, "Specialized Treatment Approaches: Problems in Rehabilitation," provides guidelines for intervention of a variety of problems ranging from minor treatment complications to malingering. It includes recommendations for the management of muscular bracing/guarding, poor compliance, personality conflicts, traumatic conditioning, and chronic pain and injury syndrome. There is also an overview of the concept of the addicted athlete.

In chapter 14, "Case Studies: Professional Issues for the Treatment Provider," a panel of sport psychologists offer their personal reactions to a series of injury situations. The issues addressed include fear, assessing readiness for return to play, steroid use, fear of success, eating disorders, and pain control. Steroid use and eating disorders have well-documented direct medical consequences, and they indirectly increase injury risk. Because of their potentially disruptive psychological impact, they constitute psychological injury.

10
CHAPTER

A Comprehensive Approach to Injury Management

John Heil

Neil Bonnett (personal communication, March 11, 1990) describes his experience with rehabilitation from a severe injury:

> Following a leg injury in a wreck at Charlotte, I was experiencing pain like I never knew existed, and I was really low. [Fellow race-driver] Bobby Allison came for a visit. He had been hurt severely twice in his career. I asked him how he overcame it . . . He said I needed to set a goal and he defied me to quit.

> After I left the hospital I put all the physical therapy equipment in my den. I worked out from 8 to 10 A.M. then from 12 to 1 P.M., then from 5 to 6 P.M. All around the room was trophies and pictures of race cars, reminders of everything I wanted to do. Everytime I would get to hurting so bad I did not think I could lift the weights, I would stop and get my breath and look up and see what I wanted to continue to do in front of me. The only thing stopping me was me quitting. I would really concentrate. I could almost sit there and see the tendons and stuff in my leg. I have never been psychic by any means but I get to thinking you can make some things happen like that. I turned my rehabilitation into the race.

This straight talk from Neil Bonnett points a way to recovery that makes sense. It highlights the benefits of social support, goal setting, knowledge about injury, and treatment procedures and advocates the use of mental training.

The scope of psychological services for the injured athlete is broad relative to other treatment groups. Diversity of these services is reflected by the suitability of both traditional clinical and performance-enhancement intervention; the differing treatment settings in which services may be provided (competitive environments, the training room, medical settings); severity of injuries treated and level of psychological adjustment; and other special considerations regarding development, sport, and lifestyle. This chapter identifies principles that guide psychological intervention for injury in general, while focusing on specific methods suitable for the routine management of uncomplicated injury. Subsequent chapters offer guidelines for management of problem injury situations due either to severity or to difficulties in psychological adjustment.

The Foundations of Injury Management

An athlete's ability to avoid injury initially, to return to play quickly after injury, and to cope with setbacks as they occur significantly impacts overall athletic success. When injury occurs it is useful for the athlete to think of rehabilitation as part of the game that she or he must play well in order to succeed. The goals of routine psychological intervention with athletic injury are as follows:

1. Facilitation of the rehabilitation process
2. Maintenance of emotional equilibrium
3. Mobilization of existing coping resources
4. Enhancement of mental readiness for performance
5. Promotion of a sense of self-efficacy

These goals define a performance-enhancement model of intervention that emphasizes support and skill-based approaches to treatment. It is proactive, conceives of rehabilitation as a sport performance challenge, and encourages the use of psychological skills already developed for sport performance. This approach is motivated by the fact that as medical recovery is speeded (by advances in sports medicine), there is correspondingly greater pressure for quick psychological recovery. It also recognizes the other stringent performance criteria that make the athlete's world such a challenging one. These include the following:

1. The psychological stress of performance
2. Training strategies that push physical limits
3. Risky health practices in which athletes feel pressure to engage (e.g., substance use, extreme weight loss measures)

4. Reliance on highly refined sport-specific mental skills (e.g., concentration, information processing) for effective performance
5. The life-absorbing nature of serious athletic participation

A team approach to treatment is advocated because it provides some comprehensive care and facilitates synergism among treatments. Quick physical recovery and mental readiness for return to play involve more than simple compliance by the athlete; they demand vigorous physical effort and mental tenacity (Steadman, 1982). Presenting treatment as a collaborative effort between sports medicine providers and the athlete encourages active participation by the athlete and fosters a sense of personal responsibility. Steadman (1982) called attention to the ability of some athletes to demonstrate innovation in their personal approaches to rehabilitation. Neil Bonnett's description (personal communication, March 11, 1990) of his recovery from a broken wrist illustrates this point.

Later the doctor told me with that type of break I would probably lose 40 percent mobility. After the doctor put the case on the thing got to bothering me. I went back and he changed it. I came home and it got to bothering me, so I took a pair of snips and cut the cast off. . . and moved my thumb a small bit. Then I bought a case of fiberglass cast material. I would put a case on, and take it off every day. At night I would work at moving it a little bit. I started to race with the cast still on. The doctor said he had never seen that much mobility after a break like that.

Few athletes are as masterful at the process of rehabilitation as Neil Bonnett. The purpose of the treatment approach described in this chapter is to help athletes strive for this same level of excellence.

Education, social support, goal setting, and mental training are the key elements in a comprehensive approach to injury management. Goals define the task, and education provides an understanding of how to proceed. Mental training (the subject of the following chapter) and social support are the coping resources on which the athlete may draw to remain on task in the face of adversity. Putting the key elements together points the athlete toward a remarkable recovery from sport injury.

Education

Underlying successful treatment is sensitivity to the athlete's readiness for a particular intervention. This enables the psychologist to identify and seize the opportunity provided by the "teachable moment," a time when the athlete is uniquely ready for integral understanding and personal change. The primary goal of education is to help the athlete understand in detail the processes underlying injury and rehabilitation. Education is the foundation upon which the alliance of the athlete with the sports medicine team is built. It can also serve as a basis for ongoing dialogue regarding that essential but elusive injury management skill— differentiating pain and injury.

The athlete cannot give optimal effort to something that he or she does not understand. An active approach to education counters the notions held by many that medical treatment is something that a practitioner administers and a patient passively receives, and that healing is a process of waiting. Injury provides a timely opportunity for learning about the body and physical performance. The sport emphasis is simply shifted from performance skills to health and safety. This refined understanding of the body's limits that is gained through rehabilitation can play an important role in preventing future injury.

Athletes who address physical performance from the perspectives of skill development and health maintenance improve their chances for lon-gevity and success in sport. At age 44, Nolan Ryan continues to be one of the best pitchers in major league baseball. Many assume this is just a fortunate accident of inheritance. However, he has for many years per-formed a daily, year-round strength and conditioning program. His per-sonal physician attributes Ryan's longevity and success to an approach to sport that incorporates performance in a broader context of fitness and health maintenance (Shepard & Pacelli, 1990).

Following an injury, its cause and physical consequences should be described in terms that the athlete can understand. Treatment providers should also give the athlete a sense of how the injury will heal and specific information about methods of rehabilitation and how they aid healing. Explanations presented in pictorial language creating vivid visual and kinesthetic images enhance understanding and facilitate the application of mental training to injury. Treatment providers should also describe the timetable of rehabilitation and the expectations they have of the athlete. Special concerns such as anticipated plateaus in progress and tolerance of pain may be discussed as necessary. A list of these and related factors to be addressed is presented in Table 10.1.

This list calls for treatment providers to make a significant commitment to education. In actual practice, many of the items on the list are taken care of routinely as a natural part of the treatment process. Yet often patients appear to have unanswered questions or an apparently inade-quate understanding of injury and treatment. In general medical practice, compliance with medication use and with prescribed independent activi-ties is known to be poor; treatment providers use medical terminology and provide brief explanations that patients often simply do not under-stand. This confusion may be compounded by the stress of injury and a poor understanding of medical practice on the part of the athlete. The antidote to this is the treatment provider's consistent, systematic attention

---

Table 10.1
Injury Education Guidelines

Basic anatomy of the injured area
Changes caused by injury
Active and passive rehabilitation methods
Mechanisms by which rehabilitation methods work
Description of diagnostic and surgical procedures (if necessary)
Potential problems with pain and how to cope with these
Differentiation of benign pain from dangerous pain
Guidelines for independent use of modalities (i.e., heat, cold)
Plan for progressing active rehabilitation (e.g., resistance training)
Anticipated timetable for rehabilitation
Possibility of treatment plateaus
Purposes of medication with emphasis on consistent use as prescribed
Potential side effects of medication with encouragement to report these
   to the physician
Rationale for limits on daily physical activities during healing
Guidelines for the use of braces, orthotic devices, or crutches
Injury as a source of stress and a challenge to maintaining a positive
   attitude
Rehabilitation as an active collaborative learning process
Methods of assessing readiness for return to play
Deciding when to hold back and when to go all-out
Long-term maintenance and care of healing injury

---

to education and explicit efforts to determine whether the athlete understands the information provided. A survey of athletic trainers showed that the importance of educating athletes about the nature of injury and rehabilitation was broadly recognized (Wiese, Weiss, & Yukelson, 1991).

One of the most important elements in safe rehabilitation and in injury prevention is the ability to differentiate pain and injury. However, this is probably the most poorly articulated of injury management skills, no doubt due to the inherent complexity of this task. The athlete must learn to differentiate performance pain from injury during performance—and benign pain (that occurring routinely) from harmful pain during rehabilitation. There is no simple or straightforward way to do this; it appears to be a subtle process cultivated over time and based on experience with healthy performance and injury. As the athlete learns more of the rehabilitation process from the sports medicine specialist, an ability to differentiate pain and injury will be fostered.

In summary, the recommended educational approach sets up injury rehabilitation as a learning process, encourages the active participation of the athlete, and serves as a foundation for goal setting.

Goal Setting

The importance of setting and striving for goals has long been recognized in sport (Carron, 1984; Locke & Latham, 1985) and rehabilitation (Danish, 1986; Fordyce, 1976). Goal setting links motivation to action. In rehabilitation, goal setting should parallel the treatment plan, establish an implicit statement of commitment by the athlete, and identify treatment as a collaborative process.

Setting and pursuing goals is a pragmatic process. The goals of "being a winner" or "getting back to 100%" following injury are worthwhile. However, until the athlete can understand what it takes to do this and can measure progress, such goals are of limited value. A general summary of guidelines for goal setting is presented in Table 10.2.

In addition to setting goals, identifying barriers to goal attainment is also important. Factors that may interfere with effective rehabilitation include the following (Danish, 1986):

- A lack of knowledge about the rehabilitation process
- A lack of skill at a particular rehabilitation task
- A perception that the risks of treatment outweigh the benefits
- Lack of social support

By identifying barriers to goal attainment, treatment providers can identify reasons for noncompliance other than poor motivation. Fear of reinjury, concern regarding pain, and other inhibitions in risk taking often underlie poor compliance.

For many athletes, goal setting for rehabilitation will be a novel application of a familiar concept. A goal program may be relatively simple and informal or complex and multifaceted. The specifics of a goal-based program will vary depending upon the following:

- Length and intensity of treatment
- Urgency of speedy return to play
- Level of commitment to sport
- Initial psychological adjustment to injury
- Difficulties in rehabilitation

The more problematic the injury and the greater the athlete's commitment, the more intense the approach to goal setting.

Goal setting is most readily applicable to active rehabilitation; however, it can be extended to include any of the elements of rehabilitation. Goals

Table 10.2
Guide to Goal Setting

Specific and measurable

The athlete must know exactly what to do and be able to determine if gains are made.

Stated in positive versus negative language

Knowing what to do guides behavior, whereas knowing what to avoid creates a focus on errors without providing a constructive alternative.

Challenging but realistic

Overly difficult goals set up failure and pose a threat to the athlete. The lower the athlete's self-confidence, the more important success becomes and the greater the importance of setting attainable goals.

Timetable for completion

This allows for a check on progress and evaluation of whether realistic goals have been set.

Integration of short-, intermediate-, and long-term goals

A comprehensive program links day-to-day activities with expectations for specific competitions and with season and career goals.

Outcome goals linked to process goals

Process goals (what to do) define the pathway to outcome goals. Outcomes are influenced by a variety of factors, many of which may be beyond the athlete's control. Process goals direct the athlete's focus to those factors most readily controlled.

Personalized and internalized

The athlete must embrace goals as his or her own, not as something imposed from outside.

Monitored and evaluated

Feedback must be provided to assess goals. Goals should be modified based on progress.

Sport goals linked to life goals

This identifies sport and rehabilitation as life learning experiences and helps the athlete put sport in a broader perspective. This is especially important for athletes whose return to sport is doubtful.

may be set for use of medications and modalities as well as braces or orthotic devices. They can also be set for important behaviors to avoid (e.g., for maintaining activity limitations) during the healing process. Simply listing such goals and recommending that they be followed as prescribed is an affirmation of their importance.

Goals can be set for coping with the psychological challenges that rehabilitation poses, such as boredom, impatience with maintaining activity limits, frustration with pain, or feelings of being down. Setting such goals implicitly acknowledges the suffering of injury, identifies it as a normal or ordinary behavior, and characterizes effective coping as an achievement. Where psychological adjustment problems are evident, training in coping techniques can be provided and goals set for their use. (See the section on rehabilitation rehearsal in chapter 11.)

Where progress is painstakingly slow, the treatment provider may take a more fine-grained approach to goal monitoring, calling greater attention to relatively small gains and demonstrating that progress is being made. Some rehabilitation gains are beyond the athlete's ability to observe. Through the hands and eyes of the sports medicine professional and through diagnostic imaging, gains may be noted that are not otherwise apparent. It is beneficial for the practitioner to share these observations with the athlete and explain their meaning relative to the healing process.

Where treatment plateaus occur, the athlete can supplement performance goals with effort goals using the Rating of Perceived Exertion Scale initially developed by Borg in the 1960s, which continues to be investigated and refined (e.g., Borg & Ottoson, 1986). This scale has been used to monitor a wide range of performance and rehabilitation activities (Monahan, 1988). Perceived exertion can safely guide those who adhere too vigorously to a "no pain, no gain" philosophy, helping such athletes maintain appropriate limits. Athletes engaged in protracted rehabilitation can become easily discouraged when they compare their current levels of ability to preinjury levels. When this occurs the athlete should be refocused toward goals attained thus far and to those to be met next.

Global goals that extend beyond day-to-day rehabilitation can be identified. Examples include improving knowledge of the body and of principles of rehabilitation, refining skill in differentiating pain and injury, decreasing future injury risk, and improving stress coping. This approach recognizes the enduring importance of injury avoidance and coping as essential athletic skills. It also relates sport skills to other life challenges, enhancing the potential for their use after the athlete retires from sport.

The process of setting, monitoring, and refining goals clarifies communication between the athlete and the sports medicine treatment provider. The effectiveness of this communication will influence the quality of treatment relationship and often will impact treatment effectiveness. A well-planned goal program identifies the challenges of rehabilitation, treats injury as a learning experience, and helps maintain a performance-enhancement orientation to injury rehabilitation.

Social Support

Social support is a form of interpersonal connectedness. It encourages the constructive expression of feelings, provides reassurance in times of doubt, and leads to improved communication and understanding. Social support is one of many needs that can be met by sport participation, through camaraderie with other athletes and team membership. Social support is also a vehicle for increasing athletic performance as well as enhancing the athlete's well-being (Richman, Hardy, Rosenfeld, & Callanan, 1989).

The general medical literature offers empirical endorsement for the psychological and medical benefits of various forms of social support (Taylor, Falke, Shoptaw, & Lichtman, 1986; Wallston, Alagna, DeVellis, & DeVellis, 1983; Williams, Ware, & Donald, 1981). Social support buffers the effects of stress on health and enhances the prospects for recovery of those who are ill or injured. Those who possess a strong sense of social support demonstrate greater self-efficacy, lower anxiety, better interpersonal skills, and more risk-taking behavior (Sarason, Sarason, & Pierce, 1990). In his review of adjustment to combat, Kardiner (1959) emphasized the importance of social support and team identity both as buffers to mental disorder and key components of treatment when problems occur. The sport psychology literature consistently notes the benefits of social support in helping cope with injury (e.g., Danish, 1986; Rotella & Heyman, 1986). Research has also shown social support to be related to compliance with rehabilitation following injury (Duda et al., 1989; Fisher et al., 1988). Unfortunately, the injured athlete tends to be separated from the team and to lose this source of support at a time when it is most important.

The anecdote that follows emphasizes the intangible yet fundamental nature of social support. Bob was a college teammate who suffered a series of chronic injuries that necessitated regular treatment over a long period. One day he arrived at the therapy center to be told that he didn't need treatment any longer. At first he looked surprised and a bit disoriented. Then he lay down on a treatment table and let himself drift off into a relaxed state, as he usually did during therapy. When he got up he looked rested, refreshed, and quite a bit less tense. He then talked for a while with the trainer, thanked him, and left. I noted this at the time with a great deal of curiosity but little understanding. Eventually I realized how much I looked forward to treatment as a time out from the hustle of the day and how the training room was such a comfortable place to be—a lot of which had to do with how well-liked and respected the trainer was. In retrospect, I believe that Bob benefited that day from the supportive milieu of the training room that had been established over months of treatment. Even in the absence of the need for treatment he got a psychological boost from just being there.

Just as support is beneficial, pressure or confrontation regarding injury is potentially detrimental. In a study of over 500 female intercollegiate volleyball players from 65 schools (Hankins et al., 1989), researchers noted that challenges to the validity of the subjects' injuries and pressure to return to play from coaches and other players produced psychological distress. In a well-researched journalistic look at youth tennis, McDermott (1982) graphically illustrated the devastating consequences for athletes of the absence of social support in times of emotional difficulty.

Rosenfeld et al. (1989) identified a model that includes six forms of social support: listening, technical appreciation, technical challenge, emotional support, emotional challenge, and shared social reality. These are elaborated in Table 10.3.

Table 10.3
Elements of Social Support in Athletic Environments

Listening

Listening in a nonjudgmental way to the concerns and feelings of another, as well as emphatic sharing of joys and sorrows

Technical appreciation

Acknowledgment of good performance, based on technical understanding of the tasks in question

Technical challenge

Encouragement to meet performance goals by those who have a technical understanding of the tasks in question

Emotional support

Active support of an athlete through emotionally demanding circumstances (without necessarily taking his or her side)

Emotional challenge

Encouragement to meet and overcome obstacles that are emotionally demanding

Shared social reality

Sharing of similar experiences, values, and views that provide a basis for self-evaluation through social comparison

There are three distinct segments of the injured athlete's support system: the sport team, the sports medicine team, and parents, spouses, and friends. All of these people, by virtue of their knowledge and their relationships with the athlete, provide certain forms of social support; no single group appears to provide all forms of support in practice. Technical appreciation and technical challenge can only be provided by those with a significant understanding of sport performance (i.e., coaches and teammates) or rehabilitation (i.e., sports medicine team). Emotional challenge can be provided by those with personal concern for the athlete. Shared social reality can be provided only by those with similar life experiences, such as friends and teammates. Rosenfeld et al. (1989) found that teammates and coaches provided little listening, emotional support, or emotional challenge and concluded that coaches believe that emotional distance is necessary to maintain the role of authority. Rosenfeld et al. speculate that competitiveness (of teammates with the injured athlete) and the task orientation of sport shape the forms of support received from teammates.

Richman et al. (1989) offered the following recommendations regarding social support: It is best provided by a network of individuals; it needs to be developed and nurtured; and it functions best as part of an ongoing program rather than simply a reaction to crisis. Specific recommendations offered for treatment providers include: be a willing listener, acknowledge both effort and mastery, and balance the use of technical appreciation and technical challenge.

Social support is most needed and least available with injury requiring surgery and lengthy rehabilitation. The athlete is taken out of the sport system, limiting the opportunity for contact with coaches and fellow athletes. Visits by teammates to peers hospitalized for surgery are quite valuable, especially when family is not conveniently located. Routine consultation-liaison intervention is also beneficial in this regard. The Social Support Functions Questionnaire (Pines, Aronson, & Kafry, 1981) may be modified for use with athletes to identify their support network and to provide direction to formal supportive efforts.

Continuing team contact is a natural way for the injured athlete to gain support and carries a host of other benefits. Attending practice and games keeps the athlete current with changes in plays and team strategies, helps the athlete stay in touch with the rhythm of the season, and continues established relationships with team members. It also provides the athlete an opportunity for continued visual learning, which can be supplemented by formal mental training. Continued involvement with the team has been reported to provide a feeling of being needed and a sense of security (i.e., reassurance that the coach has not given up on the injured athlete) (LaMott & Petlichkoff, 1990; Wiese et al., 1991).

Injury support groups and peer modeling are useful interventions. An injury support group brings athletes together to deal with issues of mutual concern (Wiese & Weiss, 1987). Support groups can provide coping models in the form of athletes who have recovered from serious injury. Formal support groups are most appropriate for athletes facing long rehabilitation, especially those feeling depressed or isolated. A buddy system of peer modeling involved matching an injured athlete with one who has recovered from injury. This is particularly helpful where injury occurs at a sport-life transition, for example, in the case of an athlete who is injured at the start of a college career and consequently is poorly integrated into the sport program and is also faced with other social and lifestyle changes. Flint (1991) created a videotape of athletes demonstrating coping behaviors at various stages of recovery from serious injury. In related research, she found that injured athletes who viewed this videotape demonstrated more positive attitudes about recovery and better knowledge of rehabilitation. Where injury leads to career terminations, support is of great importance (Botterill, 1982).

Social support can be provided in a variety of ways by a diverse group of individuals. Its effects, though intangible, are significant. Much work remains in determining how to provide effective social support for a particular athlete in a specific situation. Injury severity, psychological adjustment, developmental status, existing modes of social support, and the meaning of sport to the athlete are key considerations.

Remarkable Recovery

Remarkable recovery is that notable for speediness, for triumph over great physical odds, or for movement to a higher level of performance following injury. The pursuit of remarkable recovery defines the quest for excellence in athletic injury rehabilitation. The comments of Neil Bonnett (in this and preceding chapters) offer insight into the personal perspective that underlies remarkable recovery. Steadman (chapter 3), from his perspective as an orthopedic surgeon specializing in athletic injury, notes the ability of many athletes to recover quickly and efficiently relative to the norm. He also comments on the resourcefulness that athletes often show in guiding rehabilitation and on the ability of some to return to higher levels of performance following injury. Steadman speculates that those who return to higher levels of performance have gained significant knowledge from their injury experiences. Drawing on his clinical insights regarding the interplay of mind and body, Steadman has designed a program that motivates athletes into action through a combination of education, goal setting, and social support.

In applied research on the speed of injury rehabilitation, Ievleva and Orlick (1991) found that those who recovered more quickly had adopted positive mental sets toward rehabilitation and had assumed active, involved roles. Goal setting and self-directed practices resembling mental training led the way in this process. Ievleva (1988) also commented on the abilities of some athletes to return to higher levels of performance following injury, noting that this occurs with athletes who describe injury as a learning experience.

The goal of routine intervention with uncomplicated injury is to bring the level of excellence noted in remarkable recovery more frequently to rehabilitation. This approach rests on education, goal setting, social support, and mental training—the four pillars of injury management outlined in this chapter and chapter 11. When treatment providers present injury rehabilitation as an aspect of the game that the athlete must master in order to succeed, he or she may proceed on the continuous quest for a personal best whether in injury or in health.

Concluding Comments

This chapter has identified a comprehensive program for the routine management of athletic injury. The program includes education, goal setting, and social support, as well as mental training (which is discussed in chapter 11). When these interventions are applied in the context of a carefully designed and systematic program, the health and well-being of the athlete are enhanced and speedy return to optimal functioning is facilitated. This is most effective when there is a team approach and when psychological principles guide all aspects of treatment.

The approach recommended is performance oriented, proactive, and preventive. When treatment takes such an approach, psychological adjustment problems are less likely to develop. Where problems do occur, they can be identified and treated in a timely fashion, thereby limiting their overall impact.

11
CHAPTER

Mental Training in Injury Management

John Heil

Mental training techniques have been used widely to improve sport performance. This chapter provides guidelines for use of mental training to help the athlete meet the performance demands of rehabilitation and to prevent injury.

Over 80 years ago the United States Olympic team traveled by ship to the 1912 Games in Stockholm, Sweden. Among this group was Jim Thorpe, who would eventually win the Olympic gold medal in the decathlon. Following his impressive victory he was described as the world's greatest athlete by the King of Sweden, who presided over the games. A Native American, Jim Thorpe would eventually be recognized as one of the greatest athletes of the century for his achievements in track and field, professional baseball, and other sports.

It is easy to imagine the extent to which travel aboard ship limited training opportunities and served as a great source of frustration to the athletes as they slowly made their way to Sweden. One day Jim Thorpe was observed sitting quietly on deck, his eyes cast downward, seemingly lost in thought. He was asked if there was a problem. He responded that there was not and pointed out that he had made two marks on the deck separated by a carefully measured distance. He added that this was his goal for the long jump at the Olympic Games and that he was preparing mentally for the jump. He went on to jump this same distance at the Games as he had mentally trained to do.

This anecdote is related by John Steckbeck (1951), a friend of Jim Thorpe and chronicler of the exploits of the Carlisle Indians (as the members of the athletic teams of the College of American Indians in Carlisle, Pennsylvania, were known). It illustrates one athlete's creativity and resourcefulness in coping, through mental training, with the problems imposed by travel by ship. The more closely sport psychologists work with athletes, the more apparent it becomes that most athletes engage in similar procedures as part of their preparation for competition. This practice seems to arise naturally out of the demands of sport performance, and it reflects the mental commitment of serious athletes to their sport. The often repeated maxim that sport is "some large percent" mental supports this. However only recently, with the emergence of sport psychology, have systematic training principles been applied to these naturally occurring and instinctive methods, thus rendering them more effective and efficient.

Mental Training and Sport Performance

The benefits of the use of a broad range of psychological self-regulation procedures in athletic settings are generally well recognized. Although generally regarded as a contemporary phenomenon, mental training has roots in the ancient meditative traditions (Heil, 1984). The use of Zen-based techniques of mental training with the martial arts is most well recognized. Although some mental training approaches use traditional meditative methods, techniques have been drawn largely from the methods of behavioral and cognitive psychology initially developed for clinical populations. From whatever tradition derived, mental training methods usually include some combination of the following:

- Relaxation training, which develops increased body awareness, deepens muscular relaxation at rest (general relaxation), and increases muscular efficiency during performance (differential relaxation).
- Mental imagery, which uses the imagination to create a private "theater of the mind" where sport situations can be rehearsed and replayed. For example, a person is able to rehearse a key play at a critical moment during competition, or review a prior performance error, to gain insight into more effective future performance.
- Self-talk, whereby a person uses usually cryptic assertive statements or affirmations to improve confidence or focus attention. Alternately, self-talk may be used to stop or modify thoughts that are detrimental to performance.
- Biofeedback, which typically relies on psychophysiological instrumentation to provide quick, accurate feedback about subtle changes in muscle tension or other autonomically mediated events (e.g., heart rate, brain activity). This increases self-awareness and helps the user develop a greater sense of self-control.

- Hypnosis, which relies on careful focusing of attention so that the practitioner can use suggestions about confidence, coping with stress, and athletic performance to guide behavior. Autogenic training is a popular variant of hypnosis.

With increasing use and specific adaptations to meet the demands of sport, mental training methods have evolved a distinctive quality well suited to performance enhancement.

The use of psychological self-regulation skills as mental training is a cornerstone in the emergence of an applied sport psychology. Mental training techniques have been found to influence metabolic parameters, endurance, and muscular strength as well as motor skills, presumably through effects on the cognitive-symbolic processes that underlie these skills (Dishman, 1987; Druckman & Bjork, 1991). Their enthusiastic application is based on their practical appeal and their effectiveness as perceived by athletes and coaches (e.g., Orlick & Partington, 1988; Partington & Orlick, 1987). A number of well-designed practically oriented training programs are available in both audiocassette (Unestahl, 1982) and written formats for sport psychologists (Orlick, 1986, with coaches guide) and for coaches (Martens, 1987; with study guide, Bump, 1989). The use of mental training is growing not only with athletes but with other performance-oriented populations such as performing artists.

These same self-regulation procedures are of demonstrated utility in the management of pain and the psychological sequelae of injury in general medical populations (e.g., Turk et al., 1983). However, within the sport setting relatively little attention has been devoted to the use of these methods in injury, although interest is increasing (Samples, 1987).

The use of self-regulation skills described in this chapter assumes that sport performance goes on even during injury, although the type of activity (sport-specific training vs. rehabilitation) and setting (performance arena vs. training room) change. Continued use of psychological training methods during injury recovery helps the athlete maintain mental skills, provides a sense of continuity with athletic performance, and is a key element of a vigorous proactive, psychologically based rehabilitation program.

Theoretical and Practical Considerations

The fundamental skills upon which virtually all mental training is based include manipulations of behavioral processes (breath control and muscle tension control) and of cognitive processes. It is useful to think of cognition as composed of two distinct modes: "picturelike" and "wordlike" thought. In most sport and injury situations there is a practical advantage to the use of picturelike cognitions (imagery) as opposed to wordlike cognitions (Orlick & Partington, 1988). The picturelike mode allows the athlete to focus on relevant visual and motor cues as they unfold in the moment; thus it is useful to conceive of this mode as a "language for action." Imagery-based methods essentially cultivate the creation of an inner theater where any of life's dramas, including rehabilitation, may be played. The richer and more personalized the imagery, the more effective the "suspension of disbelief" upon which this inner theater depends.

Combinations of techniques with varied applications to different sport and rehabilitation situations constitute a mental training program. This program must be individualized to suit the constraints of the injury situation and the mind-set of the athlete.

Generalization and automatization are essential elements in the development of a systematic mental training program. The athlete must generalize mental skills from the ideal condition under which they are most easily learned and are typically practiced to the more challenging situations presented by sport or rehabilitation. Although mental training skills are most easily learned during conditions of autonomic and motoric quiet, they must be used in high stress, action-oriented situations. The athlete must also automatize skills so that their application becomes a natural aspect of performance. In addition to longer massed practice routines, brief spaced practice approaches are recommended. Multiple brief applications of mental skills blend more naturally into the ecology of the sport or rehabilitation performance situation. The use of cue-controlled methods, for example use of fearful cognitions to cue thought stopping, assists in automatization.

Approaches that incorporate variety, novelty, and a progressive approach to skill learning help maintain interest and motivation. Careful attention to coaching philosophy in the design of mental training programs is also important. A final crucial consideration is the setting of realistic limits for mental practice. The athlete simply may not maintain a program that is too complex or time-consuming, however well conceived in theory.

Mental Training Approaches to Injury Management

A variety of methods for work with the injured athlete are available. This section provides rationale and recommendations for the use of continued performance-enhancement training, rehabilitation rehearsal, healing imagery, and biofeedback. Pain management and fear of injury are presented in detail in subsequent sections.

Continued Performance-Enhancement Training

Steadman (1982) emphasized the importance of maintaining continuity of training during injury. For example, a skier with a knee injury should be encouraged to continue strength training with the uninjured leg and to maintain aerobic conditioning while working directly on injury rehabilitation. Continued mental training is a natural extension of this principle; it helps the athlete maintain a performance-oriented mind-set and facilitates mental readiness for return to play. This is most easily accomplished if the athlete is already involved in a mental training program. When injury provides the athlete with some free time, he or she can take the opportunity to accelerate the intensity of mental training. For the previously "mentally untrained" athlete, the downtime of injury presents an excellent opportunity to develop self-regulation skills at a time when they are particularly useful.

The athlete can maintain fundamental arousal control and attention control and psychomotor skills through continued routine mental practice, which also helps take her or his mind off pain and fear. The athlete can practice specific sport-related applications as if he or she were still playing. Mental rehearsal can be conducted in conjunction with review of films or videotapes of prior performance. This approach to skill rehearsal when focused on the review of particularly successful performances can help maintain an ideal performing state (e.g., Unestahl, 1982). Special opportunities for maintaining the mental aspects of sport performance are available to the athlete who continues to attend team meetings, practices, and competitions. The athlete remains current with team plays and strategies, and continued visual learning is facilitated. Athletes can rehearse sport skills in "real time" while on site at practice or competition by projecting themselves into the performance situation as it unfolds before them.

Rehabilitation Rehearsal

Mental rehearsal techniques can help athletes anticipate and deal with the challenges of rehabilitation (e.g., Rotella, 1982). Rehabilitation rehearsal may be used early in the treatment process in anticipation of a particularly challenging course of rehabilitation or where early signs of difficulty in psychological adjustment consistently occur. Alternately, this approach may be used during the latter phases of rehabilitation in response to specific problems.

Typically, the psychologist verbally guides the athlete in the use of imagery and subsequently encourages the athlete to master the mental rehearsal through independent practice. Rehearsal per se is typically preceded by a relaxation procedure that calms and quiets the athlete and enables him or her to focus intently on the mastery or coping imagery. In the mastery style approach, events are rehearsed with a favorable process and outcome, that is, as occurring without problem or setback, just as one would hope they would proceed. In the coping style approach, anticipated problems in the process are introduced into the rehearsal scenario, and the athlete uses coping techniques (e.g., refocusing of attention and self-affirmation) to produce a positive outcome. Both mastery and coping style approaches are confidence building; the coping approach in addition helps the athlete build the ability to use the specific coping skills that are rehearsed.

Consider an athlete hospitalized immediately following knee surgery who anticipates a long and uncertain course of rehabilitation and who demonstrates anticipatory anxiety regarding the demands of rehabilitation and uncertainty regarding successful return to play. The psychologist constructs a mastery rehearsal scenario, based on information provided by the athlete, that focuses on key transitions during rehabilitation. The scenario describes the situation that the athlete is likely to encounter in multisensory language (i.e., sights, kinesthetic feel, sounds). A positive confident feeling is cultivated as the athlete rehearses these in a relaxed state of mind, typically with eyes closed to help create the sense of inner theater. The list of situations follows:

1. Leaving the hospital
2. Beginning of active rehabilitation
3. Removal of braces or other immobilizing devices
4. Beginning of on-site involvement at practice
5. Return to limited practice
6. Return to full practice
7. Experience of a high-risk situation for reinjury
8. Return to competition

This approach treats rehabilitation as a protracted multistage process and illuminates the path to recovery by highlighting key events. It educates the athlete about rehabilitation milestones and calls attention to intermediate and long-term goals. This rehearsal builds confidence by fostering a sense of control at a time when this is disrupted by the limitations imposed by injury.

Treatment providers can use an adapted version of the technique later in rehabilitation by combining a prospective look at the rehabilitation challenges remaining with a retrospective look at the stages successfully passed. Treatment providers can use the mastery approach without directly challenging denial, where it is present. Alternately a coping-style rehearsal can challenge denial when this appears to be necessary. For this purpose, coping-style rehearsal can be used to call attention to problems the athlete is likely to encounter or is experiencing but not acknowledging.

Problems that occur during rehabilitation may be addressed directly with a coping-style approach. Consider the athlete who had knee surgery and is now well into the rehabilitation process. He is on crutches but is involved in vigorous rehabilitation, attending classes at college, and observing occasional team meetings and practices. The following four recurring situations are identified as being stressful to the athlete.

1. Still on crutches, the athlete is irritated by his need to rely on others for transportation and help with daily activities that were performed independently prior to injury. He feels weak and inadequate.
2. The athlete dreads his rehabilitation. He finds it boring and simply wants to get it over with. However, because the training room is so busy, he often has to wait for access to equipment. As he waits he grows increasingly impatient and angry.
3. When attending meetings and team practices as a prescribed part of his continued performance-enhancement training, he at times feels both helpless because he is unable to actively practice and hopeless about return to play.
4. A popular student athlete, he is often asked about his injury and is encouraged to be tough. Although these encounters are initially enjoyable, their continued occurrence leads him to feel isolated and frustrated.

The coping rehearsal is preceded and followed by a relaxation procedure designed to create a calming, stress-management effect. The scenarios that summarize the recurring situations identified above are imagined in sufficient detail to create the feeling of being there. This is followed by rehearsal of selected coping methods such as deep breathing, positive imagery, and self-talk (including thought stopping and self-affirmation). For example, the athlete imagines himself to be at a team meeting discussion of an upcoming competition. He sees himself sitting on the bench feeling helpless and hears himself say, "I'll never get back to my old form." He then rehearses the coping strategy beginning with the statement "Stop!" followed by a relaxing breath and a positive image of himself back at play feeling strong and confident.

Alternately, the athlete imagines meeting an acquaintance who says hello and encourages him to be tough. He feels himself tighten his grip on the crutches and become irritated. He then rehearses taking a deep breath, relaxing his grip on the crutches, and affirming his mental toughness with the self-affirmations, "I am focused and in control." For recommendations for converting negative thoughts to self-affirmations, see Harris and Harris (1984).

Psychological preparation for surgery and other invasive procedures, introduced in chapter 9 and presented in detail in chapter 13, is a special adaptation of rehabilitation rehearsal.

Healing Imagery

Whether the way one thinks about injury influences the healing process is a matter of long-standing speculation. It is intuitively held that those with hopeful, positive attitudes tend to recover more quickly and completely. Research in psychoneuroimmunology and the disease-prone personality has raised interesting questions regarding the role of psychological factors both in resistance to disease and in the healing of active disease states (Friedman & Booth-Kewley, 1987; McCabe & Schneiderman, 1984).

Reported benefits from the use of "healing" images in the management of cancer have created a great deal of interest (Achterberg & Lawlis, 1978). This method uses vivid images to represent disease or injury, the physiological coping mechanisms, and the effects of treatment. These images are presented in a drama of healing played out in the inner theater of the mind. This method essentially involves the creation of a metaphorical anatomy that may be either relatively realistic or more personalized and fantasy based. For example, the patient can imagine chemotherapy either as a series of molecular structures flowing through the bloodstream that tear down and wash away cancer cells or as cavalry attacking an enemy force with sabers. Patients can imagine radiation therapy as a force disintegrating cancer cells, or alternately as a Pac-man figure or a biological "Rambo" attacking them.

There is controversy regarding the mechanisms underlying healing imagery. However, whether use of healing images has the desired biological effect is a separate question from whether it is simply useful to entertain the notion that what is imagined is possible. If the individual who practices such as technique finds it stress reducing, then it is appropriate and useful. In fact, anxiety reduction appears to be the most likely and frequent benefit of healing imagery. Themes of power and control that are inherent in the imagery scenarios probably produce a sense of self-efficacy. When used during the course of rehabilitation, these themes also function as competing responses counteracting pain and limiting spontaneously arising anxiety or fear.

Images that anticipate reinjury and those that recall the injury negatively affect recovery (Grunert et al., 1988; Ievleva & Orlick, 1991). Fearful images of reinjury can severely disrupt rehabilitation. For example, a persistent image that an injured Achilles tendon is like a frayed rubber band ready to snap in the course of rehabilitation will evoke fear and reluctance.

Intrusive recollections of traumatic events are a key diagnostic criterion in posttraumatic stress disorder and signal incomplete psychological recovery (American Psychiatric Association, 1987). These occur most vividly in the form of flashbacks during waking hours and as dreams during sleep. Less disruptive but also of concern are brief, recurrent, intrusive recollections of the circumstances of injury. The amount and psychological impact of intrusive recollections decrease as recovery occurs (Grunert et al., 1988).

Preliminary research with athletes shows that spontaneous use of positive imagery is greatest among those who recover most quickly (Ievleva,

1988; Ievleva & Orlick, 1991). This includes images of the healing process itself as well as images of healed injury. However, the beneficial effects of positive imagery were negated where extensive negative imagery was reported. See Table 11.1 for a brief listing of healing and healed images.

Table 11.1
Imagery for Rehabilitation

Healing images

Treatment modalities
 Ultrasound as creating a healing glow
 Therapeutic application of ice as freezing up and shutting down pain receptors

Rehabilitation activity
 Blood surging to the muscle and rebuilding it at an accelerating rate during resistance training

Medication
 Nonsteroidal anti-inflammatory medication as sponges absorbing local tissue irritants

Mental training
 Deep breathing as infusing the body with a healing energy
 Deep concentration as opening gates that release endorphins

Healed images

Shoulder injury
 Ligaments as a combination of wound steel and rubber, strong but flexible

Knee injury
 The meniscus as smooth as teflon following surgery

Foot injury
 The bone structure as internally buttressed by a new network of bone, strong yet yielding like a suspension bridge (following stress fracture)

Back injury
 The spinal column supported by tendon, ligament, and muscle like the rigging of a great sailing ship

The fundamental assumption underlying the use of this approach is that the healing image in some way empowers the organism. Creation of effective healing and healed imagery scenarios is facilitated by the following:

- Use of the athlete's personal imagery of injury and pain
- Use of the athlete's imagery of the healing process
- The athlete's knowledge of the biological mechanisms of injury and healing, and the ability to describe these as vivid images
- The athlete's knowledge of the mechanisms of action of treatment modalities, and the ability to describe these as vivid images
- Identification of coping strategies that the athlete uses intuitively

Biofeedback

Biofeedback is a self-regulation technique in which auditory or visual feedback provides information about biological functions not usually available to a person's awareness (e.g., Schwartz, 1987). These functions include autonomically mediated activity as well as skeletal muscular function lost or diminished through injury. Commonly used measures include muscular activity, skin response, peripheral temperature, respiration rate, heart rate, and brain wave activity. Timely and precise feedback of fluctuations in these biological functions increases the person's awareness of the specific circumstances and behaviors that lead to change. However, biofeedback is of only limited utility in the absence of a specific cognitive strategy that guides change (Meichenbaum, 1976). Biofeedback may be used readily as an adjunct to other techniques.

Application of biofeedback to sport performance is growing (Petruzzello, Landers, & Salazar, 1991; Sandweiss & Wolf, 1985; Zaichowsky & Fuchs, 1988). Electromyographic (EMG) biofeedback offers varied applications with the healthy and the injured athlete. It has brought about improvements in both fine motor and gross motor performance, probably through reduction in the psychomotor manifestations of performance anxiety. EMG biofeedback applications with injury include muscular relaxation (reduction in muscle tension), muscle reeducation (increase in muscle activity with sensory motor deficits), and discrimination training (relaxing one muscle or muscle group while another is tensed). However, only muscle reeducation has a well-developed tradition of research and application with injury (Fernando & Basmajian, 1978).

Using muscular feedback to reduce tension can speed recovery. For example, it can optimize recovery between repetitions and sets during rehabilitation activity. It also can serve as an antidote to muscular bracing or guarding, which commonly are seen in injury and which diminish performance and increase injury risk. A generalized global relaxation (e.g., frontalis feedback) or feedback from specific muscle groups allows more efficient use of muscles through improved awareness and reduction of chronic tension-holding patterns. The athlete may generalize skills to sport or rehabilitation by using EMG biofeedback in conjunction with an imagery-based coping rehearsal of circumstances that elicit bracing or guarding.

In discrimination training, simultaneous feedback is presented from two or more muscles or muscle groups. This enhances body awareness and fine-tunes muscular response. For example, adjacent muscle groups that typically function in unison can be trained to function more independently. Patellofemoral pain syndrome is a dysfunction of the patella's ability to track in the femoral groove. Conservative medical treatment typically focuses on strengthening of the vastus medialis independently of the vastus lateralis in order to achieve balance between these two muscles (Wise, Fiebert, & Kates, 1984). However, resistance training typically increases strength uniformly in both muscles, thereby maintaining muscle imbalance. Biofeedback-assisted discrimination training circumvents this by training the athlete to work the muscles independently.

Bill is a 28-year-old who injured his shoulder and back in a motorcycle accident. After a 6-month recovery he has returned to many of his previous activities but pain and fatigue continue to be problems. Pain gradually increases through the day from his work as an electronics technician. Pain and fatigue limit his ability to play the drums (he performs with a local rock group) as well as his ability to participate in recreational sports. I monitored right and left trapezius EMG activity at rest, during drumming drills, and during rest intervals between drills and found baseline levels for left and right trapezius to be equivalent. Quicker onset of fatigue in the injured shoulder relative to the uninjured shoulder appeared linked to greater effort expenditure during drumming. As the injured shoulder approached the fatigue point, there was a remarkable increase in effort expenditure and contralateral shoulder involvement. During rest intervals between drumming drills, EMG levels on the injured shoulder returned to baseline at a remarkably slower rate compared to that of the other shoulder. In sum, the injured shoulder worked and rested less efficiently.

This insight into the muscular dynamics of drumming and rest guided problem solving for Bill. He was assigned a comprehensive mental training program that included EMG biofeedback, controlled breathing, muscular relaxation, and imagery rehearsal. He practiced EMG-assisted relaxation at rest intervals and differential relaxation during drumming.

Although clearly in need of further development, the use of biofeedback training in the rehabilitation of athletic injury offers significant promise. A novel approach to EMG monitoring in injury risk assessment has been proposed by Andersen and Williams in chapter 5.

Mental Training Approaches to Pain Management

Pain is the most common and compelling aspect of rehabilitation. Pain and to a lesser extent fear are always on the psychological agenda of rehabilitation. How well the athlete deals with these is a good measure of how effective rehabilitation will be. The critical importance of coping with pain and fear is most apparent at return to play. Following are guidelines for pain management that are based on an understanding of the pain-sport attentional matrix.

Pain in Sport

There are many varieties of performance pain ranging from the brutal impact of collision sports to the sustained effort of aerobic activities, and from routine muscular soreness to the generalized somatic discomfort of performance anxiety. Response to pain is highly personalized and subject to a wide range of influences. That children are often less willing than adults to report pain related to injury and illness has been noted in medical settings (McGrath, 1990). Researchers have noted that broadly based cultural factors influence pain tolerance (Kiesler & Finholt, 1988; Wolff, 1985) as do experimentally created team norms in sport (Johnston & Mannell, 1980). Muscular endurance and tolerance of fatigue related pain were enhanced when a physical task was performed conjointly with others as compared to solo performance (Martens & Landers, 1969). How sport culture shapes pain attitudes and coping is an interesting but poorly understood issue. A study of distance runners (Peterson, Durtschi, & Murphy, 1990) revealed that some elite runners choose to reject the word *pain* in favor of *exertion* when describing the sensations associated with maximum running effort.

Laboratory-based pain research suggests that athletes generally are more pain tolerant than nonathletes. Furthermore, some studies have found differences between collision-sport and noncollision-sport athletes (Jaremko, Silbert, & Mann, 1981; Nowlin, 1974; Ryan & Foster, 1967; Ryan & Kovacic, 1966; Walker, 1971). It is unclear to what degree pain tolerance is a natural selection factor (i.e., those who tolerate pain poorly are less likely to succeed at sport) versus a learned aspect of sport participation. Ample evidence suggests that pain tolerance can be improved (Turk et al., 1983). Scott and Gijsbers (1981) found that elite swimmers tolerated pain better than recreational swimmers and that pain tolerance was greatest at times of heavy training. Athletes have demonstrated the ability to reduce minor aches and pains associated with sport performance following instruction in a simple pain control technique (Gauron & Bowers, 1986).

Differentiating Pain and Injury

Playing with pain is often expected, whereas playing with injury is generally discouraged—but the distinction between these two situations is often unclear. The importance of differentiating routine pain and injury pain is frequently noted in sport settings; however, little is offered in the way of systematic recommendations about how to do this. Routine performance pain is usually of relatively short duration and does not indicate danger. Injury pain indicates danger to the athlete's physical integrity and.threatens his or her ability to perform. Consequently an individual who can cope effectively with routine performance pain may have more difficulty with injury pain. However, even where playing with injury carries significant risk, many athletes choose to do so (e.g., Nideffer, 1983) as do some dancers (Clanin et al., 1986) and musicians (Rozek, 1985).

In routine sport performance the key question is, When does pain move beyond simply limiting performance and signal imminent injury? Following injury, the most important question regarding pain (e.g., in conjunction with rehabilitation) is its status as benign or, alternately, as a signal of danger. This objective medical decision falls to the sports medicine professional and serves as the basis for prescription of physical activity. Until this question is answered and safe limits of behavior are determined, the utility of psychologically based pain management methods is severely compromised.

Generally, pain that is dull, does not persist after activity, and is not accompanied by swelling or increased tenderness is benign. In contrast, harmful pain is more often localized to the site of injury, is sharp, occurs during therapeutic exercise, persists after activity, and is accompanied by swelling and increased tenderness (Rians, 1990).

Pain Management Strategies

A broad variety of self-regulation skills have proven beneficial in pain management. Turk and his associates (Fernandez & Turk, 1986; Wack & Turk, 1984) identified six categories of pain management techniques: external focus of attention, pleasant imaginings, neutral imaginings, rhythmic cognitive activity, pain acknowledging, and dramatized coping (see Table 11.2). The external focus of attention strategy involved directing one's attention away from pain and toward environmental events. In pleasant imaginings the patient employs an internal focus of attention on pleasant imagery. In the neutral imaginings strategy, there is an internal focus on neutral events. With rhythmic cognitive activity the patient engages in a repetitive or systematized mental task, which can include the use of repetitive phrases. The pain-acknowledging strategy involves a reinterpretation of pain or a shift away from an ordinary style of attention; for example, the patient may focus closely on the sensation itself and attempt to accentuate its multisensory quality, may imagine anesthesia at the site of pain or may cultivate a sense of detachment from the pain. In dramatized coping, the patient creates a fantasy scenario, imagining pain as occurring in different circumstances than is actually the case.

Table 11.2
Cognitive Pain Control Strategies

External focus of attention

General—Listening to music; focusing on the horizon

Sport—Concentrating on the ball; attending to environmental cues that are related to sport performance

Pleasant imaginings

General—Imagining relaxing on the beach; imagining being at a favorite place or with a favorite person

Sport—Imagining the feeling of having performed a task well; imagining celebrating with others following a victory

Neutral imaginings

General—Thinking of a routine activity like walking up the steps, or imagining nonemotive events

Sport—Imagining calmly dressing before or after a competition or practice

Rhythmic cognitive activity

General—Counting backward from 100; repeating a neutral mantra or self-affirmation

Sport—Coordinating breathing with activity; making repetitive performance or pain coping self-affirmations

Pain acknowledging

General—Imagining generalized feelings of anesthesia; imagining pain being moved away from an area of the body through circulation of the blood; observing pain with a sense of emotional detachment

Sport—Imagining lactic acid buildup as inducing numbness without pain; perceiving pain as a positive sign of effort

Dramatized coping

General—Seeing oneself in pursuit of a heroic task in which tolerance of pain is associated with personal triumph

Sport—Imagining pain experienced during rehabilitation as occurring in conjunction with outstanding athletic achievement

Association-Dissociation: Pragmatic Value. Pain management techniques have been most parsimoniously categorized (e.g., Morgan & Pollock, 1977) as either associative (focused on pain) or dissociative (focused away from pain). Four of the techniques described by Fernandez and Turk (1986) have a dissociative quality (external focus of attention, neutral imaginings, rhythmic cognitive activity, and pleasant imaginings), whereas two are associative (pain acknowledging and dramatized coping). Dissociative strategies are most commonly used because of their diversity and because they are relatively easily learned. They also appear to be most effective for most of the people most of the time. Of these, pleasant imaginings is most efficacious (Fernandez & Turk, 1986). Dissociation seems to work by decreasing sympathetic nervous system response and reducing muscle tension, changes that simultaneously inhibit the biological transmission of pain impulses and have a calming effect, thus reducing the overall bothersomeness of pain. Where a dissociative method increases danger or otherwise interferes with proper execution of a rehabilitation skill, its use must be carefully limited.

In clinical settings, associative methods of pain control see far less application. In situations of severe pain in which dissociative methods are ineffective and may even be frustrating to the patient, an associative strategy can be used as an alternative. Associative techniques are most effective when part of a multifaceted pain-management strategy that incorporates dissociative techniques as well. One of many possible approaches is the "pain focus," in which an intentionally vivid multisensory image of pain is derived from a personal interview. Following an introductory relaxation procedure, the patient focuses on the distinct sensory qualities of pain, as described by the practitioner. The patient's attention is then drawn to the inevitably changing nature of the pain image. The practitioner follows this with systematic attempts to modify any of the sensory elements of the pain image beginning with those that naturally fluctuate the most. From this, follows attempts to develop a new, more positive image of pain. As a way of pacing the athlete's mental effort, the practitioner shifts from this associative focus to a restful dissociative focus and then back. This enhances the athlete's sense of mental control of the image and hence of the pain as well. Eventually the athlete learns to perform the technique independently.

Consider a distance runner who reports effort-related chest pain that interferes with her ability to sprint at the end of a race. She describes the pain as red-orange and as swirling, burning, and stinging with a hissing sound. The runner is trained to respond to pain with a close focus on its sensory quality and to look for fluctuations or changes in the picture of pain. Eventually the runner shifts to the image of pain as a meteor hurtling her toward the finish line. Actual training is accomplished through a multistep process that begins with guided practice of imagery rehearsal and proceeds to a self-directed in vivo performance, first in training and then in competition.

One may wonder how focusing on pain can reduce it. The associative approach is paradoxical in this regard. Severe pain often may seem uncontrollable, leading the pain sufferer to feel like a helpless victim. The benefits of the associative approaches seem to derive from the patient's gaining a sense of control over the uncontrollable, thus decreasing the related sense of helplessness. For example, mindfulness meditation, which uses an associative focus while simultaneously cultivating a sense of emotional detachment (Kabat-Zinn, 1982), has been shown to reduce pain related to diverse medical problems. It is hypothesized that the detachment upon which this technique relies leads to an uncoupling of the sensory dimension of the pain experience from the reactive component. This reactive emotional component of pain is a significant source of its aversiveness. Thus, by using this technique, the patient attenuates the aversiveness of the pain by emotional dissociation while associating with (focusing on) the sensory component. A "pain metaphor" associative method (e.g., in *30 Scripts for Relaxation, Imagery, and Inner Healing Vol. 2* Lusk, in press) functions in a similar manner.

Association-Dissociation: Clarifying the Concept.   Although the association-dissociation concept has pragmatic value, it is an oversimplification. Research using this paradigm (primarily with distance runners) has yielded inconsistent and confusing results (Peterson et al., 1990). At the heart of this is the problem of generating operational definitions that clearly and consistently differentiate mental strategies according to this typology (Heil, 1990). There are also critical differences in the optimal uses of pain management strategies with clinical populations as opposed to athletes. Most clinical pain management methods are not designed for use in conjunction with skilled activity. Sport-related applications must not only address pain but also athlete safety and performance effectiveness.

Despite its obvious importance in sport, the relationship between pain and performance is poorly understood. Studies have examined the cognitive strategies used by distance runners to cope with the discomfort of pain, fatigue, and exertion (Masters & Lambert, 1989; Morgan, 1978; Okwumabua, Meyers, Schleser, & Cooke, 1983; Peterson et al., 1990; Schomer, 1986, 1987). Although limited by methodological problems, this work is an important beginning, characterizing the successful distance runner as having a rich and varied set of attentional strategies including the ability to tune into performance cues despite pain. However, although some mental strategies are clearly associative (monitoring breathing, muscle tension, and sense of effort) or dissociative (imagining building a house), others are not so simply classified.

Consider the following coping strategies derived from work by Morgan and Pollock (1977):

1. Focus eyes on a distant location toward which you are running, and coordinate running rhythm and respiration. Repeat the word *down* in conjunction with your breathing.
2. Imagine that your body is a steam engine with your legs working like powerful pistons and your lungs exhaling steam as you move steadily uphill.

Independent groups of pain management specialists and sport psychologists were unable to consistently identify these and similar strategies as either associative or dissociative (Heil, 1990). I suggest that underlying this conceptual problem is a widely held fallacious assumption regarding the relationship between performance and pain; this assumption is that attention to pain and attention to performance are yoked, covarying in a predictable way. Actually, attention to performance and attention to pain vary independently. In practice, pain management methods must address two distinct contexts—pain and sport. However, in keeping with established convention in sport, the following text uses the terms *association* and *dissociation* to refer respectively to two attentional directions—"toward" or "away from" a specific context. From this a conceptualization scheme is recommended in which attentional context (sport and pain) and attentional direction (association and dissociation) are addressed simultaneously.

Pain-Sport Attentional Matrix

The interrelationships of attentional context (pain and sport) and attentional direction (association and dissociation) define the pain-sport attentional matrix (see Figure 11.1). Its four quadrants can be combined in four combinations: pain association/sport association; pain dissociation/sport dissociation; pain association/sport dissociation; and pain dissociation/sport association. In this way associative and dissociative techniques are presented not simply as pain management but more broadly in terms of attention control.

It is important to differentiate general attentional state from the intentional use of an attention-control technique. There is an obvious difference between unplanned, spontaneous, obsessive rumination on pain and the use of an associative technique, although each involves a focus on pain. Technique by its nature is systematic, purposeful, and disciplined. In this instance, it is an attempt to gain a sense of control over pain (if only through a modulation of the reactive response to pain). This sense of control is in marked contrast to the sense of helplessness that usually accompanies a ruminative focus on pain. The element of self-control is crucial in determining the relative effectiveness of a specific pain-sport attentional focus, whether elicited intentionally as a technique or occurring spontaneously.

Sport

	Association	Dissociation
Association	Pain association Sport association	Pain association Sport dissociation
Dissociation	Pain dissociation Sport association	Pain dissociation Sport dissociation

Pain

Figure 11.1   Pain-sport attentional matrix.

A cognitive strategy may be quite useful under one set of performance conditions but not under another. In designing a pain management program the sports medicine professional must consider the nature of pain, its relationship to the proper execution of physical technique, and the performance demands of the particular athletic activity. For example, a pain management strategy for a particular injury will vary according to whether the activity is continuous (sprint or swimming) or intermittent (bowling, football), interactive (football, basketball) or solitary (golf, basketball free throw), automated (distance running or swimming) or skill based (golf, football). The practical utility of each of the four pain-sport attentional combinations is reviewed next.

Pain Dissociation/Sport Association.   As a general attentional state this is ideal for sport performance under most situations. As a technique, it is the prototypical approach for benign injury pain and is also appropriate for routine performance pain. A simple example of the practical use of technique to elicit this attentional set is to let awareness of pain be a cue to redirect attention to an appropriate sport-related focus. For example, when thoughts of pain occur during performance the athlete immediately refocuses attention on the ball, on the center of action, on an immediate performance goal, or on a sense of mental readiness. This method may be used during the flow of performance as well as at pauses in activity.

Pain Association/Sport Dissociation.   Because this attentional combination is characterized by a persistent focus on pain and away from sport, its use is very limited. It can easily result in diminished performance and in increased likelihood of acute injury, especially in high-risk sports. This method is most appropriately used at naturally occurring breaks in activities (e.g., between pitches in baseball, between offensive and defensive rotations in football, or between bouts in tournament fencing or wrestling), especially when pain becomes more prominent. When a rest interval is relatively lengthy, the athlete may use a correspondingly lengthy pain association/sport dissociation technique. When the break in activity is brief, a simple technique of shorter duration is recommended. Upon return to performance at the end of a rest period, the athlete will need to shift focus away from pain and back to performance by redirecting attention technique (as described in the preceding example of an athlete using pain as a cue to refocus attention).

When injury pain is relatively minimal and the attentional demands of sport are high, pain may be neglected leading to increased injury risk especially for chronic overuse syndromes. In this case, the systematic use of a pain association/sport dissociation technique can limit injury risk. The athlete may use a brief self-monitoring procedure periodically either at natural breaks in activity or during highly automated sports to help attend to and modify activity in a way that will decrease injury risk. For example, a distance runner may systematically scan her body to attend to general muscle tension and to painful areas and then modulate muscle tension or correct faulty biomechanics. This method may also be used to limit the habitual bracing/guarding response that often follows injury.

Pain Dissociation/Sport Dissociation. As a general attentional state during performance this is problematic, because it allows the athlete to control pain at the expense of attention to sport. However, techniques characterized by this attentional focus can be very powerful for pain management and can be used at natural breaks in sport activity. Athletes can best use pain dissociation/sport dissociation methods with injury-related pain away from sport settings, for example, at bedtime when pain interferes with sleep. However, judicious use of this attentional focus can be beneficial also with automated or overlearned sports (e.g., distance running or swimming; Schomer, 1986, 1987; Peterson et al., 1990). Overuse of this method will have a deleterious effect on performance and will increase injury risk.

Pain Association/Sport Association. As an attentional focus this presents some interesting theoretical possibilities. For example, when the pain message is a cue to proper execution, the athlete must attend to both pain and performance. When the athlete uses muscular guarding/bracing to avoid pain, effective performance is limited because pain is reduced at the expense of the proper execution of technique. Alternately, a willingness to tolerate pain and to use it as a cue to proper technique can help enhance performance. This approach significantly challenges sensory motor awareness and concentration. Fordyce's (1976) behavioral-shaping program to correct gait deviation is an example of a rehabilitation technique that requires simultaneous attention to pain and performance.

A perspective that identifies the discomfort of exertion as a positive factor linked to maximal effort may simultaneously improve pain tolerance and performance. The work of Peterson et al. (1990) with elite distance runners supports this. There is also potential for the use of pain acknowledging and dramatized coping methods as well as mixed associative-dissociative approaches to improve pain tolerance during sport performance.

Mental Training Approaches to Managing Fear of Injury

Piano virtuoso Byron Janis's career was marked by remarkable success and resiliency in the face of injury until he was debilitated by psoriatic arthritis. He described his realization that managing fear is necessary for effective rehabilitation:

> The first thing I had to conquer was fear. I realized what a debilitating thing fear is. It can render you absolutely helpless. I know now that fear breeds fear. If you think something terrible is going to happen, it frequently does. Apprehension makes you tense enough to force it to happen. (Goldsmith, 1985, p. 5)

Fear of injury spans healthy sport performance as well as injury. Like pain, fear has adaptive value but is a potential source of problems. Fearful thoughts are powerful intrusions on consciousness that athletes cannot and should not categorically ignore. Consequently, fear should be treated as a mental element of performance that must be understood and managed. In high-risk sports, fear can contribute to a respect for dangerous conditions and can limit dangerous behavior. Alternately, fear can disrupt concentration and interfere with skill execution (via increased muscle tension), thereby increasing injury risk. Fear of reinjury can limit the athlete's tendency to return to play too soon or take inappropriate risks. However, fear of reinjury can seriously inhibit performance. As with pain, an athlete must learn to determine whether fear is relatively benign or dangerous.

High-Risk Sports

Olympic skiing gold medalist and sport psychologist Kathy Kreiner-Phillips (1990) described the fear that skiers at all levels of ability can experience as they stand poised to start a run that challenges their limits:

> Your mind is racing . . . you feel your heartbeat pounding in your chest. Your focus is on the heaviness of your breathing and the stream of negative thoughts running through your mind. . . . The image of

you falling all the way to the bottom is foremost in your mind. (p. 114)

In her ski training workshops, she combines technical coaching and mental training to improve performance and assure safety. She encourages skiers to accept their anxieties as normal and to eliminate fear through a combination of relaxed breathing, positive self-affirmation, and mental rehearsal.

Fear may also be an intrinsic element in the appeal of a particular sport to an individual. The surge of adrenaline that comes as one attempts to challenge limits in the face of risk provides a sense of vitality and vigor not readily accessible in daily activity. When effectively harnessed this extra energy can enhance performance.

Based on his work with gymnasts, Feigley (1988) suggested that athletes may attempt to hide their fear because they feel coaches view fear as a weakness, because they are afraid of looking foolish, or because they perceive themselves to be the only ones who are fearful. Athletes may display fear indirectly through constant complaints of fatigue or minor injury that are without apparent basis. Also seen are inconsistent or erratic emotional responses and various forms of avoidance including absenteeism and lack of readiness to perform during practice. Readily observable fearful behavior that is denied by the athlete and the apparent absence of fear where fear is appropriate are both cause for strong concern. Guidelines for the management of fear are summarized as follows (Feigley, 1988). Practitioners should

1. identify the appropriateness of the fear response and its adaptive value,
2. identify the nature of the fear as specifically as possible through careful observation of performance and discussion with the athlete,
3. adjust training to strengthen the specific skill element most closely linked to fear, and
4. use mental training techniques (such as described by Kathy Kreiner-Phillips, 1990).

As an alternative, more free-form and intuitively based approaches may be attempted as well. *Zen in the Martial Arts* (Hyams, 1979) describes a martial arts master who while growing up in Korea was terrified of tigers. As a martial arts student he was encouraged to visualize battling a tiger as part of his martial arts meditation. He spent time in zoos studying the tiger's habits and movements; then he began to work out strategies for imaginary bouts with the tiger to find ways of exploiting its weaknesses. Throughout his life the master continued to imagine himself in conflicts with a tiger—sometimes winning, sometimes losing, but no longer afraid. He stated, "In the heat of combat I am calm which is as it should be because I have discovered that fear is shadow not substance" (p. 113).

Fear of Reinjury

The prospect of reinjury or failed recovery is one with which all injured athletes must deal. Most do this well; some do not. Athletes may fear being injured either during rehabilitation procedures or with return to play. In a survey of collegiate women volleyball players, 22% reported fear of reinjury (Hankins et al., 1989).

Fear of reinjury can range from a normal recovery behavior to a subclinical syndrome. It is distinct from traumatic conditioning, which is relatively more severe and psychologically disruptive (see chapter 13 for more detail). Fear of reinjury is distinct from sport performance phobia, with which there is fear of failure to perform a specific skill without the implication of injury (Silva, 1989).

Underlying fear of injury is a series of interrelated psychological and physiological responses that can slow rehabilitation, inhibit performance following return to play, and increase risk of reinjury. For a detailed explanation see "The Psychophysiological Mechanism of Risk" in chapter 1.

The fear of reinjury is always present to some degree. As a normal recovery behavior it demands that the athlete mobilize coping resources. Such fear may show itself as a sense of cautiousness during rehabilitation and in return to play, a mild and transient effect that eventually resolves with return to play. Where the effects of fear are greater or more enduring they may result in a subclinical psychological adjustment syndrome. That is, they may be disruptive enough to affect the speed of recovery or mental readiness without undermining eventual recovery.

Two case reports follow. The first illustrates how fear of reinjury can slow return to play even where there is eventual effective recovery. The second illustrates how lingering fears can continue to inhibit performance.

Bob was a college basketball player who suffered an ankle injury during practice. He progressed routinely through the early rehabilitation stage. Following return to practice, he showed good ankle mobility and strength based on performance in drills. However, in practice scrimmages Bob did not make moves commensurate with his level of recovery, stating he was not able. The sports medicine specialist could not offer an objective explanation for Bob's behavior. Eventually Bob was ready to make the necessary moves again (without any apparent change in functional ability) and returned to competition. Despite his eventual effective recovery, fear of reinjury apparently prevented him from making as prompt a return to play as his injury physically allowed.

Ming was an experienced white-water canoeist who took a kayak class in order to learn the Eskimo roll, a challenging maneuver that involves righting the kayak once it has tipped over. Many find this to be an awkward experience—strapped in a boat upside down while working on a new and complex motor skill in the space of time that they can hold their breath. Using her existing white-water skills, Ming had shown exceptionally good boat control during on-the-surface maneuvers practiced in the initial class meetings. Very early in the process of learning the Eskimo roll, Ming found herself upside down, unable to right the boat and unable to bail out because of faulty placement of equipment. After a few anxious moments she was able to kick loose. Following this she experienced a significant setback in learning the Eskimo roll and also in general boat-handling ability. Although not readily obvious to others, this setback was very apparant to Ming. Although she eventually learned the Eskimo roll, progress was clearly slowed by the incident.

In each of these situations, the athlete's confidence in his or her ability to perform was diminished by injury or by the prospect of injury. Bob's problem was more evident but resolved naturally, whereas Ming's was more subtle and enduring. These examples are typical of situations in which the athlete would benefit from psychological intervention but in which it is seldom provided. In everyday life, problems of this degree are relatively inconsequential. However, in the intensely competitive world of sport they are clearly significant.

A rehabilitation program that incorporates goal setting and social support will work proactively to limit fear of reinjury. Where this fear is displayed, the practitioner should initially conceptualize it as a confidence issue, with which the athlete questions his or her ability to perform safely and effectively. The following list describes an approach to the management of fear of reinjury. The sports medicine professional should

1. "normalize" the athlete's response; that is, let the athlete know it is normal to experience some fear;
2. reassure the athlete that fear itself is not a problem, although how it is dealt with can be;
3. emphasize the adaptive value of fear in setting safe limits;
4. reframe the arousal component of fear as the body becomes energized and ready for performance;
5. clarify the current status of injury, emphasize progress since the start of treatment, and present realistic expectations for continued recovery;
6. reassure the athlete of the benign nature of associated pain;
7. identify safe limits for performance as clearly as possible; and
8. introduce mental training approaches as appropriate.

These steps (except for the last regarding mental training) can often be accomplished within one or two meetings, and they may be all that is necessary. Where the athlete expresses significant concern or evidences problems in technique or concentration, the treatment provider should initiate a mental training program. In this context, the management of fear should be regarded as a problem in attention control. A fear-performance attentional matrix, similar to that proposed for pain, provides the basic structure for the design of a mental training skills program. Because spontaneous fear of reinjury distracts the athlete from performance and increases reinjury risk, the primary task of mental training is to help the athlete refocus attention appropriately. For example, a coping rehearsal scenario can be constructed to help the athlete practice refocusing attention following fearful cognitions. Refocusing techniques can be gradually incorporated into performance. Following confrontation with a feared situation, the practitioner should provide the athlete with feedback about performance and reassurance of safe physical status.

Concluding Comments

This chapter outlines the roles of mental training methods and a performance-enhancement philosophy in the management of athletic injury. Avoiding injury when healthy, coping with rehabilitation when injured, and managing pain and fear are skills essential to athletic success. These abilities are rooted in a finely tuned sense of body awareness and no doubt are related to the often-noted importance of differentiating pain and injury. A comprehensive performance-enhancement approach to injury management and intensive use of mental training reduces the psychological distress of injury and increases mental readiness for return to play. This approach also promises to help unlock the riddles of pain and injury that pervade sport and medicine.

12
CHAPTER

Specialized Treatment Approaches: Severe Injury

John Heil

In his autobiographical work describing his career in football, defensive back Jack Tatum (Tatum & Kushner, 1979) recounted the circumstances of an injury to wide receiver Darryl Stingley:

> Darryl ran a rather dangerous pattern across the middle of our zone defense. It was one of those pass plays where I could not possibly have intercepted. . . . I automatically reacted to the situation by going for an intimidating hit. It was a fairly good hit, but nothing exceptional, and I got up and started back to our huddle. But, Darryl didn't get up and walk away from the collision. That particular play was the end of Darryl Stingley's career in the NFL. (p. 234)

The injury damaged Darryl Stingley's cervical vertebrae and spinal cord, leaving him a partial quadriplegic, his life changed forever. His struggles are recounted in the following excerpt ("The Petals Are Un-Folding for Darryl Stingley Again," 1982):

> For the first time in my life I had encountered something beyond my control. . . . I didn't like myself, I guess because being an athlete was no more. I'd been reduced to something in a wheelchair. I had lost all that I had worked for. It was more than playing football. I could take losing football. But, what about me? What about the physical me? . . . How do you explain that you just plain don't care? It took me months to stop being bitter and angry. . . . I really had what they

call an "attitude." . . . I'd call it distant and withdrawn. But, I really wanted to get in touch with myself. Initially after that accident you don't want to be involved with anybody until you come to grips with yourself. . . . I was able to see, with the sensitivity that developed over those months of frustration, that people really cared about me and it was time to make my move. . . . I said to myself, "O.K. Darryl, here it is, the challenge of your life. You can't do any of those things anymore." You just look in yourself and find out what you are all about. There is nothing shallow or superficial. You really find out. . . .

Even now it is hard to look back. . . . When I do, I relive the same pain and agony. The whole first year I was fighting for my life. The second year was a transition period. I guess it will always be a transition. It's still "why me?" You see people walking around doing things you use to do, and you say, "why me, why me?" I lost just about everything I had except my life. Then, all of a sudden, it becomes a new way of life. It's redefining who I am now. Everything that was, was. It can no longer be. When you stop asking yourself why, you start living. (p. C-6)

Injuries like that suffered by Darryl Stingley are rare in day-to-day competition. But given the magnitude of sport participation, the number of catastrophic injuries that occur worldwide is quite large.

Although most athletes accept minor injury as a part of everyday life in sport, they seldom anticipate severe injury. When it does occur, it is psychologically threatening and poses special challenges. Where injury ends a career, it is especially disrupting.

Specialized psychological approaches to the management of severe injury are presented in this chapter. There are sections on helping the athlete deal with surgery, sport-disabling injury, and catastrophic injury. There is also discussion of fatal injury and recommendations for intervention with family and teammates following this most tragic form of injury.

Surgery and Hospitalization

Surgery is one of the marvels of sports medicine. In the skilled hands of today's surgeon, damage that was once irreparable can be repaired giving the athlete a new lease on life in sport. In contrast, there is nothing that can't be made worse by surgery (Rettig, cited in "Scanning Sports," 1990). The combination of healing power, risk, and surrender of control makes the experience of surgery particularly compelling. Athleticism is marked by control over one's body and over events as they unfold in the competitive environment. But surgery and hospitalization are the antithesis of this, often involving surrender of control over such fundamental activities as sleeping, eating, and voiding. Consequently the hospital can be a particularly threatening environment for the athlete.

Surgery and other medical procedures can be both painful and frightening. Philadelphia Flyer hockey stand out Tim Kerr was suffering from a shoulder injury late in a competitive season but continued to play. He became increasingly susceptible to minor shoulder separations; when he was bumped and his shoulder separated he would shrug it back in place and resume play. He described himself as a firm believer in concentration and mental control and attributed his ability to play in spite of injury to his ability to mentally control distress. Yet he stated in a news article that when faced with the prospect of surgery he was fearful, but not of the pain or even the outcome (Cataldi, 1987):

> The worst thing about operations as far as I am concerned is that I don't like to be put out. . . . The anesthesia—that's the thing I am most nervous about. . . . I mean you are actually putting your life in somebody else's hands. It's up to [the anesthesiologist] whether you ever wake up or not. That's a scary feeling. (p. 3-D)

As discussed in the following sections, psychological consultation can help athletes preoperatively and postoperatively.

Preoperative Consultation: Coping With Pain and Anxiety

The general strategy underlying psychological preparation for surgery (and other procedures that are painful, frightening, or otherwise threatening) is that by increasing understanding and fostering an active role in coping, practitioners can decrease the patient's feelings of helplessness and enhance the patient's sense of self-efficacy. Three general categories of psychological preparation have been identified: educating the patient about the procedure, identifying and planning the use of medical options for pain control, and training the patient in psychological self-regulation techniques (K.O. Anderson & Masur, 1983; Chapman & Turner, 1986).

In the education-based approaches, the practitioner describes operative (or other) procedures in detail. This may include a review of anatomy, a description of the actual steps involved in the procedure, and a discussion of painful and other physical sensations that may be experienced. Because uncertainty is the basis of anxiety, these approaches help to reduce anxiety. Initially, detailed descriptions should be provided by the physician or other member of the medical staff. Psychologists may follow up to assess the athlete's level of understanding and sense of self-efficacy for coping with the procedure.

A variety of medication and therapeutic modalities are available for helping the patient cope with pain and physical discomfort such as transcutaneous electrical nerve stimulation (TENS), heat, cold, and pressure point massage. Their mechanisms can be described to the patient and a plan arranged for their later use. Significant recent advances in medications, dosing strategies, and technologies for the delivery of analgesics has led to substantially reduced postoperative discomfort with only minimal side effects (Stanley, Ashburn, & Fine, 1991).

The acute pain that accompanies medical procedures leads to sympathetic excitation and increased muscle tension, responses that may increase the patient's pain. Emotional arousal and pain can generate a vicious cycle through their common effects on the sympathetic nervous system (Chapman & Turner, 1986). Psychological self-regulation techniques reduce subjective emotional distress and limit the sympathetic nervous system and muscle tension responses to pain, anxiety, and fear. A broad range of procedures has been found to be useful. These are described in detail in chapter 11. The nature of the invasive procedure, preexisting self-management skills, and time constraints on training are considerations that the practitioner needs to address in designing mental training approaches to psychological preparation for invasive procedures.

The diagnostic interview conducted before psychological preparation techniques are developed should identify the following:

- The athlete's general concerns regarding injury or illness
- Specific questions or concerns the athlete has regarding the particular procedure
- The athlete's prior experience with invasive procedures
- The degree of anticipatory anxiety associated with the procedure
- The athlete's personal coping strategies (formally trained or inherent) that are suitable for use in conjunction with procedures
- The athlete's motivation for taking an active (vs. passive) approach to coping with medical procedures

The preoperative use of psychological preparation techniques has reduced reports of pain and psychological distress, decreased the length of hospital stays, and reduced medication use (K.O. Anderson & Masur, 1983; Chapman & Turner, 1986; Mumford et al., 1982). These procedures have been found to be effective not only with adults but also with children (McGrath, 1990).

Psychological evaluation can identify patients who despite good operative results are likely to experience problems with rehabilitation following surgery (Ransford et al., 1976; Spengler & Freeman, 1979; Wiltse & Rocchio, 1975; Wise et al., 1979). The psychological evaluation should include consultation with the physician regarding her or his concerns about the athlete as well as diagnostic review and psychological testing. This evaluation process parallels the chronic pain and injury assessment protocol presented in chapter 9.

Circumstances that signal the possible need for this preoperative psychological evaluation include prior rehabilitation problems, current psychological adjustment problems, or a history of drug dependence. Where evaluation supports the likelihood of problems with rehabilitation, the practitioner should provide a vigorous program of psychological preparation for surgery (such as previously described) supplemented by a detailed description of the rehabilitation tasks to be faced following surgery. This should be followed postoperatively by an intensive goal-oriented program that includes psychological coping skills training (Fordyce et al., 1986). This should include careful specification of guidelines for the use of medication and other pain-control modalities with a goal of limiting potential dependence.

Preoperative Consultation: Clarifying Costs and Benefits

A preoperative assessment is also beneficial when the decision to undergo surgery is particularly complex. This may be the case where surgery is not necessary for daily activities but is primarily a means of maintaining athletic performance, and where there is either marginal likelihood of success or a significant probability of complications. The goal of the intervention is to crystalize the athlete's understanding of the relative balance of the costs and benefits of surgery. There are four interrelated questions that the athlete must be able to answer thoroughly and precisely.

1. What are the benefits of surgery and their degrees of probability? That is, what is the likelihood of complete or partial recovery?
2. What are the costs of surgery and their degrees of likelihood (e.g., failure to return to play, surgical complications that may worsen the condition, the length of downtime for rehabilitation)?
3. What are the benefits of not having surgery and their degrees of probability? (e.g., full or partial recovery through rehabilitation, less disruption of current lifestyle)?
4. What are the costs of not having surgery and their degrees of probability (e.g., lengthy period of rehabilitation, increased injury risk)?

This approach requires careful input from medical personnel and coaching staff. It also may be useful for the athlete to discuss his or her situation with others who have been in similar circumstances. Although additional medical opinions may be beneficial, at some point these can complicate the decision-making process (as suggested by Petrie in chapter 2). The psychologist must act as facilitator, actively listening and clarifying the athlete's understanding of the potential outcomes and his or her feelings about these.

Recovery from surgery following injury can have unexpected twists, as the following case report illustrates. As a high school basketball player,

Paul was nationally ranked. However, toward the end of his high school career he suffered recurrent knee injuries that limited his play in the latter part of high school and over his first year of college. During this period he developed a more cautious style of play, which together with injury limited his effectiveness as an athlete. He eventually considered the possibility of surgery and was offered a 40% chance of full medical recovery with the absence of pain. However, he was told that a long period of rehabilitation would be necessary following surgery. What Paul failed to realize at that time was that medical recovery did not mean skill recovery. The long downtime for surgery and rehabilitation, which was compounded by a prolonged period of ineffective play preoperatively, left Paul with a long way to go in recovering his skill level and mental readiness. He also felt he had never gained the confidence of his collegiate coaching staff because of his problems with injury. At the point he sought psychological consultation, he was weighing the benefits of continued work toward skill recovery and toward gaining the confidence of his coaches versus the benefits of devoting additional time to alternate career pursuits.

Postoperative Consultation

As a routine intervention, postoperative psychological consultation provides support and encouragement to the athlete during a difficult time. Postoperative consultation also allows treatment providers to easily identify any problems the athlete has adapting to injury. When problems are identified, timely psychological counseling may be initiated. Visits by the coach and teammates to the hospitalized athlete also provide support and encouragement as well as distraction from the aversive elements of hospitalization.

The more severe the injury and the greater its psychological impact, the more urgent and intensive intervention should be. Postoperative assessment should follow the guidelines for consultation-liaison assessment presented in chapter 9. Treatment providers may encounter a wide variety of intervention scenarios and must always operate under the assumption that the goal of intervention is to help the athlete cope with both the trauma of injury and the trauma of treatment.

In the immediate postoperative period the athlete will often benefit from help in coping with the aversive elements of hospitalization. Pain, disruption of sleep, and anxiety associated with hospitalization can be managed with mental training methods (see chapter 11 for more information). Discomfort with things such as drainage tubes, monitoring equipment, and bloody bandages can be managed with techniques similar to those designed for coping with invasive procedures (see the preceding section in this chapter). Activity limitations can be particularly frustrating. For example, following knee surgery patients often undergo passive movement of the knee through a specific limited range of motion. In this procedure, the injured leg is harnessed to a motorized device and is moved in a tracking mechanism. The continuous and almost inescapable (for a time) nature of this procedure can be frustrating for many.

The following case study underscores the benefits of timely intervention. Louis was a university baseball player hospitalized for shoulder surgery, which was successful. Although the immediate postoperative rehabilitation of the shoulder appeared to be on course, Louis experienced the onset of hypertension following surgery. This was particularly distressing in light of the recent death of a parent by heart disease. He was prompted to use mental training procedures (which he had learned previously to enhance his sport performance) to help manage his hypertension. Louis was also supported and encouraged regarding his rehabilitation goals. He appeared reassured, the hypertension resolved, and rehabilitation continued on course. To what extent the hypertension responded to prescribed medication versus this supportive and skill-based intervention is unclear. What is noteworthy is the positive emotional response of the athlete to this intervention and the appreciation he subsequently expressed.

Career-Ending Injury

Injury plays a significant role in the closing of athletic careers. This is most evident where severe injury prohibits the athlete from returning to sport; however, the problem is far broader than this. When injury causes an athlete to miss a critical competition or otherwise interferes with the athlete's ability to be in top competitive form, he or she may fail to make the team or otherwise move to a higher level of competition. Research shows that injury is a factor in dropout from youth sport (Gould, 1987). The repeated stress and strain of injury affect longevity in sport for recreational as well as highly successful athletes (Svoboda & Vanek, 1982).

The consequences of career-ending injury are potentially severe from a psychological point of view. The athlete is more likely to experience difficulties in adjustment than would be the case in injury of comparable severity where return to play is anticipated.

Elite Athlete

The prospect of giving up a beloved sport activity can be difficult, whether the athlete is young or old and whether a highly successful competitor or a modest achiever. The more abrupt and unanticipated the ending of a sport career, and the greater the athlete's commitment, achievement, and rewards for success, the more difficult the adjustment. Consequently, career-ending injury for the elite athlete is the most potentially traumatic example of injury-forced retirement. For this reason the discussion that follows focuses on career-ending injury in the committed and successful athlete, while recognizing that the general principles of intervention are valid to some degree for all athletes.

In many circumstances career termination is a group phenomenon (e.g., at the end of each competitive sport season in high school or college), and in such cases there is a natural mechanism of support based on the shared experience. With injury-forced retirement this support is not so readily available.

The relative ease or difficulty an athlete has in coping with career-ending injury is a reflection of the relative balance of coping resources and sense of loss. The athlete with greater personal and social resources and life skills will best be able to adjust to career-ending injury.

However, the importance of one's sport experience is a relative measure, balanced against other life experiences, opportunities, and resources. This is well reflected in the comments of one alcohol and drug counselor who works in a blue-collar town with a faltering economy, where high school football is an important social and emotional aspect of community life (A. Davis, personal communication, 1988). From the many former football players numbered among his clients he has observed that most appear to have reached the culmination of their existence playing high school football. When unemployment, divorce, or other life problems leave these former athletes with little else to look forward to, they spend a great deal of time drinking and reliving their glory days to their continuing misfortune.

For the professional athlete, career-ending injury poses special problems. In *Sports in America*, Michener (1976) described professional athletes as a privileged class often ill-prepared for life after sport. Former professional basketball player and now Senator Bill Bradley offered a similar perspective, suggesting that once a professional or similarly successful athletic career ends the athlete must face a world where failure to perform well in other areas of life will no longer be overlooked because of athletic performance. Bradley described a worst-case scenario wherein the athlete falls victim to a "Faustian bargain": Some athletes, without quite realizing it, sacrifice exquisite physical prowess in a few years of intensified youth, living the rest of life unable to recapture the feeling of those few special years. Bradley (1976) even compared the athlete to a warrior, suggesting that "it is the fate of the warrior class to receive the awards, plaudits, and exhilaration simultaneously with the means of self-destruction" (p. 204).

Psychological Counseling

Counseling of the athlete who suffers career-ending injury should address three issues: the trauma of injury, the loss of the athletic career, and reorientation to a new lifestyle. The first two of these are more immediate and potentially urgent, whereas the third is more protracted and multi-faceted.

A general outline of treatment approaches follows:

1. Supportive counseling to help the athlete cope with injury and the loss of sport.
2. Insight-oriented therapy to help the athlete gain an understanding of the meaning of sport to the athlete and the role of sport as a vehicle for building life skills.
3. Problem-solving therapy aimed at helping the athlete cope with injury and lifestyle change. This may include stress management skills training, recommendations for resumption of physical activity and the establishment of social support networks, and vocational exploration and goal setting.

This therapeutic strategy aims to "normalize" dysphoric emotional responses by characterizing these as natural reactions to a difficult set of circumstances. It emphasizes a problem-solving approach to help the athlete identify needs previously met through sport and to reorient his or her lifestyle to continue to meet these needs.

Although the focus of competitive sport is typically on prowess and achievement, physical activity can also be a means for coping with stress, an outlet for emotional tension, or a source of enjoyment. Consequently, the athlete should be encouraged to continue physical activity as a means of stress management and for its inherent pleasure. In a study of professional baseball players, Lerch (1979) found that life satisfaction following retirement was most significantly related to health, which, in turn, is related to maintaining a physically active lifestyle. Because retirement limits the opportunities for contacts between former teammates and undermines the basis of their own common interests and experience (Lerch, 1979), adjustment to retirement may be eased for the athlete who remains involved with former teammates or with sports. The athlete can become involved in related sport activity (e.g., seminars or training camps for developing athletes), participate in special "veterans events" (where former players come together to compete), or establish a more or less formalized support network for retired athletes (Botterill, 1982).

Because retirement typically occurs during the years of early adulthood, it is prudent to think in terms of career change as opposed to retirement. This is a more apt characterization, because the athlete will probably need to continue to earn a living (which is not implied by retirement). Counseling should focus on the skills developed in sport and the application of these to other career pursuits; motivation, goal setting, time management, concentration, and teamwork are valuable in any of a broad variety of pursuits. The United States Olympic Committee has recently developed a career counseling program for athletes who are former members of Olympic or Pan American teams. In preparing this program, organizers discovered that athletes were concerned less with basic career counseling needs (e.g., resume preparation, job search) and more with identifying special qualifications gained through sport and understanding how to apply these in other career activities (Petitpas, Danish, McKelvain, & Murphy, 1992).

Catastrophic Injury

Catastrophic injury includes trauma that results in permanent functional disability, typically from damage to the head and spinal cord, and other injuries of comparable severity. The occurrence of permanent functional disability is infrequent relative to all sport injury, but the actual number of such injuries yearly is large. The effect of catastrophic injury on lifestyle is profound, potentially touching on all aspects of behavior—physical, mental, emotional, and social. The development of injury-monitoring systems and increasing epidemiological research are leading to a better understanding of the frequency, type, and causes of catastrophic injury. These efforts have also led to the identification of high-risk sports and specific high-risk situations within sport. This in turn has resulted in improved treatment approaches as well as preventive efforts designed to limit risky situations.

A growing number of sports-monitoring systems ranging from the National Safety Council to the National Football Head and Neck Injury Registry are establishing injury databases ("Injury Statistics Groups," 1991). The National Center for Catastrophic Sports Injury Research (NCCSIR) has monitored traditional high school and college sports since 1982 and has calculated the incidence of catastrophic injury to be 1.5 per 100,000 participants per year in high school football and 8.8 per 100,000 participants in collegiate football (Mueller & Blyth, 1987). Relatively high rates of severe injury also have been noted in men's and women's gymnastics (at both high school and college levels), in high school wrestling, and in ice hockey. There is also a significant amount of catastrophic injury among cheerleaders, apparently because cheerleading requires more athletic skill and holds more inherent risk than meets the eye.

The risk of brain injury from boxing has long been apparent (Casson et al., 1984; Lubell, 1989a; Maliszewski, 1990), with awareness of this risk dating to when Martland (1928) first described "punch drunk syndrome" (dementia pugilistica). The more prevalent problem, chronic damage, appears linked to the cumulative trauma of years of training and competition in boxing; in short, the more punches received the greater the risk of injury. However, most attention has been directed to incidents of fatal injury due to acute brain trauma, which though rare tend to be highly publicized. The 1985 position statement of the American Psychological Association (cited in Maliszewski, 1990) encourages periodic neuropsychological evaluations of boxers and ring-side evaluations performed by neurocognitive specialists during bouts.

The potentially tragic impact of even minor brain injury is nowhere more poignant than in Muhammad Ali (Schaap, 1984), one of the greatest and most well-known athletes of this century. The cumulative effect of too many punches has undermined his effectiveness as a spokesman and role model—and the privilege he earned as a champion. This is a source of sadness for those who consider him "The Champ."

In comparison to sports performed on the playing fields and in the arenas, athletic activities that take place on racetracks and in the natural environment carry even greater risk. Heights and high speeds are the key elements that contribute to increased catastrophic injury in these settings. Careless diving into pools and natural bodies of water accounts for approximately 1,000 of the 10,000 spinal cord injuries that occur annually (Samples, 1989); 9 out of 10 of these injuries result in quadriplegia. Outdoor activities such as mountain climbing, hang gliding, and recreational skiing as well as motor sports such as automobile, snowmobile, and motorcycle racing carry relatively high risk of severe injury (Reif, 1986).

Psychological Intervention

The psychological impact of catastrophic injury is broad and deep. It involves the immediate trauma of injury, the continuing trauma of hospitalization and treatment, the loss of sport activity, the loss of the ability to engage in ordinary activities, and the disruption of long-term life plans (e.g., social and career). Intervention begins with an assessment of what has been lost and the cost of this loss to the athlete. The loss of physical ability is likely to have a much greater impact on an athlete than on a sedentary person. Physical function loss needs to be considered in conjunction with the emotional impact of injury and its interpersonal effects. Where there is head injury, treatment providers must assess emotional and intellective functioning with attention to the direct effects of physical trauma and to its reactive consequences. Sorting these out is both important and difficult.

The brief model of athletic injury presented in chapter 4 is relevant here. Initially the athlete is likely to react to injury with shock and disbelief. In varying degrees denial will be exhibited throughout the rehabilitation process, and depression is also common as a natural reaction to loss. Intervention should initially focus on helping the athlete cope with the trauma of injury and treatment; the general guidelines presented in the preceding section on surgery and hospitalization are applicable. The psychologist should address concerns regarding the pain accompanying injury and fears of exacerbating injury in the course of treatment.

Subsequently, the psychologist should focus attention on issues related to the loss of sport and on the need to establish a new lifestyle that includes physical activity. Guidelines presented in the preceding section on career-ending injury offer a general framework for this component of treatment.

Less readily apparent but of great significance are the interpersonal effects of severe injury. The deep and pervasive disruption of the athlete's life influences spouse, family, and close friends as well, who share the athlete's grief. Family and spouse often must make significant life adjustments to help accommodate the athlete. They may also become the inadvertent victims of the athlete's grief, especially when it is exhibited as frustration, irritability, and anger. A treatment plan that does not incorporate family and intimate friends is incomplete. Social support from family, friends, and teammates is clearly important, yet their support can be as demanding of them as it is potentially beneficial for the athlete. As a consequence, those in the athlete's social sphere may benefit from guidance from the psychologist in their interactions with the injured athlete.

Sport After Disability

Sport offers the same benefits to the person who is disabled as to the one who is not (Asken, 1989). There are opportunities for the casual recreational athlete who wants and needs an outlet for physical activity. The seriously committed athlete has the opportunity to pursue competitive excellence through specially organized sport activities for people who are disabled. Probably most relevant and important, however, are the direct benefits of physical activity as part of the rehabilitation process.

Although the benefits of existing sport programs for people who are disabled are great, there are problems as well. Despite the recent growth of such programs, there is limited awareness about them. For the athlete who was highly successful prior to injury, the adaptation to sports for people who are disabled can be difficult, especially when participation renders the athlete's deficits all the more apparent.

At 41 years of age, Michael Goodling is a highly successful disabled athlete competing in wheelchair sports (Asken, 1989). He is internationally ranked in archery and has had significant success in national and regional competitions in a variety of other sports. As an occupational therapist on a rehabilitation unit, he helps others learn to perform activities of daily living in spite of their physical limitations. As a college freshman he was in a motor vehicle accident that severed his spinal cord in the thoracic region, paralyzing both legs and leaving him wheelchair bound. Before his injury he had been an avid recreational athlete and a high school varsity golfer. Goodling describes himself as fortunate to have been in a collegiate setting (University of Illinois) where there is a well-developed sport program for people who are disabled. He continues to enjoy the opportunity for socialization and stress management that sport provides him, and he appreciates the opportunity to push his physical limits in a competitive environment.

Goodling is a strong advocate for the use of sport psychology with athletes who are disabled (Asken, 1989). However, he cautions that psychologists may need to take special care to adapt mental training to the limits imposed by the athlete's disability. For example, progressive muscle relaxation must be modified for practice by a paralyzed athlete. Goodling also advocates the application of sport psychology techniques such as goal setting and mental preparation to rehabilitation populations, based on the success he has had with these methods in his work as an occupational therapist. Accessibility to a sport psychologist can help athletes who are disabled deal with the psychological aspects of disability that many carry throughout their lives. Goodling's concern that sport psychology for those who are disabled has not kept pace with other developments in sports medicine has been echoed by sport psychologists (e.g., Sachs & Henschen, 1988).

Fatal Injury Risk

On March 4, 1990, Hank Gathers walked onto the basketball court as a top-ranked college player with a promising professional career awaiting him. He was known to suffer from cardiac arrhythmia, which had apparently precipitated a fainting episode earlier in the season and for which he had been prescribed medication (Munnings, 1990). While being treated for the arrhythmia he had been identified as a potential risk for sudden death syndrome. There can be little doubt that the promise of glory was a factor in his presence on the court that day. During the game he suffered a fatal myocardial infarction, a shocking event that was all the more horrifying for being so highly visible. This story calls attention to the risk-taking inherent in sport and the related compulsion some athletes feel to compete against and sometimes tempt the odds.

In most sport settings fatal injury is infrequent; when it does occur it is typically attributed to extraordinary circumstances or to an unlikely chance occurrence during routine activity. Yet, in some sports (e.g., mountain climbing), the specter of death is ever present. From an epidemiological perspective injury is an inevitable consequence of the dangers inherent in sport, and fatal injury is a concomitant. Ryan (1973) noted the work of the National Safety Council, which states the following:

> One accidental death occurs for every 100 disabling injuries, 1 disabling injury for each 29 accidental injuries, and 1 accidental injury for each 300 unsafe acts. Since the practice of sport is replete with unsafe acts, the approximately 900,000 unsafe acts statistically necessary to produce one accidental death is frequently attained. (p. 106)

Absolute numbers of fatalities are difficult to calculate, especially when one considers the broad range of competitive sport and recreational activity. Drawing on multiple sources, Kraus and Conroy (1984) offered a "conservative" estimate of over 6,000 deaths in the United States in 1978 from athletic and recreational activities. A large percentage of these are due to small boat accidents, drownings occurring during recreational activity, and the use of recreational vehicles (motorized and nonmotorized).

Two categories of fatal injury are typically identified: direct, resulting from participation in the sport, and indirect, caused by systemic failure from exertion or due to a complication of a nonfatal injury. To this a third category may be added: fatal injury due to sport-motivated risk behaviors, such as drug use and extreme weight loss measures. Wadler and Hainline (1989) compiled from news headlines a list of 14 athlete deaths due to drug use since 1980. However, the full effects of drug use, eating disorders, and failure to adjust to the pressures of competition remain unknown.

Reif (1986) calculated risks for a wide variety of highly skilled athletic activities. Fatal injury is more likely to occur in boxing than in any other (nonmotorized) competitive sport, with college football a distant second followed closely by ski racing; motor sports also carry significant risk of fatal injury. However, outdoor adventure activities are most dangerous. For example, fatalities per year in hang gliding and parachuting are approximately 1 in 500 to 600 participants. Many outdoor activities can be pursued with significantly low risk; however, as individuals push the limits of sport performance, the danger increases. For example, among all mountain climbers risk of death is estimated to be at 1 in 1,750 per year. However, among dedicated experts the risk rises to 1 in 167. For climbers on a single Himalayan climb the risk grows to a chance of 1 in 20.

Coping With Fatal Injury

Fatal injury creates an emotional shock wave that ripples outward through the athlete's social sphere and leaves a legacy of sadness. Not only is the athlete a victim, but family, teammates, and friends are victims as well. Counseling can help them cope with their loss, and circumstances will dictate whether this is best done formally or informally, individually or with others who share in the grief.

Death may raise questions about the role of the sport activity in the participant's life. This is especially so with activities for which the threat of death or severe injury is well recognized. For family and friends it can be important to know that death was not a result of some aberration in personality but rather was an unfortunate consequence of participation in a highly regarded life-enhancing activity. The deceased athlete's peers in sport may have questions about the role of sport in their lives and may find it appropriate to review their attitudes toward risk taking. Preferably directed by a psychologist, the athletes should be provided with an opportunity to deal with these issues individually or in a group. For more information on risk taking, see the subsequent section on sensation seeking.

As physician for a high school hockey team, Peter Karofsky was present when a 15-year-old was struck in the chest by a puck during a game and died. He described the reactions of those present (Karofsky, 1990):

> Immediately after the incident both the students and the adults who attended the game were in need of help. The players discussed their own vulnerability and their guilt at feeling relieved that their parents didn't have to suffer the loss of a child. Many cried openly. Some players expressed fear that a similar event could happen to them. Others felt guilty that the event hadn't "hit" them yet. Parents were stunned; most said that they imagined their own sons on the ice where the victim had lain. Almost all the parents tried to sense what the event was like for the dead player's family. (p. 103)

Based on this experience Karofsky offered the following suggestions for dealing with fatal injury. Health professionals should:

- speak with the athletes, the parents of the victim, and the coaches;
- arrange a group meeting as soon as possible with the team, cheerleaders, coaches, and parents;
- speak to the media and assist the school in discouraging reporters from interviewing team members;
- attend the funeral with the team (if appropriate);
- work with school counselors in helping students cope with their concerns;
- work with the athletic director and coaches in arranging low-key practice sessions;
- work with the athletic director and team in deciding when to play the next game; and
- be available to counsel parents, coaches, and students during the remainder of the season.

The impact of fatal injury on teammates, family, and friends is not only powerful but also enduring. Dan was a freshman, Division I university football player with congenital heart disease who died suddenly shortly before the start of a game. Approximately 4 years later the remaining members of his recruiting class were interviewed regarding their recollections and reactions to their teammate's death (Henschen & Heil, 1992). Players were uniform in their retrospective reports of shock and disbelief at the time of the event, and they said they felt the emotional effects through the duration of the season. What was most remarkable, however, was the continuing impact of this event on the players years later; the interview process itself stirred deep emotions within the athletes. Many of the players indicated they had continued to think about their deceased teammate, often at unexpected times, but kept their thoughts and feelings to themselves. In an interview it was apparent the players were uncomfortable with these thoughts and feelings and did not know quite how to deal with them. About half of the players interviewed reported an enduring change in their attitudes toward life as a consequence of the event.

Fatal disease can be as unsettling as fatal injury and requires the same kind of intervention. With the disclosure of HIV-positive status by Earvin "Magic" Johnson and Arthur Ashe, the specter of AIDS has become a reality in the world of sport. Statements by the International Federation of Sportsmedicine, the World Health Organization, the United States Olympic Committee, and the National Collegiate Athletic Association have described a person's risk of being infected by the HIV virus while engaged in sport-related activities as extremely low but have added that such infection is theoretically possible (Hamel, 1992). To date there are no confirmed reports of the transmission of AIDS during athletic events. However, athletes are at risk for infection based on lifestyle factors, as has been tragically demonstrated. The outpouring of grief from teammates, competitors, and fans that has followed the disclosures of these highly esteemed athletes is likely to be experienced many times over at all levels of sport in the years to come. This crisis will eventually touch virtually everyone.

Catastrophic and Fatal Injury in Perspective

The tremendous impact of catastrophic and fatal injury calls for action that goes beyond restorative and supportive efforts after the fact and comes to grips with prevention. This requires an understanding of the actual risks involved in sport and of the motivations that guide athlete behavior (Heil, 1992), issues that are addressed in the following sections on prevention and sensation seeking.

Prevention

Risk is endemic to sport. It is influenced by athletes' risk-taking attitudes and coaches' expectations as well as by the quality of equipment and facilities. Successful preventive approaches demand multidisciplinary efforts, which require the expertise of a wide range of sport professionals. Preventive programs in diving and football illustrate the potential for effective multidisciplinary efforts (Clarke, 1989; Samples, 1989). Adams, Adrian, & Bayless (1987) offer sport-specific guidelines for reducing the likelihood of catastrophic injury. Psychology has a role in injury prevention, for example, by improving compliance with safety standards for equipment and facility use (e.g., Everett, Smoll, & Smith, 1990). Other approaches, much less well explored, include helping shape coaches' and athletes' risk-taking behaviors.

Of special concern is the growing tendency for individuals with significant health problems (such as congenital heart disease) to compete in spite of grave health risks. Recent legal developments have rendered the decision about sport participation in the face of a serious medical condition as a collaborative effort between physician, sport organization, athlete, and parents. The psychologist may use a cost-benefit analysis with the athlete to help in the decision-making process (such as described in the preceding section on clarifying costs and benefits of preoperative consultation).

Earvin "Magic" Johnson's acknowledgment of his HIV status has created a new level of awareness that in turn offers opportunity for education to overcome widespread misunderstandings about AIDS. A lack of understanding of the mechanisms of transmission and the fear of becoming infected by the HIV virus during sport can lead athletes to perceive risk where it is virtually nonexistent. This false perception of risk can and does create problems in the social sphere of the HIV-positive athlete, which can ultimately influence the athlete's psychological well-being and his or her accessibility to sport. This is tragically illustrated in a case study report of an HIV-positive dancer (Heil & Lanahan, 1992).

Precautions for coaches and athletes to further reduce the already minimal risk of HIV infection in sport are summarized in the brochure *AIDS in Sport* (Landry, 1989), available from the American Coaching Effectiveness Program. The psychologist can offer practical mechanisms to help with compliance with such behaviors (see chapter 13 for general guidelines).

Sensation Seeking

The obvious association between severe injury and willingness to take risks has raised questions about the motivations of risk-taking individuals. The focus of attention has been on high-risk sports such as mountain climbing, hang gliding, and motor sports. A variety of possible mechanisms have been postulated by Ogilvie (1974) to explain these athletes' participation in what appears to the uninformed observer to be daredevil behavior. These mechanisms include the pursuit of supermasculinity (sparked by feelings of inadequacy), counterphobic reactions (in which the individual unconsciously but repeatedly exposes himself or herself to frightening situations as a way of denying fear), and the manifestation of an unconscious death wish.

Current evidence suggests that these explanations are rarely valid. Ogilvie (1974) found that risk-taking athletes were not emotionally unstable or neurotic but were typically adaptable, resourceful, energetic, intelligent, and characterized by a high degree of emotional control. High-risk athletes' experiences were not confrontations with death or danger but were exhilarating, stimulating, and inherently sensual. Ogilvie (1974) speculated that a classic observer error led to the initially false interpretation. This occurs when the observers project themselves into the situation, monitor their own feelings about the activity, and assume these to be the same as the athletes'. The result in this case says more about the observer than the participant.

On the basis of programmatic research, Zuckerman and his colleagues (Zuckerman, 1984; Zuckerman et al., 1964) were able to place the behavior of the high-risk athlete into a broader psychological context. They proposed the existence of a "sensation-seeking" personality style rooted in neurophysiological mechanisms. The concept of sensation seeking was further developed by Farley (1990) under the label "type T personality." He identified a "T+" personality style, which includes the adventurer, scientist, and artist who take risks in generally positive, healthy, and adaptive ways, and a "T−" type, which includes criminals, drug abusers, and others whose risk taking is negative and destructive. Evidence suggests that high-sensation seekers are more resistant to the psychological impact of life stress and change, leading them to be at relatively less risk for injury (R.E. Smith et al., 1990b).

Some will continue to question the sensibilities of those who pursue high-risk activities, in some cases rightfully so. However, the choice is the athlete's and should be respected. When asked about his motivation for climbing Mount Everest, Sir Edmund Hillary replied, "If you have to ask the question you will never understand why" (Ogilvie, 1974, p. 94).

Concluding Comments

Although serious injury is relatively rare in sport, danger is ever present and some sports clearly carry more danger than others. Eliminating all danger is not only impossible but undesirable, because risk is inherent to sport. Removing risk would undermine the pursuit of excellence and eliminate the joy and exhilaration of sport. Nonetheless, severe injury is cause for grave concern, and all involved with sport have a responsibility to limit its occurrence—and to limit its impact when it occurs.

It is especially important that athletes have psychological care in times of great need, which are made all the more difficult by loss of sport. Grieving teammates, friends, and family of the fatally injured athlete may also need counseling. Although quality medical services are the norm, there is a great deal of room for growth in the psychological management of severe injury. Existing methods and procedures are not used optimally because injured athletes have limited access to psychologists.

Finally, to deal with the aftermath of injury is simply not enough; psychologists must undertake preventive efforts as well. This rests to a large extent on understanding the motivation of athletes and the pressures they are under to engage in risky behaviors.

13
CHAPTER

Specialized Treatment Approaches: Problems in Rehabilitation

John Heil

Athletes typically rehabilitate effectively from injury; however, it has long been recognized that in some cases problems will develop (e.g., Sanderson, 1978; A.M. Smith, Scott, O'Fallon, & Young, 1991; Yaffe, 1983). These may be mild and transitory or more severe and enduring. A significant factor in all rehabilitation is the sense of time urgency that pervades sport. Athletes tend to want to take shortcuts or make up for lost time caused by injury, and those who are successful at this become champions in health and injury. But the pressure for quick return to play is a potential trap; when time urgency turns to impatience and when hope prevails over good judgment, problems are in the making.

The most typical minor rehabilitation problems include slower than predicted rehabilitation, prolonged treatment plateaus, exacerbation of injury in the course of rehabilitation, and failed return to play. Such situations though potentially dangerous for the athlete generally resolve satisfactorily but slow the athlete's return to play. Most common of the more complex situations that may appear are persistent pain management problems or significant difficulties in psychological adjustment. These may be influenced by an array of factors including psychosocial stressors, maladaptive coping strategies, injury severity, the reaction of significant others, substance use, and more.

Injury chronicity is a further source of problems. Slow recovery not only places a great psychological demand on the athlete but can also result in disuse-related changes. Prolonged inactivity, whether voluntary or imposed, leads to a variety of consequences ranging from musculoskeletal and cardiovascular deconditioning to disruption of circadian rhythms and sensory acuity (Bortz, 1984), which may need to be addressed directly in treatment. When problems in rehabilitation persist, differences in understanding about the nature of injury may arise between the athlete and treatment providers. The physician and sports medicine specialist may view the athlete as a malingerer or faker. The athlete in turn may question the quality of care received and may wonder whether she or he is being returned to play before fully recovered for the benefit of the team. Should such a situation arise there is a risk for breakdown in communications, confidence, and quality of care, exacerbating an already difficult course of rehabilitation.

Problems in rehabilitation that do not resolve promptly call for specialized treatment approaches. The greater the urgency for return to play, the more important psychological management becomes. Careful monitoring and prompt response allow treatment providers to address problems early in their development, thereby limiting their impact. Minor treatment complications may be addressed and prevented from developing into more enduring problems. By optimizing athlete compliance, treatment providers can limit the most common cause of unnecessarily slowed rehabilitation. Poor compliance (including both failure to follow through on prescribed activities and failure to rehabilitate within safe limits) is also a sensitive indicator of other potential rehabilitation problems (Fisher, Domm, & Wuest, 1988). Some athletes may become overinvolved with sport, exhibiting addictionlike behavior that renders them at increased risk for injury problems. Personality conflicts will sometimes occur between the athlete and treatment providers, which will undermine effective recovery. When the circumstances of injury are particularly troubling, traumatic conditioning may occur. Poor coping ability, at its worst, can lead to chronic pain and injury syndromes. Distinct from this is malingering, a relatively rare but troubling phenomenon.

Minor Treatment Complications in Rehabilitation

Relatively minor difficulties with treatment such as treatment plateaus, pain flare-ups, injury exacerbation, and failed return to play are fairly common. These often resolve naturally but delay the athlete's return to optimal functioning. When minor treatment complications occur, treatment providers must reassure and support the athlete and use the setback in a positive way, educating the athlete about the causes of the setback and whatever related adjustments may be required in the treatment process.

Where complications are more persistent, the psychological component of injury management should be strengthened. This begins with the psychologist reviewing the rehabilitation program with attention to the four elements of comprehensive injury management: education, goal setting, social support, and the use of mental training and other coping techniques. In particular, the sports medicine team should consider a stronger goal orientation to treatment; if comprehensive goal setting is implemented, treatment providers should collaborate to redefine goals with more thoroughness and clarity. When complications call for the adoption of less ambitious goals, reassurance is especially important to the athlete. It can be useful for the psychologist to reinterpret the newly defined goals in relation to the more global objective of skill development in injury management. In cases of significant setbacks, it is important that the psychologist pay careful attention to discrepancies between the athlete's perspective and those of the sports medicine staff, and look for outright cognitive distortion (see chapter 4 for more information).

If injury is a hill (or mountain) to be crossed and if rehabilitation is the road to recovery, then the process may be viewed as a slow, steady, winding climb as the athlete negotiates the curves that are the challenge of recovery. Two of the more typical challenging scenarios unfold when the road levels off in a plateau or the athlete encounters a steep and precipitous drop, as in a treatment setback or pain flare-up. In the case of a treatment plateau, the question on the athlete's mind is likely, Why am I not progressing? It is helpful for the athlete to know that plateaus are common. It is also possible that the athlete perceives a plateau when in fact the slow, steady climb continues. Often, subtle gains that the physician or sports medicine specialist sees clearly are not perceived by the athlete. Explaining to the athlete how progress is gauged from a medical perspective and presenting the specific criteria by which progress is judged are instructive and reassuring.

In an environment where people routinely talk about giving 110%, it is not surprising that athletes often push beyond recommended rehabilitation limits. To the extent that this probes the upper limits of rehabilitation intensity, it is quite helpful. However, when the limits in rehabilitation are set only by injury exacerbation or pain flare-up, problems will evolve. A pattern of inconsistent rehabilitation performance certainly obscures and may inhibit progress, and multiple failure tends to undermine the athlete's confidence.

To help the athlete set limits more effectively and better cope with the psychological consequences of flare-ups, through collaborative effort the sports medicine team should

- temporarily reduce rehabilitation activities (if indicated), then gradually return the athlete to prior levels of activity;
- attempt to identify precipitating factors and modify athlete behavior accordingly;

- reassure the athlete when pain is benign, and caution the athlete when it signals injury exacerbation;
- temporarily increase the use of pain-control modalities (e.g., ice, heat) and medications (as prescribed by the physician);
- encourage increased use of mental training for pain, stress management, and mental readiness;
- help the athlete to avoid worrisome, catastrophic thinking by accurately describing the nature of the flare-up; and
- encourage strict adherence to the rehabilitation plan (i.e., discourage doing extra on good days).

This plan promotes a sense of self-efficacy in the face of difficulties and counters the development of a sense of helplessness. It draws from the lapse-relapse work of Marlatt and his associates (Brownell, Marlatt, Lichtenstein, & Wilson, 1986).

Muscular Guarding

Muscular guarding (also called bracing or splinting) is a natural protective response to injury that isolates or decreases the mobility of the injured area through postural adjustment. This is an adaptive response during the initial phase of injury; however, it leads to increased muscle tension locally and regionally and shifts the dynamic balance of the body. Guarding can become habitual, leading to increased injury risk. Injury may result either directly through improper technical execution or indirectly as a consequence of preoccupation with injury that distracts the player from other risk factors inherent in sport.

Following return to play, even modest amounts of guarding can inhibit the body mechanics of optimal performance. John Elway, quarterback for the Denver Broncos, suffered acute traumatic bursitis in his elbow following impact with another player early in the 1988 season. Continued play and subsequent reinjury led this acute problem to become a chronic one. As a consequence, Elway threw more interceptions than touchdowns for the first time in 4 years. The winningest team in professional football the preceding 4 years fell to an 8-8 record. Elway responded in a newspaper interview, "It wasn't so much the tenderness, it was just that I was always a little leery of it. I was always protecting it" (McCarthy, 1989, p. 116).

Where injury is prolonged and bracing is persistent, secondary pain syndrome may develop. (See chapter 17 for more information on myofascial pain syndrome.) Jane was a golfer who injured her shoulder in a motor vehicle accident. Her recovery was slow, marked by a series of treatment setbacks and by development of myofascial pain syndrome with related sleep problems. She showed significant guarding, and her sport performance was severely hampered. A worrier by nature, she ruminated on the circumstances of her injury and on her inability to perform well. She also reported feeling especially tense and nervous while driving her car. When these concerns were discussed in detail during conversation, guarding behavior visibly increased.

Jane underwent a comprehensive treatment program that included psychological counseling and mental training. Mental training focused initially on developing skills in general relaxation, which led quickly to improvements in sleep. Differential relaxation and EMG biofeedback were then introduced to help reduce the bracing behavior. Diagnostic EMG monitoring revealed high levels of resting muscle tension in the injured shoulder girdle. Monitoring also showed excessive increase in muscle tension with the use of adjacent muscles (the forearm and hand of the injured arm) and the contralateral muscles (the noninjured shoulder). Dual-channel EMG monitoring (of the injured and noninjured shoulders) provided feedback about the response of the injured shoulder with adjacent or contralateral muscle use, and guided Jane in the practice of differential relaxation. Supervised training was supplemented by an independent practice regimen that included three elements. The first was a daily differential relaxation training protocol of 20 to 30 min duration. In addition, Jane practiced a brief relaxation session of approximately 1 min duration each time she got in and out of her automobile. This inhibited both the situational anxiety that was associated with driving and the tendency to increase tension in the shoulders because of the hunched posture that Jane (like many people) assumed when driving. Jane was also instructed in a quick relaxation technique (approximately 5 to 15 s duration) that she used whenever intrusive ruminative thinking occurred. This combination of methods helped her to reduce muscle tension, generalize differential relaxation to daily activity, and reduce the bracing response.

Poor Compliance

Poor compliance merits special attention because of its relative frequency, its potential for leading to treatment complications, and its tendency to occur in conjunction with psychological adjustment problems. Poor compliance with medical regimens ranging from medication use to exercise programs is widely recognized as a factor limiting effective recovery (Dishman, 1988).

The most fundamental element of compliance (and the most easily monitored) is attendance at treatment sessions. However, there is more to rehabilitation than simply showing up; the completion of exercise protocols with proper form and good intensity is essential as well. The term *adherence* has been used to denote this broadened definition of compliance (e.g., Duda et al., 1989). The formula Compliance + Alliance = Adherence (Meichenbaum & Turk, 1987) emphasizes the importance of providing the athlete with a sense of active involvement in treatment. This is advocated by Steadman (in chapter 3) and others (e.g., R.J. Johnson, 1991). In the wake of failed efforts to identify a noncompliant personality type, noncompliant/nonadherent behavior is best regarded as a person-situation interaction. To simply dismiss the noncompliant athlete as suffering from a bad attitude is to fail to appreciate the scope and complexity of athlete behavior and response to injury. Even the highly motivated athlete may demonstrate a mild degree of noncompliance; this is most likely when the athlete does not understand the value of particular therapeutic recommendations. Where rehabilitation is unencumbered by problems, noncompliance is not cause for great concern. However, it does tend to slow the speed of recovery and return to play.

In many cases, poor adherence is a sensitive early indicator of psychological adjustment problems due to injury or other life circumstances. Research with athletes shows nonadherers to be more anxious somatically, less confident about treatment, lacking a sense of social support, less independently motivated, and less explicitly goal oriented (Duda et al., 1989; Fisher et al., 1988; Wittig, 1986).

A number of psychological models of compliance/adherence have been developed. A synthesis of the health belief model, the self-regulatory model, and the decision-making model identifies a set of factors that predict adherence (Knapp, 1988; Sonstroem, 1988). These include the patient's perception of need for a given intervention, expectation for a positive outcome, and belief that the benefits of participation outweigh the costs, as well as the presence of a series of tasks that seem reasonable and capable of completion as prescribed. With poor adherence the treatment provider should first look for issues such as scheduling problems, financial concerns, or poor understanding of the rationale for treatment. When this approach is not fruitful, a more in-depth review is suggested to determine if the athlete understands the connection between the short-term goals of rehabilitation and the long-term goal of recovery, has sufficient trust and confidence in the rehabilitation specialist and physician, feels confident in his or her ability to achieve the goals that have been set; or is experiencing psychological adjustment problems (related to pain, fear of reinjury, or other issues).

Special Circumstances

Adherence is sometimes a problem even when the athlete understands the approach, is self-confident, is motivated to participate, and trusts treatment providers. This occurs when rehabilitation tasks are unusual in some way, for example, when tasks involve ongoing self-monitoring or multiple brief rehabilitation activities.

In rehabilitation from back injury, ongoing self-monitoring of proper posture is necessary, especially in the period immediately following exercise. To change even simple behaviors that are as highly automated as posture is quite difficult. The commonness of poor back posture makes this more likely to be a problem. Another unique compliance challenge occurs when rehabilitation is not "massed" in one or more regular, relatively lengthy treatment sessions but is "spaced" at brief intervals throughout the day. For example, a recommended treatment protocol for anterior knee pain (chondromalacia patellae) includes 15 to 20 brief (approximately 30 s) daily trials of isometric quadriceps contraction. Although this requires only a total of 10 min of activity per day, individuals may forget to do this activity as often as required (Garrick, 1989). To facilitate adherence, the activity may be cued or triggered by naturally occurring events during the day. One simply needs to identify activities that occur as frequently as the rehabilitation activity needs to be performed. For example, students could be asked to do repetitions at the beginning and ending of each class, before and after each meal, and at arising and bedtime. As an alternative, the treatment provider may arrange some regularly occurring signal to serve as a cue to practice, such as the half hour or hour chimes that are provided on multifunction watches. Reminder dots (colored paper stick-ons) can be placed at key locations to cue the athlete to practice. Keeping a checklist of completed tasks also helps call attention to consistent practice and provides a tangible record of compliance.

Overcompliance

For the committed athlete, the pressure to return to play is great. Deeply held notions in sport regarding risk taking and pushing limits may be transferred to rehabilitation. Athletes may also experience pressure from coaches and teammates to return to play quickly (Hankins et al., 1989). As a consequence athletes may overdo prescribed physical rehabilitation protocols and ignore recommended limits on daily activities. In some cases this leads to faster rehabilitation—and if so, all the better. However, it can also lead to treatment setbacks and reinjury.

Setting limits on athletes' behavior can pose a dilemma to the sports medicine team, because speedy return to play is fundamental to sports medicine. Steadman (see chapter 3) encourages treatment providers to give the athlete some degree of freedom in setting limits, based on his observations of the remarkable resourcefulness of some athletes. The rehabilitation performance of stock car racer Neil Bonnett (recounted in chapter 10) exemplifies the potential of the resourceful athlete to recovery quickly. Those who approach rehabilitation with similar intensity and insight may well push limits to their benefit. Those who have the intensity but lack the finely tuned sense of limits may fail—and some may fail miserably.

Problems with overdoing activity or with overcompliance most often reflect stubbornness or a mild degree of denial regarding the limits imposed by injury. When rehabilitation is particularly lengthy, impatience may prompt the individual to overdo. More persistent problems with overcompliance, especially those that persist despite corrective actions taken by treatment providers, may reflect a pervasive maladaptive element of personality such as obsessive-compulsive tendencies or impulsiveness. Overcompliance may also reflect excessive risk-taking behavior. Two poorly adapted risk-taking styles were described by Ogilvie and Tutko (1966): counterphobia, where the individual takes risks as a way to deny an underlying fear, and a self-punitive orientation, which is motivated by a poor sense of self-worth. A particularly unfortunate scenario can evolve in which the athlete perceives injury as proof of effort; individuals who have low self-esteem and for whom the fear of failure is greater than the desire of success may succumb to this trap.

The following list contains guidelines for the management of persistent over-compliance problems. Treatment providers should

- educate the athlete about the mechanisms of injury and rehabilitation;
- emphasize that the prescribed amount of activity is the best amount and that overdoing prescribed activity may aggravate injury and slow recovery;
- present the goal as a bull's-eye, a target to be hit with precision. This counters the notion that a goal is a line to be crossed, the further the better;
- support consistency and accuracy in goal attainment;
- consider having the athlete use the Rating of Perceived Exertion Scale (Borg & Ottoson, 1986) to identify and maintain appropriate levels of effort during rehabilitation;
- develop a flare-up plan for helping the athlete cope with treatment setbacks (see the preceding section on minor treatment complications); and
- redirect the athlete's desire and energy for more work at rehabilitation into mental training (as presented in chapter 11).

The overall objective of managing overcompliance is to help the athlete learn that smart rehabilitation (i.e., sometimes less rehabilitation) is better than more rehabilitation.

The "Addicted" Athlete

In addition to its traditional application to substance abuse, the term *addiction* is often used metaphorically to describe intense involvement with any behavior. This term has been applied colloquially to a wide variety of activities ranging from watching soap operas to wearing lucky socks. Positive addiction refers to the dedicated practice of behaviors that are generally regarded as constructive and health enhancing. This includes physical activities ranging from a daily morning walk to formal competitive sport (Glasser, 1976). Subsequently, the term *negative addiction* has been used to describe a pattern of behavior whereby the excessive practice of potentially health-enhancing behaviors comes to have a significant negative effect (Morgan, 1979).

The fundamental characteristic of the addicted athlete is the need to perform a given activity regularly in order to maintain emotional equilibrium. The syndrome is most frequently seen in recreational athletes, especially runners (Layman & Morris, 1986), whose enthusiasm for sport grows beyond the capability of their lifestyles to support it. The negatively addicted athlete will continue training even when it is contraindicated for medical, interpersonal, or work-related reasons. The addicted athlete is at substantial risk for injury and rehabilitation problems because of the tendency to overexercise. Even where the intensity of training is within reasonable physical limits, overinvolvement may lead to family, work, or other interpersonal problems. The key feature appears to be not the absolute volume of training per se but the compulsive style with which it is pursued even in the face of obvious negative consequences. Withdrawal-like symptoms typically appear when the individual is unable to train; these include depression, anxiety, irritability, and interpersonal discord as well as sleep disturbance and other vegetative signs. Unable to sustain desired training intensity and unable to tolerate inactivity, the athlete experiences intense emotions.

The psychological dynamic underlying exercise addiction is hypothesized to be diminished self-esteem (e.g., Hays, 1990), which is bolstered by the progressive gains in performance that come with continued training. As participation grows beyond manageable levels, resulting in physical, psychological, or interpersonal problems, gains made in self-esteem are diminished. Although treatment practices recommended in the preceding section on overcompliance are beneficial, successful treatment outcomes rely on psychological counseling designed to address self-esteem and other underlying psychological issues.

The case study that follows demonstrates the complexity and potential depth of dysfunction of the addicted athlete. Annie was a highly successful advertising executive who began a jogging program to help cope with the stress of work and family life. She approached jogging with the same intensity with which she pursued her job and made relatively quick gains in performance. This success and the boost in mood she experienced from running fueled her enthusiasm and led her to consistently increase her training load. She began to experience hamstring problems, sought treatment, and then resumed her training regimen only to aggravate her injury.

Over the 1-1/2 years, she experienced a continuing cycle of injury, recovery, and reinjury. Each setback left her more determined to return to her prior level of performance. When unable to run she suffered depression, which was alleviated with return to activity but was redoubled by reinjury. She vigorously pursued a variety of physical treatments that allowed her to continue training. Eventually an Achilles tendon injury (in the leg that was not initially injured) and severe side effects from an aggressive elective medical procedure left her unable to run.

By the time she was referred to a multidisciplinary rehabilitation program she was wheelchair-bound periodically throughout the day, severely depressed, and suffering significant marital problems. Psychological evaluation revealed an emotionally disruptive childhood and resulting poor sense of self-esteem. Hard work and determination had led Annie to a series of achievements, first in school and then at work. These bolstered her self-esteem and convinced her of the necessity of pushing hard in the face of obstacles.

A comprehensive psychological treatment program was devised that incorporated insight-oriented psychotherapy, family involvement, intensive goal setting, and mental skills training in conjunction with physical rehabilitation. Strict adherence to a gradually progressing goal-oriented program countered her tendency to push into pain and thus exacerbate injuries. Annie was chronically muscularly tense and failed to use rest periods during her rehabilitation regimen for optimal recovery. Her mental skills training program included regular practice of relaxation and visual imagery (about 20 to 30 minutes per day) to facilitate recovery from the day's activity and frequent but brief use of relaxation techniques during rehabilitation sessions to help pace activity and maximize physical recovery. She showed significant gains in activity, mood, and family relations during this intensive course of treatment. But in the follow-up period she failed to adhere to treatment recommendations and slipped back into a pattern of overactivity, which was followed by a severe physical and emotional crash. She resisted efforts to reinstitute her recommended rehabilitation program and eventually dropped out of psychological treatment, again seeking acute medical interventions.

A tendency to overexercise in conjunction with compulsive adherence to activity regimens may be seen in patients with anorexia nervosa and bulimia. Consequently, when dealing with addicted athletes, treatment providers should explore for the possibility of eating disorders (especially for those in high-risk sports). For more information on the identification of eating disorders see chapter 15.

Personality Conflicts

The importance of social support in recovery from injury is widely recognized. The relationship of the patient with treatment providers is the cornerstone of support for the injured athlete. If personality conflicts arise within these relationships, this base of support is disrupted.

Fortunately, such conflicts are far more the exception than the rule. When a personality conflict occurs it is best conceptualized as a problem of trust based on misunderstanding. The source of many such problems can be traced to the differing points of view held by the athlete and treatment provider. Sports medicine professionals and the athlete share the common goal of quickest safe return to play. However,the physician's or the sports medicine specialist's point of view is objective, reflecting a normative standard of rehabilitation based on clinical experience. The athlete's point of view, in contrast, is subjective and may often be skewed from normative standards. This perspective may be due to a compelling need to return quickly to play or unresolved concerns regarding injury or ongoing pain. Failure by treatment providers to be sensitive to the athlete's urgent need for speedy return to play and willingness to assume risk for reinjury—and failure to address these concerns directly—can lead to problems.

Communication that is clear, consistent, and ongoing is the first line of prevention of personality conflict. Treatment providers should always be sensitive to cultural differences between themselves and the athletes they treat. Working through personality conflicts should begin with an attempt to identify and resolve any misunderstandings between the athlete and the treatment providers, perhaps through a detailed review of the course of injury and rehabilitation. There should be clarification of treatment providers' expectations for the athlete (e.g., compliance, procedures for resolving questions and concerns) and of the athlete's expectations for treatment providers (e.g., clear information regarding treatment, participation in the treatment process).

When problems persist a more systematic approach is required. Although any of a variety of approaches may be taken, those that are most likely to be successful will share some common elements; they will frame concerns in the context of misunderstood expectations and communication problems between treatment providers and the athlete, avoid placing blame on any party, focus on specific and practical solutions, and treat this intervention as a trust-building exercise.

If the situation is not resolvable, the treatment provider should consider referring the athlete to another sports medicine professional who can provide the same treatment. This can be useful even where it appears that the athlete's issues are clearly ill founded or unrealistic; a similar experience with another treatment provider may help the athlete realize this. If the athlete has an established history of personality conflict or ongoing behaviorally based health risks (such as substance abuse or eating disorders), the referral process is more complicated. If it appears that the athlete is seeking referral in order to avoid appropriate treatment or to mask relevant elements of current status or personal history, special caution is urged. It may be appropriate in situations such as this for the physician not to surrender the attending role and to opt instead for additional medical opinion on a consulting basis. At any point in this process, the physician or sports medicine specialist may consult a psychologist to provide an impartial viewpoint or to work directly with the athlete.

With a team approach to treatment, personality conflicts are less likely to occur and are more easily managed when they do occur. This is a consequence of the broader range of perspectives available from which to assess the conflict as well as the greater variety of potential problem-solving options.

Traumatic Conditioning

Traumatic conditioning is a maladaptive psychophysiological response to a specific traumatic event such as injury. Its manifestation may be glaringly obvious or deceptively subtle, and onset may be immediate or delayed. It may be manifested by an increase in fear and anxiety as one approaches situations that resemble the situation in which the trauma occurred, or it may be characterized by spontaneous intrusive recollections in which circumstances of injury are replayed often with exaggeration of the actual outcome. Traumatic conditioning exists on a continuum from mild to severe. In mild form, it appears as a subclinical syndrome, interfering with performance and resulting in substantial discomfort but not meeting diagnostic criteria of the diagnostic and statistical manual (DSM-III-R) of the American Psychiatric Association (1987). More severe manifestations meet diagnostic criteria for either phobia (Mavissakalian & Barlow, 1981) or posttraumatic stress disorder (Saigh, 1992). Traumatic conditioning is distinguished from fear of reinjury, which is relatively less severe, enduring, and psychologically disruptive (see chapter 11).

Traumatic conditioning is best viewed as a "one-trial," Pavlovian, classically conditioned response (see Figure 13.1). Anxiety, pain, and fear are natural consequences (that is, unconditioned responses) of trauma (or unconditioned stimuli). Traumatic conditioning occurs when the setting or circumstances associated with injury (conditioned stimuli) continue to elicit anxious, painful, or fearful responses (conditioned responses) that are typically associated with actual injury and that persist in spite of their perceived irrationality. Insight by the athlete into the underlying dynamics of classical conditioning is not adequate to ameliorate this traumatic response. The athlete, like "Pavlov's dog," is unable to inhibit the conditioned response once it is established without a formal and systematic approach to its elimination. Research on this classically conditioned response phenomenon has emphasized its biological underpinnings. It is

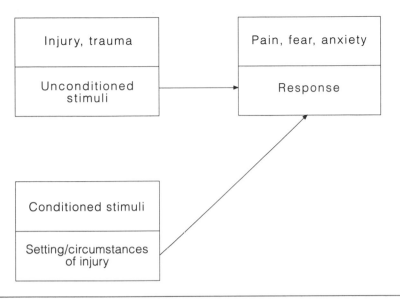

Figure 13.1   Traumatic conditioning.

hypothesized that an "organ conditioning" takes place whereby psychological and somatic factors are maintained in a mutually reinforcing cycle (Dlin, 1985). Phobiclike symptoms as well as intrusive recollections may exist in varying degrees singly or in combination.

Phobic Response

A phobic response to injury typically manifests itself as fear or anxiety when the athlete encounters situations resembling those in which injury occurred. Phobic response may be manifested more subtly as unexplainable difficulty in rehabilitation. At times a phobic response may be managed marginally by the athlete and may only become apparent at return to play. The extent to which phobic response to injury leads to attrition from sport and therefore goes unrecognized is not known.

The assessment of phobic response should begin with a behavioral analysis of the performance context (sport or rehabilitation) in which fear or anxiety occurs. This assessment may be conducted "in vivo," that is, situations where the athlete demonstrates fear or anxiety. Alternately, psychologists can use imagery-based rehearsal of the threatening situation. Both approaches facilitate recall of details and put the athlete in touch with the specific manifestations of the fear response, including images, thoughts, and sensations. This can be supplemented with a "How bad could it get?" questioning strategy designed to identify existing catastrophic images and cognitions.

As a general rule, intervention should examine and clarify the reality of the images, the probability (of occurrence) of the fearful thoughts, and the meaning of the sensations associated with phobic response. Distinguishing the rational and irrational elements of fear is especially important given the prevalence of true risk in sport. A management plan for the rational elements of fear should be devised as a component of an overall treatment plan. Treatment providers may take a variety of specific treatment approaches for the management of phobic response; systematic desensitization, stress inoculation training, and related cognitive behavioral approaches have been shown to be valuable (Beck & Emery, 1985), their effectiveness being based on their enhancement of coping skills in attention control and arousal control. As initially developed by Wolpe and Lazarus (1968), systematic desensitization is based on the use of relaxation training for the reciprocal inhibition of anxious response in conjunction with the presentation of progressively more challenging fearful images. Research suggests that success is related most directly to maintenance of a relatively long duration of relaxed attention in the face of the feared situation (Mathews, 1978). Stress inoculation training is relatively more dynamic in its use of imagery, emphasizing shifts in images that demonstrate enhanced coping. It is also broader in scope, facilitating more systematic attention to images, thoughts, and sensations (Meichenbaum, 1985). Among the related cognitive behavior approaches, the self-control triad is a three-step covert conditioning procedure; the user begins by saying or thinking "stop," then takes a deep, relaxing breath, and concludes by imagining a positive scene (Cautela, 1983). This method is brief enough to be used "in vivo," helping generalize cognitive coping skills to the sport environment.

The case presented next illustrates the enduring effects of fear of injury and the benefits of appropriate treatment. Jeff was a 12-year-old competitive springboard diver who hit the board while practicing a newly learned reverse somersaulting dive. He was frightened and experienced some physical discomfort but sustained no significant or enduring injury. After that incident he continued to have difficulty with reverse somersaulting dives, although he made progress with other skills. While trying reverse somersaulting dives in practice he often demonstrated long delays before execution as well as occasional balks. At times he would spontaneously do a simple reverse dive in lieu of somersaulting. Despite persistent work by the coaching staff, 1 year later he was unable to consistently perform somersaulting dives. This situation met the diagnostic criteria for phobia as detailed by the American Psychiatric Association (1987):

- The person persistently fears a specific activity.
- The person experiences anxiety in anticipation of this activity.
- The activity is avoided or endured with intense anxiety.
- Fear interferes with the individual's ability to complete the activity.

- There is related distress about the fear itself.
- The athlete recognizes fear as excessive in light of ability and prior skill level.
- Fear persists in spite of significant ameliorative efforts.
- The fear is circumscribed, not interfering with the ability to perform other sport skills.

In addition to its impact on competitive ability, the distracting effect of fear also increases injury risk. Jeff was introduced to relaxation and visual imagery training in conjunction with supportive counseling. He practiced three visual rehearsal techniques with varying speed of imagined movement and with differing degrees of attention to kinesthetic and visual cues. In a slow speed rehearsal, Jeff studied "snapshotlike" images (provided by the coach) of key segments of the reverse somersaulting dive, focusing on both correct technique and positive outcome. The athlete focuses more intently on the visual aspect of the image (relative to the kinesthetic). Initially this method was used diagnostically to identify components of the dive where there was a breakdown in appropriate mental focus. Subsequently, Jeff used this method in extended home-practice sessions. Jeff was also trained in a "near real-time" (15 to 60 s) mental rehearsal of the dive with equal attention to visual and kinesthetic cues. This rehearsal was brief enough for Jeff to use intermittently in practice at his or the coach's discretion when there were balks or hesitation. In addition, Jeff practiced a "faster than real-time" (1 to 3 s) mental rehearsal, focusing on the overall feel of the dive. This was of brief enough duration for him to use immediately before the execution of the dive to help prompt readiness to perform. Substantial gains followed.

Intrusive Thinking

Intrusive thinking of a disruptive or disturbing nature often occurs with injury. Usually it is a relatively mild and normal response. Spontaneous catastrophizing cognitions of injury and treatment outcome are common examples of intrusive thinking. The frequency and intensity of intrusive recollections tend to diminish over time, especially as physical recovery progresses.

Traumatic intrusive recollections of injury are much less common, more disruptive, and of greater concern. They are notable for their spontaneous yet persistent occurrence and their dystonic quality. They are more related to the psychological trauma of injury than to its severity (Grunert et al., 1988). Recollections may be elicited by exposure to circumstances associated with injury or may occur independently without apparent triggering stimuli. They may manifest as spontaneous daytime thoughts or as night dreams. The visual, kinesthetic, and visceral components vary in their vividness and their sense of reality in the moment. At their most intense they create a feeling of "being there" again, like a flashback.

Ultimately, the impact of intrusive recollections is a function of their intensity and frequency as well as the type of replay. Three types of intrusive thinking have been identified: simple replay, perseverative replay, and catastrophic replay (Grunert et al., 1988). Simple replay involves a recreation of events immediately preceding and including injury. Simple replay serves a positive purpose by identifying ways in which the athlete could have altered the event, thus preventing subsequent occurrences. This promotes a sense of mastery and decreases anxiety. In perseverative replay, the athlete recreates the same events but places a persistent and prolonged focus (like a "stop action" photo) on the injured area of the body. In catastrophic replay, the athlete recreates events but imagines an injury of greater severity than the one that actually occurred. In perseverative and catastrophic replay, the athlete tends to perceive little control over the injury and to reexperience the fear of injury. From this follows a fear of reinjury and tendency to avoid situations that resemble the one in which injury originally occurred.

Athletes may be reluctant to report intrusive thinking, feeling that they may be perceived as strange or unbalanced. This is unfortunate, because simply discussing its occurrence is beneficial, especially in a supportive context where intrusive recollections are regarded as a normal response to difficult circumstances. Whenever circumstances of injury are traumatic or otherwise frightening, treatment providers should inquire about the occurrence of intrusive thinking.

Supportive counseling, reassurance regarding recovery, and mental skills training will limit the impact of intrusive thinking and hasten its resolution. Cognitive-behavioral approaches such as the self-control triad, systematic desensitization, and stress inoculation training can be used to combat intrusive thinking. The athlete may rehearse the feared events, imagining alternate positive outcomes. This may be supplemented by rehabilitation rehearsal and healing imagery (see chapter 11). Intrusive recollections may be treated as a trigger or cue to elicit positive images regarding rehabilitation and performance. This approach automatically adjusts the intensity of intervention to the severity of the problem and generalizes the treatment effect to the performance situation.

Full-blown posttraumatic stress disorder (of which intrusive recollection is a key symptom) is far less common than intrusive recollection alone. In addition to stressors such as combat or natural disaster, injury may elicit this disorder (Fordyce, 1979). Those who experience poor recovery from injury are at increased risk for posttraumatic stress disorder. Its occurrence in conjunction with chronic pain syndrome has been described (Muse, 1985). In addition to intrusive recollections, a numbing of responsiveness to the environment and significant anxiety in conjunction with chronic pain (described in the subsequent section) characterize injury-related posttraumatic stress disorder. Because onset of the symptoms of posttraumatic stress disorder may be delayed, its timely identification is important.

Treatment should incorporate approaches for the management of intrusive recollections as well as those presented subsequently for the management of chronic pain.

Chronic Pain and Injury Syndrome

Chronic injury syndrome, characterized by lifelong limited physical ability, is an unfortunate consequence of an athletic career that happens all too often. This is graphically portrayed in the video production *Disposable Heroes* (Couturie, Else, & Witte, 1986), which examines the impact of injury on professional football players. Most athletes manage the long-term residual effects of sport injury with remarkable effectiveness, although the continuing stress that it causes can severely undermine their quality of life. This is illustrated by the experience of ironman Jim Otto, formerly of the Raiders Football Club. Although he has established a successful business career, Otto has undergone 13 surgeries, lives in constant pain, and even has difficulty getting dressed in the morning. Some people will not be able to manage chronic injury effectively and will succumb to full-blown chronic pain syndrome, leading lives of diminished effectiveness and unnecessary suffering.

Chronic pain syndrome constitutes the worst-case scenario of problems in adapting to injury. It occurs where injury and its subsequent effects on psychological well-being and lifestyle precipitate a cycle of progressive decline. Societally, chronic pain syndrome is a problem of tremendous proportion, with total cost in medical expenses and lost productivity in the United States estimated to be approximately $65 billion yearly (Association for the Advancement of Behavior Therapy, 1990). However, the greatest cost is in human suffering. Chronic pain syndrome is differentiated from uncomplicated chronic injury by the degree of its psychological impact on the athlete and by the role of psychological factors in undermining quality of life. The following sections focus primarily on chronic pain syndrome.

General Concepts

To understand chronic pain, practitioners must appreciate the connection between the nociceptive barrage that is the neurochemical basis of pain and its eventual effects on behavior. Pain begins as a series of sensory inputs that move from the periphery of the nervous system to multiple brain sites, where they are integrated and perceived as pain. Pain, in turn, elicits suffering. As pain becomes chronic, it leads to problems that can include deconditioning, musculoskeletal deficiencies, sleep disturbance, depression, traumatic conditioning, interpersonal problems, and substance abuse. These factors, which alone are independent problems, add to the overall suffering and may indirectly exacerbate the pain itself. In the end, the severity of chronic pain syndrome is defined not by the intensity of the sensory input but by its ultimate impact on behavior. (See chapter 17 for a more detailed treatment of the biology of pain.)

The scope of chronic pain is graphically portrayed in Figure 13.2. What is noteworthy is that the overall impact of pain on lifestyle is greater than would be expected from medical evaluation alone. Because of the self-perpetuating nature of this syndrome and a tendency toward progressive decline, it rarely resolves spontaneously. Pain syndromes are universally regarded as chronic when they last 6 months or more, although in athletic populations they may begin to be evident as early as 8 weeks following injury (E.W. Johnson, 1987). Generally, the more severe the injury, the greater the psychological cost, and the more prolonged the recovery, the greater the risk of chronic pain. The sooner treatment is provided the more favorable the prognosis.

The athlete is also at greater risk for failed rehabilitation when injury and overtraining syndrome occur in tandem. Ford (1983) described the "humpty-dumpty" syndrome, which includes elements of chronic pain and overtraining. Failure to account for the overtraining syndrome may lead treatment providers to underpredict recovery time. This causes the athlete to strive for unrealistically high goals in rehabilitation, setting up

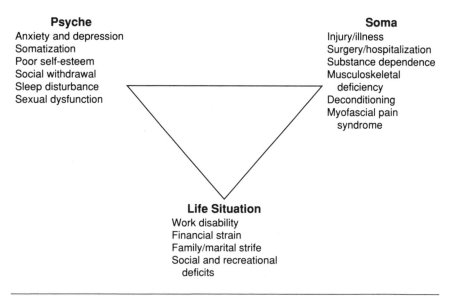

Figure 13.2   Chronic pain syndrome.

rehabilitation failure and exacerbating existing overtraining syndrome. In that overtraining in itself indicates problems in setting appropriate limits, identifying and helping the athlete accept a realistic timetable for recovery is all the more important.

The assessment of chronic pain should be comprehensive, encompassing the broad range of risk factors and using the methods and measures described in Part III. Because of the multifaceted nature of this problem, a comprehensive team-based approach to evaluation and treatment is necessary.

Adequate assessment and treatment of chronic pain are often beyond the expertise of those who lack specialized training; hence, referral to designated pain-treatment centers should be considered. The treatment that has evolved for chronic pain is interdisciplinary and intensive. The core treatment team at a pain-treatment center includes specialists in medicine, psychology, physical therapy, occupational therapy, and nursing. In the true interdisciplinary approach care is carefully coordinated, in contrast to an assembly-line approach in which each provider works independently.

The goal of treatment is to return the athlete to a healthy, productive lifestyle and to restore emotional equilibrium, as opposed to simply reducing pain. Treatment is simultaneously directed toward pain, suffering, and the behavioral consequences previously noted. Once chronic, pain will often fail to diminish totally, and the individual must be prepared to face life with pain. Treatment includes a strong, goal-oriented approach to rehabilitation to encourage carefully paced, steady progress and to supplant pain as the primary determinant of activity level. For example, rest follows goal attainment and is discouraged as a response to routine pain.

Practitioners may identify problems with alcohol, recreational drugs, prescribed medications, or illicitly acquired medications, which may necessitate a detoxification protocol. Treatment also aims to systematically reduce reliance on medical appliances (canes, braces) and dependence on passive treatment modalities. Because pain flare-ups are inevitable it is important to develop a systematic approach to limit their physical and emotional impact. A flare-up plan specifically for chronic pain sufferers is presented in Table 13.1.

A synergistic effect results from carefully coordinated interdisciplinary treatment as individual treatment approaches influence multiple problem behaviors and as multiple treatments work collectively on the same problem. For example, a program in aerobic conditioning not only improves endurance but also improves mood and muscular function and provides a variety of other health benefits (Russell, Heil, & Milano, 1986). Multiple treatments such as therapeutic exercise, relaxation training, postural monitoring, and the use of physical therapy modalities can work collectively to eliminate patterns of muscular guarding that maintain pain. For more

Table 13.1
Lewis-Gale Pain Center: The Flare-Up Dozen

1. Do not be surprised if you experience occasional flare-ups; they happen.
2. Stay active and maintain control. Do not give up and lie in bed, and do not become a slave to your pain.
3. Ask yourself, "What do I need to do differently now to cope with the pain and in the future to avoid flare-ups?"
4. If symptoms are different from the past and you are concerned that there is a new problem, contact one of your health care professionals.
5. Do not worry. It will only make things worse.
6. Remember, this happened before and you recovered. It will not last forever.
7. As a general rule, try all activities with caution.
8. Temporarily decrease by about one half the number of repetitions of activities that are a problem. Continue with the others. At the same time, double the amount of relaxation/coping techniques.
9. Avoid pain talk; focus instead on your emotions.
10. Take medications only as prescribed.
11. Try to have some fun within your limitations. Treat yourself in a special way.
12. Following the flare-up, do not try to make up for lost time. Gradually increase your activity to previous levels.

on psychological approaches to pain treatment, see Fordyce (1976) and Sternbach (1987).

Chronic Pain and the Athlete

The role of chronic pain in sport is poorly understood. Chronic pain syndrome appears to be rare among elite and highly achieving athletes. This is likely due in part to a natural selection process that weeds out those prone to injury problems, preventing them from reaching the highest levels of competitive achievement. However, the public tends to forget yesterday's heroes, who once out of sight are out of mind. The full impact of injury may not be seen until long after sport careers are over; for some, sport participation stops but problems with pain go on. Football player John Matuszak was a headliner as an athlete, but news of his death from an accidental overdose of pain medication was only briefly noted on the back pages of the sports section ("Overdose Caused Death," 1989). This incident underscores the potentially tragic consequences of chronic pain, especially where medication use (such as opioid analgesics or anxiolytics) is involved. People also tend to maintain idealized images of sport heroes and don't want to see these images tarnished. Many baseball fans may simply prefer not to know that baseball legend Mickey Mantle has been unable at times to play golf or even walk steps because of the lingering consequences of his sport injuries. Fortunately, with a vigorous rehabilitation program he can continue to play golf and engage in other normal activities (Cinque, 1989).

Enthusiastic and skilled recreational athletes are greater in number than their elite counterparts, and as a consequence larger numbers of recreational athletes suffer chronic pain. Among this group are potentially elite individuals whose athletic abilities have gone unrealized as a consequence of injury. Among the many whose athletic talents are modest, sport may still play a highly valued role. This group is vast in number, with participation estimates in the United States of 26 million in swimming, 17 million in running, 20 million in bicycling, and 28 million in aerobic or related exercise programs (Koplan, Siscovick, & Goldbaum, 1985). Practitioners typically observe the loss of this valued recreational activity as part of the overall presentation of chronic pain in the general medical population. However, this loss pales in comparison to the loss of ability to be gainfully employed, which is a frequent consequence of chronic pain. Inability to compete in sport, to hunt or fish, or to engage in recreational activities with children can be sorely felt. Consequently, returning a patient to enjoyable recreational sport activity is an important aspect of treatment.

Malingering

A sports medicine professional will face no more difficult and potentially disruptive situation than the prospect of a malingering athlete. It is difficult to know with certainty that a given situation is in fact malingering and not a misdiagnosis. Misdiagnosis may occur when problems such as myofascial pain syndrome or sympathetically maintained pain syndromes occur secondary to injury (see chapter 17 for more information). Because malingering is such a compelling condemnation, the falsely accused athlete stands to be devastated emotionally and the treatment relationship undermined, perhaps irreparably. But if malingering is in fact occurring and is not addressed, a significant behavior problem is allowed to continue. Even when malingering is present and is confronted appropriately, it constitutes a significant treatment challenge, a problem made all the more complicated because this term is both overused and misunderstood. *Malingering* tends to be generically applied to a variety of situations in which recovery from injury is fraught with problems, medical evaluation deviates from patient report, or the patient is resistant or uncooperative. In fact, each of the problems in rehabilitation presented earlier in this chapter tends to raise suspicion of malingering.

The DSM-III-R of the American Psychiatric Association (1987) defines malingering as the intentional production or gross exaggeration of symptoms motivated by external incentives for personal gain. Unfortunately, *malingering* is frequently and erroneously used to describe any illness that appears to have a significant psychological component. Malingering is mistakenly used to refer to a factitious disorder for which symptoms are intentionally produced but in the absence of external incentives and without a clear understanding on the part of the individual as to the motivation for the behavior (see chapter 14, situation 4, "Dealing With Fear of Success," for an example). *Malingering* is also used incorrectly in reference to the broad category of somatoform disorders, in which there is a significant interplay between somatic and psychological symptoms but with which intentional symptom production and motivation for gain are absent.

Overuse of the term *malingering* fails to provide adequate recognition for the broad role that psychological factors may play in contributing to problems in injury rehabilitation. The term explicitly suggests that there is no physical problem and that the athlete is not motivated to rehabilitate or return to play. From this follows the assumption that further treatment is not indicated, when in fact a problem may exist for which there are appropriate psychological interventions.

Malingering is most frequently seen in prison and military populations. Although its incidence in the general medical population is low, it is observed in workers' compensation injury and motor vehicle accidents where litigation and other financial incentives are present. Its presence in sport population has been noted (Ogilvie & Tutko, 1966; Rotella & Heil, 1991). In this setting it is assumed by these researchers to be motivated either by fear or by the need for attention. It is used by athletes who have learned from experience that they can use complaints of pain and injury to their advantage: They may gain relief from the drudgery of practice or avoid a feared or otherwise undesirable situation. Malingering may even be used by gifted athletes who realize that even if their motivations are discovered their behavior will be tolerated because of their outstanding athletic talents and their importance in future contests.

Diagnostic strategies based on client behavior, psychological testing, and physical examination have been devised (Staats & Reynolds, 1990), but their use is controversial. Specialized approaches to physical examination have been devised to help the physician better understand the large gap between uncomplicated organic disease and malingering. The work of Waddell, McCulloch, Kummel, and Venner (1980) on nonorganic physical signs in low-back pain is one such example.

Once treatment providers have ruled out all alternative explanations, they should initially deal with malingering as a "crisis of trust" (Ogilvie & Tutko, 1966). The recommended treatment approach is similar to that previously described for dealing with personality conflicts. Specific guidelines follow (Rotella & Heil, 1991). The treatment provider should

1. treat the intervention as an exercise in trust building;
2. acknowledge her or his confusion and bewilderment in attempting to understand the athlete's situation;
3. present concerns honestly and openly;
4. avoid attacking or accusing the athlete;
5. avoid taking the athlete's apparent deceptive behavior personally;
6. seek a mutually agreeable resolution for the situation;
7. clearly define boundaries of acceptable behavior (agreeable to coach, athlete, and all treatment providers) and consequences for their violation; and
8. follow up with a focus on reinforcing change in behavior to the positive.

Under limited circumstances malingering is appropriate and is actually a demonstration of adaptive behavior (American Psychiatric Association, 1987). One such possible scenario may occur when a young athlete sees no way out from adult-imposed standards of mental and physical toughness. As undesirable as such behavior may be as a problem-solving strategy, there may simply be no other alternative for a youth who is truly unable to choose whether to participate. In this situation, modification of coach or parent behavior should be the goal of treatment.

When intervening in a case of suspected malingering, a treatment provider must be prepared for the possibility of being wrong. I have had the unfortunate experience of being part of a medical team treating a patient suspected of malingering. Because there was a definitive and dangerous medical condition that appeared without apparent alternative explanation, it became essential that we share our suspicions with the patient. Although the physician sensitively approached the patient with the question of malingering and accepted his statement of denial, there was a disruptive effect on the treatment relationship. During a psychological consultation with the patient following the physician-patient meeting, I emphasized that when alternate explanations for a condition are unavailable, the physician is compelled ethically to present the question of malingering. I indicated that as health professionals, we had previously placed our trust in patients' behavior only to have this trust broken, and that these experiences had left us with an appreciation of our limitations in assessing honesty. Fortunately, the relationship between the patient and the treatment team was maintained and continued to be productive as this immediate problem resolved. Weeks later we discovered a medical explanation—a previously unknown side effect of a medication that we thought was benign.

Concluding Comments

This chapter has identified a broad spectrum of potential rehabilitation problems including minor treatment complications, muscular guarding, compliance problems, personality conflicts, traumatic conditioning, chronic pain and injury, and malingering. These problems may be precipitated by a wide array of factors ranging from an athlete's "no pain, no gain" philosophy to her or his poor understanding of the interplay of mind and body in injury. The relationship between psychological factors and injury is clearly a complicated one, and interaction between these elements can lead to a vicious cycle of mutually reinforcing negative effects. Specialized treatment approaches to the management of these problems are available. Although of narrower applicability than routine treatment interventions, specialized approaches are important because of the gravity of the problems they address. The specialized treatment skills upon which these approaches rely raise questions regarding limits of expertise. In some circumstances (e.g., chronic pain), treatment providers should carefully consider referral to a specialist and should explore the potential for a collaborative treatment relationship.

14
CHAPTER

Case Studies: Professional Issues for the Treatment Provider

Keith Henschen

With contributions by
Bruce Ogilvie, Robert Rotella, James Reardon, Wesley Sime,
David Yukelson, Deidre Connelly, and Shane Murphy

The genesis of injuries is a fascinating, multifaceted field of study. It is exceeded only by the complexity of how to work with athletes once they have been injured and are attempting to address their pain. Even as medical practitioners apply their expertise, the challenging processes of rehabilitation and reintegration commence. Concurrently, the psychological professional is frequently confronted with a number of ethical and controversial issues in facilitating an appropriate recovery.

We'll take a practical look in this chapter at the difficult issues relating to pain and injury that a psychologist might face, including limitations in use of pain control techniques, the psychologist's role in helping determine an athlete's readiness to play, steroid use and injury, methods for handling general fear, handling specific fears (such as of injury), and other health-related behaviors (such as eating disorders) and their effects upon injury. We'll use a case study approach to examine these issues.

Situation 1: Handling Fear

Marsha is a 12-year-old diver whose progress has plateaued because of her general fear of all back dives. In a practice just a few days before a major competition, Marsha executes a back dive poorly and lands on the board; she is not seriously injured but her fear response is noticeably increased. The coach keeps putting pressure on her to attempt the dive; on her next try she nearly hits the board. What would you do? Marsha exhibits excellent potential as a diver, but going backward is essential to her progress.

Reaction—Keith Henschen

Marsha is experiencing a rather common type of fear (a learned fear of harm) that usually starts in childhood and fades away by early adulthood. Because the athlete cannot wait for the fear to subside, the psychologist needs to accelerate the phobic reduction process. Because different athletes, problems, and situations require different treatment strategies, the psychologist who works with fearful athletes must be conversant with a variety of intervention procedures. A number of cognitive behavioral techniques are widely used to treat fear (i.e., modelling, systematic desensitization, stress inoculation, covert conditioning, systematic distraction, etc.). Each has its advantages and can be used effectively in certain circumstances. There is one feature common to all effective fear-reduction procedures—the athlete is exposed to the fear-eliciting stimuli.

Reaction—Robert Rotella

The most important information I would gather relates to Marsha's level of fear. How fearfully has she responded to pressure from the coach in the past? Does she focus and easily use the occasion, or does she get more scared, distracted, and tentative? Does she have a positive rapport with her coach? And, finally, is she technically ready to *consistently* perform the dive in practice? If not, it is foolish and dangerous to intervene psychologically for Marsha to try the dive in competition. If the dream is for Marsha to be great in 5 to 15 years, she must be brought along slowly, gently, and patiently. Total trust is crucial in diving, and anything that erodes it can destroy an athlete forever. The upcoming competition must not be made more crucial than it really is. I would emphasize having Marsha focus on executing dives she knows she can do, even if the lower difficulty will keep her from being the champion.

I would anticipate analogies being made to Greg Louganis's 1988 Olympic dive in which he hit the board but returned to nail the same dive a day later. I would emphasize the 15 years' age difference between the two as well as the inexperience and past success. Even at his advanced age, Louganis had time to physically perform the dive several times before his championship dive. It still took him years to get to this point.

Nothing is worth the risk of destroying a career, a mind, or a body at 12 years of age. Being able to deal psychologically with such a dangerous fear takes time and experience, not a quick fix.

Reaction—David Yukelson

Marsha seems to be experiencing a lot of pressure from her coach to compete too soon when obviously she is not physically or mentally ready for the upcoming major competition. Trying to live up to her coach's expectations may be causing her to tighten up, try too hard, or fear failure, which in turn may exacerbate the frightening situation itself and indirectly undermine her motivation, self-confidence, and self-esteem.

I would encourage her to set performance or technique goals that are within her reach and developmental capabilities, help her identify sources of stress in her life that may be undermining her motivation and confidence (i.e., social evaluation and social comparison processes, unrealistic expectations), teach her coping skill strategies, and make sure she is intrinsically motivated and feels good about her goals. I would also attempt to identify the root cause of her fear and isolate the point in her dive in which she feels she is losing control.

Situation 2: The Role of the Sport Psychologist in Determining Readiness to Play

Shane is an excellent high school basketball player who is a potential all-state prospect. Early in the season he experienced a back injury that requires rest in order to heal properly, according to an orthopedic evaluation conducted when the injury occurred. His back injury is sporadically painful but his family physician has prescribed pain-killing medication, which he uses as prescribed. His parents are very success oriented (especially the father), and they and the family physician feel that rest for Shane's back can wait until after the season ends. The family physician notes that her evaluation of Shane is the most current and indicates that on the basis of her knowledge of the patient (she has been the family physician for years) she feels confident in the current course of treatment. A psychologist with

whom Shane has worked closely for 2 years is against Shane's playing this year due to confidential information she and Shane have
shared, this being Shane's unrealistic desire to always please his
father.

Reaction—Keith Henschen

A person's reaction to pain depends upon the sensory experience of the
pain, the nature of injury, individual psychological factors, and cultural
factors. In this case the question is not whether Shane can handle the pain
but whether he should even attempt to play. Parents and physician seem
to give cautious approval to Shane's participation, as do Shane and his
coach (by their failure to raise any objections). The only dissenting voice
is the psychologist's. This is an interesting scenario, because if any of the
other characters involved (with the exception of the athlete himself) had
voted not to allow Shane to play, he wouldn't. Has the psychology profession progressed to the point that psychologists' professional judgments are
valued to the same degree as those of the rest of the sports medicine team?

Of those making recommendations, the psychologist probably has the
most crucial information on which to base a decision. The psychologist
believes that Shane is willing to continue to play only because he is afraid
that his father will be ashamed of him if he doesn't; Shane would prefer
to worsen his injury rather than disappoint his father. The psychologist is
probably the only one who is not so emotionally involved that her judgment
is biased. Shane, his father, and his coach all have very strong vested
interests that could affect their decisions. The family physician is a general
practitioner, not a sports medicine physician. She can legally prescribe
medication but is limited in her understanding of sport-related injuries.

After working closely with Shane for 2 years, the psychologist understands Shane's personality, goals, motivations, fears, and mood states.
The psychologist's decision is based on all of these factors as well as an
understanding of Shane's potential as a future athlete if he is physically
healthy. Since Shane has been identified as an all-state prospect, this
ability will very possibly garner him a college scholarship even if he
doesn't finish this season, but he could jeopardize his future if he aggra-
vates his back injury by playing out the season. The father, coach, and
athlete are thinking about the present; the physician's motive is unclear;
but the psychologist is thinking about the future of this athlete.

Reaction—Bruce Ogilvie

The brief description of this young athlete's situation reminds us of the
frequency with which we must hunt for solutions outside the sport experience. Frequently sport represents the theater in which family dynamics
are acted out.

Before medical or psychological strategies can be examined and a treatment program implemented, Shane must learn how to hold his father out of his life. I would ask Shane to evaluate the extent to which his father should intrude upon his goals and his personal life. I would ask him also to determine the extent to which he is obligated to fulfill his coach's needs and aspirations. I would push him to the limits in deciding what are his most valid obligations to others and what choices he has every right to make for himself.

To create an environment that will permit this course of action, a group meeting, where the athlete, coach, physician, parents, and psychologist express their concerns, will be necessary. Before this meeting, a first step would be referral to a sports medicine physician who would outline the probability of risk should Shane continue to compete. I would use this information to test the extent to which both father and coach are truly interested in Shane's welfare.

Should formal rehabilitation be determined as necessary by the sports medicine physician, parents, coach, and others should receive objective information about Shane's rehabilitation progress, because this will help them identify with this young man away from competition. Every graph, scale, or posted record of his physical improvement could be used to divert their attention toward rehabilitation rather than competition.

I believe that problem resolution is not possible without supportive family collaboration. Shane will benefit most by having a family that behaves as a true supporting ally.

Reaction—David Yukelson

The number one priority for psychologists is to protect the welfare of the athletes with whom they work. The goal of intervention is to help athletes gain control over their lives by providing them with skills that will help them direct their futures.

If the only reason Shane is willing to risk further injury is that he is afraid his father will be ashamed of him if he doesn't compete, then this should be communicated to his father. In most situations, parents mean well but do not understand the subtle pressures they place on their kids to succeed. Winning is too highly valued in our society, and all too often we exploit our athletes in pursuit of a winning season and the accolades that come with it. Shane is more than just an athlete; he is a young man who has his future ahead of him. Sport is not and should not be the only avenue in which an individual derives a sense of self-worth.

Situation 3: Working With Steroid Use

The Olympic Trials are in 5 months and Mike, a 27-year-old shot-putter who is the defending American champion, has just suffered a minor tear of the pectoralis major. He has a history of steroid use and now desires to gain strength again quickly. Currently Mike is moody and depressed and is separating from his wife. In all reality, the upcoming trials could be Mike's last attempt at Olympic gold.

Reaction—Keith Henschen

This is a very tricky situation. It is apparent that no matter what the advice of the psychologist, Mike has a very high probability of returning to steroid use. Mike feels that he can use steroids effectively to gain strength, and he has just enough time to complete a cycle of use that will not be detected by drug testing at the Olympic Trials. In this situation it is imperative that the psychologist not impose his or her moral feelings concerning steroid use on Mike. The psychologist should instead educate this athlete about the possible effects of steroid use and mental interventions that can be used in place of steroids to enhance performance.

Mike should be told that many of his current problems, including his recent injury, are common side effects of steroid use. He needs to know that strength gains do occur with steroid use, but that muscles also tear more easily after prolonged steroid use. Also, there is some evidence that these drugs can lead to violence and other potentially severe psychiatric effects. It is highly likely that this athlete's psychological and marital problems are related to drug use.

Reaction—James Reardon

A minor tear of the pectoralis major, though relatively insignificant physically, appears to be much more a psychological hurdle. Five months allows a lot of time for healing with no significant disruption of training. Mike's desire to use anabolics appears to be a reflection of insecurity about the injury, level of strength/conditioning, and ability to perform. This lack of confidence may be more significant than the torn pectoralis muscle.

The psychologist needs to discuss the side effects of steroids (especially muscle tears, mood disturbance, and overaggressiveness) with Mike in a practical, nonmoralistic manner. With only 5 months left to the trials, Mike has already established a strength base, and most of his strength work from this point on, is event related. Mike, like many athletes who have trained on anabolics, may overemphasize the value of strength as a component of performance. Especially at this late stage of preparations for the trials, even when substantial strength gains are made, there is rarely a commensurate increase in actual performance (i.e., throwing distance). Devoting excessive training time and energy to strength gain is to the detriment of other performance components such as technique, quickness, flexibility, and mental skills.

Five months of mental skills training may be more likely to stay with Mike and benefit his performance on the day of competition than a cycle of anabolics. Also, using steroids will not boost his confidence, especially as he approaches the drug test. Although he will have to be "off" anabolics for some time before the meet, he can use mental skills to enhance his performance during the meet.

Reaction—Deidre Connelly

Athletes' use of steroids for both performance-enhancement and cosmetic purposes is a behavior with which psychological consultants are confronted more and more frequently.

I agree that the psychologist must refrain from moralizing in his or her work with this athlete; unless the consultant realizes the dilemma the athlete faces in terms of the competitive realities, it is impossible to function effectively in this counseling situation. The necessary empathy will be missing if only the negative aspects of steroid use are presented.

An intervention that includes education about abusive behaviors as well as performance-enhancement techniques is appropriate. In addition, discussion of problem-solving and decision-making strategies will be helpful.

Situation 4: Dealing With Fear of Success

Missy is a 20-year-old softball pitcher who has a recurring thigh injury that does not seem to be related to her playing. She is an exceptional pitcher (or has been), but this year her injuries have prevented her from performing to her ability. The injury seems to get worse just before she is to pitch an important game. The trainers examining the injury are perplexed by the bruises which appear, heal, and then reappear again. But one of her teammates has noticed that Missy sometimes locks herself in the restroom (at night) and the next morning the injury is worse. The teammate even thinks she hears some pounding while Missy is in the bathroom. In conferences with the psychologist, Missy has indicated that she is very sensitive to social pressures and doesn't want to look foolish or embarrass herself in front of her friends and teammates.

Reaction—Keith Henschen

Athletes may face many different types of fears. This situation predominantly reflects fear of success but also includes some "fear of the unknown." Frequently the source of a particular fear is much more specific than the athlete realizes. Pinpointing the exact nature and source of fear is crucial for developing effective coping techniques. It is obvious that instead of actually performing, Missy inflicts injury upon herself to avoid her fears.

One solution is to confront Missy with the idea that her teammates and coaches believe that she intentionally injures herself and that injury appears to be more acceptable to her than performing poorly.

Reaction—Bruce Ogilvie

Whether her self-inflicted injury is motivated by conscious or unconscious fears, superficial behavioral manipulations rarely produce a modification effect.

Early in the counseling session I would explore the extent to which she is conscious of the psychological needs that her self-destructive behavior serves. The two most frequent causal forces that I have experienced with such athletes are fear of failure and fear of success. Though each results in the same self-defeating effects, the underlying psychodynamics are quite different.

I would want to gain the clearest possible picture of her early social conditioning experiences, particularly the quality and nature of the reward-punishment training employed in her childhood. I would do an extensive psychometric study before beginning the exploratory interview. If it can be documented that Missy is actually engaging in a masochistic assault upon her own anatomy, then by definition we are no longer dealing with a sport-specific conflict.

Behavioral goals and strategies have the highest probability of producing positive effects when the subject can confront rationally the source of her or his ambivalence about success or failure. I suspect that for Missy the process of change will be slow, because one does not divest oneself of such emotional baggage without a long struggle.

I have found that for such athletes, support from teammates and coaches in the treatment program contributes significantly to the process of change.

Reaction—Wesley Sime

If the psychologist confronts Missy directly with a statement that her teammates and coaches believe she intentionally injures herself, I think it could easily be too harsh and too threatening for her to handle. Apparently only one teammate has noticed the locked bathroom incidents, and it is simply not necessary or justifiable to present the issue to her with the implication that teammates and coaches all agree about the source of her injuries. It would be better to meet with her in an informal and nonthreatening way and to speak casually about the strange nature of the injury, thus allowing and encouraging her to unveil her problem voluntarily and with less embarrassment. Obviously, the psychologist may have to pursue the discussion subtly but persistently until Missy opts to unveil her secret. However, in so doing she may be reinforced positively by the encouragement given to her for seeking help seemingly voluntarily.

Situation 5: The Effects of Eating Disorders on Injury

Eschelle is an 18-year-old world-class gymnast who has recently had a series of nagging injuries that are not healing at a normal rate. For the past 3 years she has shown increased bulimic symptoms and moodiness as a major competition approaches. In addition to engaging in binge-purge behavior, Eschelle seems to be experiencing both intense fear of becoming obese and a disturbance of body image. Although bulimia is most apparent she appears to be suffering symptoms of anorexia nervosa as well. The psychologist, based on his assessment, believes that Eschelle seems to be practicing the bulimic behavior in response to her fear of gaining weight and also in response to a deep-seated problem of low confidence and self-esteem.

Her parents are very concerned about her, and parents of teammates are extremely concerned for their children. Eschelle is a little older and more talented than the rest of her team members and therefore serves as a role model; thus her behavior is very likely to be imitated by the younger gymnasts.

Reaction—Keith Henschen

In gymnastics today anorexia nervosa and bulimia are all too common. Anorexia nervosa can be of relatively brief duration and thus resolved or it may become chronic, which can be life threatening. Even with a single episode, the physiological damage to the individual (especially an athlete) can be awesome and usually leads to substantial injury. In addition to physical damage, social development and personal relationships are normally impaired.

Rather than concentrating upon weight changes, treatment of eating disorders should emphasize behavioral changes within the broader context of health improvement.

The potential severity of this problem calls for decisive action. I would counsel Eschelle concerning both anorexia nervosa and bulimia and their long-term side effects. I would also alert her parents about behaviors to watch for (e.g., excusing herself right after meals, or eating too much) and institute a "buddy system" (assigning someone to be with Eschelle constantly for 3 weeks prior to any competition). Love and understanding will also be beneficial.

Reaction—Wesley Sime

This scenario implies that the bulimic symptoms are "fact" and are well known to coaches, friends, teammates, and family. I will accept this premise, while postulating that most bulimics (athletes or nonathletes) are covert. Assuming that everyone knows Eschelle is bulimic, it is very important to help her analyze her behavior. Is there a rational explanation? For example, perhaps she simply cannot satiate her appetite to an acceptable comfort level without gaining weight that would ultimately impair her performance and prevent her from competing at an acceptable level. This is the most plausible conclusion drawn by a large percentage of maturing female gymnasts. Normal growth and development *are* incongruent with simultaneous elite-class gymnastic performance. For female gymnasts, the gradual increase in height and weight from puberty to adulthood confounds leverage, balance, and effective strength per pound, such that the difficult moves in world-class competition become nearly impossible to execute.

For Eschelle there may be too much liability involved in weight gain and competition. She should consider some sport-specific questions: What are you getting out of sport competition? How much longer do you want to compete? Is competing worth the relative agony of foregoing comfortable satiation of food? What options do you have in lieu of purging? Do you feel good about who you are and what you are doing?

It is critical to help Eschelle take on some new, challenging activities (behavioral strategies) to substitute for her bingeing and purging behavior. Eschelle could be drawn into a mentor/leader role with the younger gymnasts so that she clearly sees the influence she has as a role model, regardless of whether she feels her eating disorder is concealed or not. The "parent watch" and the buddy system should be used only if Eschelle can be convinced of the positive influence they may have on her success. In any case, Eschelle must consider what she really wants to do in light of her self-esteem as well as her health and well-being.

Reaction—Deidre Connelly

Eating disorders are no longer found exclusively in the sports that emphasize lean body builds; in the past several years I have witnessed these behaviors in virtually all girls' and women's sports, including field hockey, golf, basketball, and softball.

Confrontation followed by counseling is appropriate. It is critical that the athlete believes she has a trusting, protective relationship with the counselor. Informing the parents and assigning a partner to monitor behavior are risky unless the athlete wishes to bring her eating disorder out into the open and specifically desires external support. I would resort to such tactics only if other, more private means have failed.

Because these behaviors are often related to low self-esteem and/or perfectionism, the psychologist should resist pointing out that Eschelle is expected to be a role model for others on the team. The practitioner should instead deal with the overall confidence and self-esteem issues as well as eating behaviors.

Situation 6: Limitations in the Use of Pain Control Techniques

Jack is a 23-year-old All-American college football player who is in his final year of athletic eligibility. He weights 291 lb and is 6 ft 6 in. tall, with a psychological profile leaning toward overaggressiveness. Jack is in constant pain due to knee problems; he has already had an operation on each knee, and one knee needs another surgery. Jack's perception of his world, his relationships with others, his thoughts, and all his activities have changed significantly due to his preoccupation with his pain. His aggressiveness has elevated to a point that almost all social relationships have been destroyed, and he seems to be living just to endure the pain until the end of the season. Jack has another month left in the current season and refuses to have the necessary knee operation because he is convinced that he must continue to demonstrate his talents in order to be drafted into a high position. During a game Jack's current knee injury is exacerbated in the first half, and at halftime he requests that you, the psychologist, guide him through a "pain dissociation" technique (hypnosis) that he has been taught to use so he can sleep at night. Jack has never used this technique to manage pain associated with competition. You question whether using this technique will put Jack at increased risk for serious injury.

Reaction—Keith Henschen

Depending upon the psychologist's training, several kinds of psychological therapies could be administered in this situation, such as biofeedback, hypnosis, modeling, cognitive therapy, and guided imagery techniques.

Whatever the approach, there are definite limitations as to the effectiveness of the pain control technique, the foremost limitation being the ability of the psychologist. It is clear that hypnosis has been applied successfully to teach Jack to deal with continuous pain and that he believes hypnosis will control the pain of a recent injury. Even though Jack will probably be able to control his pain effectively with this intervention, the key issue is one of responsibility for the outcome.

Reaction—Bruce Ogilvie

There will be few occasions in the practice of sport psychology when one's professional integrity and ethics will be put to a test more crucial than the one represented by this case. It is difficult to educate graduate students and others about the pressures that can be placed upon the psychologist whose consultation services include the elite or professional athlete. The most important thing to remember in such a case is that any avoidance of one's ethical responsibilities in an attempt to keep an athlete competing can result in serious professional threats for the psychologist. I would not proceed with any form of psychological treatment without the absolute assurance of a qualified sports medicine physician that Jack's physical well-being was not in jeopardy. Once this *physician* and I have taken every action to educate Jack as to the responsibility that he must take for his own future, we will have lived up to the letter of our code of conduct. Should he reject our counsel, I would remove myself from the treatment picture.

Reaction—James Reardon

Like many athletes, Jack is so focused on his current situation that he is unable to look down the road. Some longer term issues need to be addressed away from the game situation. I would work with Jack on the increased fear and insecurity he shows in response to the injury. His fear of failure (i.e., not playing, lowering his draft value) overrides his ability to exercise judgment about his injury. Although Jack seems to have all the attributes for success (size, history of success, All-American status), he seems to lack the confidence that is essential in the long run. I would strongly challenge his belief about his draft status (i.e., that he must continue to demonstrate his talents in order to be a high draft choice) and his lack of trust and confidence in himself. I would encourage Jack to consult with medical personnel regarding medication only if they had already determined that the risk of more extensive/severe injury was unlikely.

Summary Reaction—Shane Murphy

This chapter presents a variety of intervention considerations found in typical psychology consultation situations, and it also offers us a chance to examine the sometimes very different approaches that different psychologists take to a case. I would like to highlight some of these differences on a case-by-case basis.

Situation 1: Handling Fear

Does the treatment of Marsha's fear really involve a "phobic reduction process"? As Rotella and Yukelson suggest, the psychologist must realize that the diver's fear in this case is realistically based. This is evidenced by the fact that she has nearly injured herself twice. Thus the analogy to a phobia (an irrational, suggested fear) is not justified. The psychologist's goals must be to help Marsha recognize her fear, help her understand how fear can increase the danger of injury, and help her cope with her anxiety so that she can continue to develop as a diver.

The consultant must be very familiar with the details of the sport context in order to identify the antecedents of fear in such situations and hence must work closely with the coach. Exactly which technical elements of the dive are giving her problems? How does the excessive tension of her fear affect the execution of the skills? Rotella hit the nail on the head here— "Is she technically ready to *consistently* perform the dive in practice?" Trying to eliminate Marsha's fear without thoroughly assessing her technical capabilities is potentially disastrous.

Situation 2: The Role of the Sport Psychologist in Determining Readiness to Play

If we examine the commentaries of Ogilvie and Yukelson, we notice an interesting difference in recommendations. Ogilvie recommends working with the athlete in order to help Shane "hold his father out of his life." Yukelson, on the other hand, suggests confronting the father and attempting to teach the parents what sport and competition are all about.

I would predict that the intervention suggested by Yukelson would be doomed to failure. As Ogilvie suggests, family dynamics are likely to intrude upon any straightforward intervention the consultant attempts. Although there will be no conscious collaboration, the family is likely to "sabotage" a well-meaning educative effort. A more systems-based approach on the part of the consultant may yield more productive results.

Situation 3: Working With Steroid Use

All three commentators recommend that the consultant avoiding bringing his or her moral feelings into this case. Unfortunately, the reality of steroid use in sports ensures that moral issues will impact the case. Because the psychologist is typically viewed as a member of the sports medicine/administrative structure, it is probable that Mike will never discuss his steroid abuse directly with the psychologist. To do so would be to risk sanctions against him as an athlete. Most often the psychologist will find out about the steroid abuse from a third source. If so, the first dilemma for the consultant is, Do I confront Mike about his steroid abuse?

The argumentative strategies suggested by the commentators are excellent. An additional possibility would be to take a realistic look at what detection of steroid use might mean to Mike. A guided imagery tour of the possible consequences of detection (as in the Ben Johnson case) might motivate Mike to refrain from steroid abuse. The psychologist must be sensitive to the competitive demands on Mike and must display empathy to his situation. However, it is virtually impossible to hide one's own feelings that steroid use and cheating cannot be condoned at any level of competition.

Situation 4: Dealing With Fear of Success

Once again, an interesting difference in approaches emerges from the reactions of the commentators. Henschen raises the question of confronting Missy with her self-injurious behavior. Although Ogilvie describes a more analytic and clinical approach to the problem, Sime bluntly states that confrontation will be "too harsh and too threatening" for Missy to deal with. A mistimed confrontation could have serious repercussions for Missy. Feeling misunderstood by the psychologist and perhaps by her teammates and coaches, Missy could easily drop out of sport and miss a valuable chance for healing. Left untreated, her inner conflicts may produce further problems for her in later life. As Ogilvie suggests, if Missy is actually engaging in self-injurious behavior, a clinical referral and intervention are warranted.

Situation 5: The Effects of Eating Disorders on Injury

The most important points in this case, which I will identify subsequently, have been highlighted by both Sime and Connelly. Although Eschelle's bulimia appears to have been triggered by sport-specific demands (the need to maintain a low weight despite passing through puberty), it is essential that the psychologist conduct a thorough evaluation with Eschelle to determine the roles of other life circumstances (e.g., family, school, peers) in her bulimia. It would be very unwise to treat Eschelle's problems differently from that of a typical bulimia referral; clinical treatment of such a problem is essential. However, it is also vital that the treating clinician thoroughly understand the sports context in Eschelle's case. Because of their important impact on Eschelle's recovery, the coach and her teammates must be included in the treatment process.

Situation 6: Limitations in the Use of Pain Control Techniques

The psychologist must act in Jack's best interests. If the consultant determines that an on-site psychological intervention (hypnosis in this case) would be detrimental to Jack, then this absolutely must not be attempted. I agree with Ogilvie that an amazing amount of pressure can be put on the psychologist for a "quick fix" in professional and elite sport situations. The word *no* must be an essential part of the psychologist's vocabulary.

Concluding Comments—Keith Henschen

What is most intriguing about this chapter is the varied ways the reactors handled the different scenarios. In most cases the basic problem was eventually identified and addressed, but the manners in which this occurred were frequently quite different. This indicates that there are many avenues available to solve problems. Each of the reactors seems to have a unique style from which they operate. As the lead author of this chapter, I would like to provide a slight disclaimer of sorts: If more information had been provided in each situation, the reactors probably would have been more in agreement. The most important point to recognize is that a problem frequently can be solved effectively via various routes.

V
PART

Psychology and the Sports Medicine Team

The value of sports medicine for the mind as well as the body is being increasingly recognized. This section provides a framework to guide the physician and the sports medicine specialist (i.e., athletic trainer, physical therapist, and other rehabilitation specialist) in the psychological management of the injured athlete. A comprehensive team-based approach is recommended, based on three fundamental assumptions: that sports medicine is a multispecialty discipline that is well suited to a team approach; that all members of the sports medicine team play a role in the psychological management of the athlete; and that careful coordination of care will optimize treatment outcome. In the preceding chapters on assessment and treatment and in the chapters that follow, recommendations are offered for psychological interventions. Some refer to the psychologist specifically and exclusively, whereas others refer to the physician or sports medicine specialist. Still other recommendations offer direction more generally to the practitioner. In a given situation, each practitioner must identify his or her levels of confidence and competence and proceed accordingly.

Chapter 15, "Patient Management and the Sports Medicine Team," provides recommendations for the identification and management of pain problems, alcohol and drug use, and eating disorders; the chapter also offers general guidelines for building rapport and communicating effectively. As team leader, the physician has ultimate responsibility for the overall management of the injured athlete. However, much of the burden for the identification of problems in adjustment to injury has typically fallen to the sports medicine specialist. The skills each provider develops are based largely on intuition and accumulated experience. This chapter is designed to supplement and refine these intuitively based approaches.

Chapter 16, "Referral and Coordination of Care," focuses on the collaborative effort of medical and psychological treatment providers. The chapter presents a perspective on referral as a process that unfolds over time and merges naturally with coordination of care. Recommendations are provided for incorporating the coach and parent into the evaluation and treatment process, and specific concerns regarding confidentiality and readiness for return to play are also addressed.

The idea of athletes as a population at risk underscores the need for a comprehensive, psychologically minded approach to injury management that includes prevention, early intervention, and treatment. Such an approach addresses not only the psychological concomitants of injury itself but also related problems that precede and contribute to injury and those that may evolve as a consequence. For example, pain problems, substance use, and eating disorders are relatively common problems with significant psychological overlay that influence injury risk and effective rehabilitation. Although the specific focus of treatment is on the injured athlete, the team-based approach presented serves as a model for the delivery of services for any of the psychological problems that athletes may face.

15
CHAPTER

Patient Management and the Sports Medicine Team

John Heil, John J. Bowman, and Bill Bean

The physician and the sports medicine specialist provide the first line of intervention when psychological adjustment problems occur, whether in relation to injury or other causes. Timely identification of problems in adjustment and psychologically sensitive approaches to intervention greatly reduce the overall impact of injury. This role has traditionally been assumed by physicians and other health care providers under a broad rubric such as "patient management" or "bedside manner." However, medical health professionals typically lack systematic training in psychological intervention. Rather, experience has served as the teacher.

The purpose of this chapter is to extend and refine those skills that practitioners have already acquired through experience. Many will no doubt feel reassured that the practices they have developed over time are reflected in the science and art of psychological practice.

The initial section of this chapter describes broad-based considerations regarding psychological triage and management. This is oriented to physicians, recognizing their leadership role on the medical team and their overall responsibility for treatment planning and decision making. The subsequent section, which focuses on developing rapport and communication skills, is directed to sports medicine specialists in recognition of the more regular and intensive contact they typically have with athletes. However, each of these sections is of relevance to both the sports medicine physician and the sports medicine specialist.

The Sports Medicine Physician

As an area of specialty practice, sports medicine is relatively new (Gayuna & Hoerner, 1986). The American College of Sports Medicine was first formed as a multidisciplinary group in 1954, with orthopedic physicians playing an important leadership role. Current sports medicine practice incorporates the full range of medical specialties and psychology. The potential scope of medical practice in competitive athletics includes the following (Gipson, Blake, & Foster, 1989):

- Provision of general medical care to athletes
- Treatment and rehabilitation of injuries
- Prevention of athlete injury and illness
- Evaluation of the safety of playing conditions
- Preparation of athletes for optimal performance
- Determination of the physical attributes of the successful competitor
- Drug (and gender) testing
- Provision of training in sports medicine

From a psychological perspective the physician needs management strategies for routine injury, injury adjustment difficulties, and other psychological problems found in conjunction with injury. Recommendations for routine management are provided in chapter 10, and the Sports Medicine Injury Checklist (see chapter 9) serves as a concise guide to identification of adjustment problems. Specific recommendations for management of pain syndromes, alcohol and drug use, and eating disorders are presented in later sections of this chapter.

The Physician and Psychology

The quality of the patient-doctor relationship is of great importance. It is related not only to patient satisfaction but also to successful outcome. In addition to providing direct medical care, the physician is also called upon in varying degrees to serve as an educator, protector, and counselor. The psychological management of the injured athlete is implemented as the physician fulfills these roles.

The role of the physician as educator is increasingly emphasized. The physician or sports medicine specialist who treats injury as a learning process for athletes by so doing encourages active involvement of athletes in rehabilitation, enhances their understanding of physical function, and helps them behave more safely in the future. Athletes need to understand the *what*, *why*, and *how* of treatment and to feel that their physicians understand them. Athletes often do not understand medical procedures and terminology, and when their medical conditions and treatment procedures are described to them they are often in a state of distress. These two circumstances can result in misunderstanding. As a consequence, treatment providers may need to repeat explanations more than once in order to be truly heard and understood. Graphic explanation of the basics of anatomy in relation to injury and the healing process, supplemented by use of medical illustrations and explanations of the methods of treatment, optimizes understanding.

The role of physician as protector is a particularly important one in sport. Injured athletes can face tremendous pressure to return to play before they are ready. It is essential that the physician be responsive to the athlete's personal goals in determining treatment course and that he or she stand firmly and resolutely on medical opinion in the face of challenge from others. The physician must also be able to keep the patient from being maligned by others when rehabilitation does not proceed as expected. Paradoxically, the physician may need to protect athletes from themselves, given that athletes face tremendous internal pressures to take risks and to return to play. National Association of Stock Car Automobile Racing (NASCAR) racer Neil Bonnett has indicated that one of the things he desires in a physician is someone who is able to hold him back when necessary (Neil Bonnett, personal communication, March 11, 1990).

The most fundamental dimension of the role of physician as counselor is in the cultivation of trust and a sense of support. This simultaneously eases emotional concerns associated with the patient's condition, and it builds the patient's confidence in the doctor. Carefully listening to an athlete's concerns and initially accepting these at face value build trust and confidence. The physician may need to take extra time and give the athlete a few moments to gather his or her thoughts. Simple things such as establishing good eye contact can make a difference. Once the physician has heard what the athlete has to say it is important that the physician not only acknowledge understanding but also to indicate what is understood, for example, the physician should reiterate to the athlete what he or she has communicated (see the subsequent section in this chapter on active listening for more information). In this way the athlete knows that the physician is listening and has the opportunity to ask questions or express concerns.

Many patients with complicated medical problems will benefit from formal psychological counseling. However, they often prefer to be counseled by their physicians, feeling awkward with the process of referral and with the stigma they may attach to psychological counseling. This can leave physicians with a dilemma in regard to the best use of their time and talents in optimal patient care. The degree to which the physician becomes involved in psychological counseling is a personal decision influenced by treatment philosophy, professional training, time, and personal inclination. Inevitably, situations will arise that require psychological referral, the process of which is described in chapter 16.

Managing Pain, Alcohol and Drug Problems, and Eating Disorders

The following paragraphs outline practical guidelines for the management of athletes suffering from pain, alcohol or drug use, or eating disorders, conditions that represent significant psychological as well as medical problems. Pain is a common sequela of injury. Alcohol and drug use and eating disorders cause a wide range of medical problems and are sources of injury risk as well. The associations of steroid use with soft tissue injury and eating disorders with musculoskeletal injury are the most noteworthy examples. Substance abuse and eating disorders may not only cause injury but may also result from injury. For example, the stress of injury may exacerbate a person's existing tendencies toward eating disorders or substance use (as a way of coping with pain, anxiety, or disappointment).

Detailed information on the diagnosis and treatment of pain and related problems in athletic injury is presented throughout the chapters on injury assessment in Part III and the chapters on the treatment of injury in Part IV. Although substance use and eating disorders are athletic problems in their own rights, an in-depth review is beyond the scope of this text. However, because of their interrelationships with injury, a brief overview is provided, and additional information is presented in other sections of the text. For a more detailed review readers are referred to Wadler and Hainline (1989) and Tricker and Cook (1990) for information on alcohol and drug use in sport and to Agras (1987) and Williamson (1990) on eating disorders. Readers may also review position papers by The American College of Sports Medicine (1976, 1982, 1983, 1987a, 1987b) and the American College of Physicians (1986).

Pain Problems. Pain management involves differentiating acute pain from chronic pain and providing treatment accordingly. In the management of chronic pain, the physician must draw on his or her diverse roles as educator, protector, counselor, and medical expert. The following list reflects basic chronic-pain management guidelines recommended by Fordyce, Fowler, Lehmann, and DeLateur (1978) and Romano, Turner, and Sullivan (1989). For additional information on pain and pain management, see chapters 4, 11 and 13. Sports medicine practitioners should

- accept pain complaints as real and determine why the athlete hurts, not whether he or she hurts;
- remember that pain is a sensory and emotional experience;
- avoid a bipolar conceptualization of pain (as either somatogenic or psychogenic);
- teach the athlete the difference between benign pain and dangerous pain;
- reassure the athlete when pain is benign (repeatedly, if necessary);
- reaffirm rehabilitation as a process toward recovery, not a cure;

- carefully differentiate situations that are "not a problem" from those for which no curative treatment approach (such as surgery) is indicated;
- avoid the use of narcotics, anxiolytics, and other psychoactive medications beyond the acute recovery period;
- prescribe psychoactive medications (when they are needed) on a time-contingent basis (i.e., at regularly scheduled intervals) rather than a pain-contingent basis (as needed for pain) and set a time limit for their use;
- be aware that pain-contingent schedules for medication and activity label pain as dangerous as well as something to be avoided;
- avoid creating dependency on modalities such as electrical stimulation or ultrasound;
- protect the athlete from invasive testing;
- emphasize personal responsibility in the treatment process;
- focus attention on what the athlete does rather than on complaints of pain; ask "What have you done?" not "How is your pain?";
- ask athletes about their psychological well-being;
- reaffirm commitment to the athlete when referral is necessary either to another medical specialist or to a psychologist; and
- educate coach and parents about chronic pain, as appropriate.

Alcohol and Drug Use.   Substance use is a societal problem of epidemic proportion. In the world of sport, drug use is a many-headed monster. The prevalence of recreational drug use, which has been widely recognized, is probably related to the adventure-seeking and risk-taking styles commonly seen in athletes. Recreational drug use also may be fueled by athletes' needs to manage the emotional ups and downs that are an inherent part of athletic competition. Ergogenic or performance-enhancing drug use, which is unique to the world of sport, is prompted by the desire to excel, which is at the heart of sport. The use of medications in injury also presents special challenges to the physician and the athlete because of the pressure for quick return to play and the willingness of many athletes to risk reinjury. (See chapter 18 for more information on the use of medication with injury.) The need to control drug use in sport has led athletic governing bodies to establish strict guidelines. As a consequence, even medication that is appropriate under usual medical conditions can be a problem for the athlete if it leads to a positive drug test.

Effective management of drug problems is based on an awareness of the symptoms of recreational and ergogenic drug use and abuse and an appreciation of the scope and complexity of drug use in sport. Recommendations to help treatment providers manage drug and alcohol use in athletes follow.

- Be aware of the tendency for athletes to deny or downplay alcohol and drug use in spite of overwhelming evidence of a problem.

- Do not assume drug problems can be solved by simply encouraging the athlete to say "no."
- Be sensitive to the pressures athletes face to use drugs.
- Be informed regarding the rules and regulations established by sport governing bodies that limit drug use, including medication prescribed for health problems.
- Be aware that athletes may have access to a mix of highly sophisticated and marginally knowledgeable sources regarding substance use, its detection, and the management of side effects.
- Establish a role as a drug educator and let athletes know that you are available for confidential consultation.
- Provide accurate information regarding recreational drug use. Overexaggeration of the negative effects can lead to lost credibility.
- Provide accurate information regarding the positive and negative effects of performance-enhancing drugs. Failure to acknowledge their positive effects can lead to lost credibility.
- Be observant of rapid changes in muscle mass or definition.
- Consider the possibility of steroid use when acute soft tissue injuries occur during routine performance.
- Be wary of athletes who present unusual symptomatic complaints and request specific medications; they may be attempting to manage side effects of illicit substance use.
- In choosing to engage in a drug-management program with an athlete, set clear expectations, carefully outline the consequences of failure to meet goals, and enforce all agreements vigorously.
- Make sure patients understand that you will not help them safely use performance-enhancing drugs under the assumption that it will be done anyway.
- When involved in formal drug testing set clear guidelines for positive results. Remember that everybody deserves a second (or even a third) chance.
- Be aware that drug testing may create an adversarial relationship between treatment providers and an athlete. This adversarial relationship evolves from the athlete's perception of the treatment provider's role as detective and conflicts with the expected role of protector.

Eating Disorders.   There is rising concern in sport over the incidence of psychological eating disorders as well as extreme weight loss measures. These practices occur with significantly greater frequency in athletes than in the general population (e.g., Burckes-Miller & Black, 1989). Weight loss measures that have been identified among competitive athletes include self-induced vomiting, fasting, fad diets, severe caloric restriction, restriction of fluid intake, enemas, excessive exercise, and the use of laxatives, amphetamines, and diuretics. These practices are most common in sports that organize competition according to weight class (e.g., wrestling) and that involve subjective evaluation of physical form (e.g., gymnastics, figure skating, and dance) (Thompson, 1987). Seriously competitive female athletes are particularly at risk.

In contrast to the isolated use of extreme weight loss measures, anorexia nervosa and bulimia are signs of a more pervasive and deeply rooted maladaptive behavior pattern (United States Olympic Committee, 1987); consequently, they are significantly more dangerous. Anorexia is marked by low weight, disturbed body image, and the persistent and false perception that one is obese, and it causes a variety of metabolic changes including amenorrhea. In contrast, bulimia is characterized by a binge-purge cycle and can exist across a range of body weights from slender to heavy.

Effective management is based on knowledge of the signs and symptoms of eating disorders and of specific weight loss practices used by athletes. A list of recommendations for practitioners follows.

- Be aware of the sports in which eating disorders and weight loss practices are most common.
- Appreciate pressures within sport that may lead an athlete to seek shortcuts to the ideal body or use extreme weight loss measures.
- Appreciate the societal pressures on women to have thin bodies.
- Be aware that eating disorders may be found in men as well as women.
- Understand the addicting nature of eating disorders and the prevalence of significant denial.
- Adopt the role of educator regarding nutrition and weight control for athletes.
- Present a balanced perspective on the benefits of weight reduction and the costs of excessive weight loss.
- Consider routine monitoring of body weight in high-risk sports.
- Be attentive to athletes whose body weights are notably low.
- Be concerned with proper nutrition when problems with stress fractures recur.
- Be attentive to signs of vomiting including deterioration of teeth enamel or the odor of vomitus on breath or clothing.
- Casually assess body image when an eating disorder is suspected.
- Work to become established as a person with whom athletes can discuss problems confidentially.
- Express concern and offer help where there is compelling evidence of eating disorders or extreme weight loss measures.
- Consider withholding the athlete from competition as a choice of last resort when other efforts at management have failed.

Eating disorders and problems with pain and substance use are multifaceted, showing significant overlay between psychological and physical factors. The role of the sport physician in prevention and early intervention is of great importance. When medical management does not yield satisfactory results, the physician should consider psychological referral. Once entrenched these problems are best managed in specialized treatment programs.

The Sports Medicine Specialist

John Heil relates the following experience:

> "As a college freshman I suffered a muscle strain necessitating many visits to the training room for treatment. Upon the first visit, I had just recovered from my initial nervousness at being in a new environment and was resting comfortably with a heat treatment when I was startled by a yell. 'Yeow! Yeow!' echoed through the training room. My initial sense of surprise gave way to puzzlement when I realized that the yell had come from the trainer. I was not sure what to think but did sense a hint of laughter in his voice and noticed the lighthearted nature of the interchange that followed between the trainer and an athlete. Some weeks later while undergoing treatment I came to a point at which I anticipated pain and was feeling both reluctant and tense. The yell came at that critical moment—and the pain and anxiety were soon quickly behind me. I found myself laughing and feeling a lot looser. As many times as I heard this yell over the years that followed, I was always left with a sense of relief and appreciation.
>
> I hope this story does not lose its meaning out of context. That trainer's yell has always struck me as the right thing for him to do in that situation. It illustrates to me the highly personalized nature of building rapport and communicating with the athlete. I am deeply grateful for the help that trainer provided me in dealing with my injury problems, and I will never forget his yell."

The sections that follow examine the role of the sports medicine specialist in the psychological management of the injured athlete and provide suggestions for building rapport and communicating with athletes.

Treatment Roles

The story of the sports medicine specialist is one of a transition from humble beginnings to a specialized profession. In the early years of collegiate sport, the role was taken on by any of a variety of individuals including masseurs, ex-pugilists, or designated assistant coaches (Gayuna & Hoerner, 1986). Developments in athletic training since the 1960s reflect the tremendous growth in the science and clinical practice of sports medicine. In 1950, the National Athletic Training Association was formed, tremendously boosting the professionalism of athletic trainers and serving as the first organization to be devoted exclusively to the treatment of sport injury. In 1974, the American Physical Therapy Association formed a special section on sports medicine. The term *sports medicine specialist*, as previously noted, is used here to refer collectively to the athletic trainer, the physical therapist, and other sport rehabilitation specialists.

The duties of the sports medicine specialist who is affiliated directly with an athletic organization has been described by Gayuna and Hoerner (1986):

- Administer first aid and therapy
- Direct and supervise rehabilitation
- Manage training room operations
- Advise on equipment purchases
- Supervise the fitting of equipment
- Conduct safety inspections of playing facilities
- Assist with medical examinations and fitness screenings
- Make services available at athletic events

The Sports Medicine Specialist and Psychology

The sports medicine specialist often counsels athletes on a variety of medical and psychological health issues, especially those that accompany injury (Furney & Patton, 1985; Wiese et al., 1991). Furney and Patton (1985) surveyed athletic trainers and concluded that "while counseling is certainly not the principle function of the athletic trainer, counseling of health related topics is perceived by the athletic trainer as an important aspect of the job" (p. 297). The sports medicine specialist typically has the most frequent contact with athletes in comparison to other sports medicine professionals, which allows the specialist to more easily identify changes in attitude and behavior. It is also the sports medicine specialist who most closely observes the athlete's struggle with the rigors of rehabilitation.

Although well trained in physical approaches to injuries, sports medicine specialists are usually left to their own devices when it comes to treating "bruised" egos or "wounded" pride. Furney and Patton (1985) suggested that training institutions need to address the counseling function more directly and to provide appropriate curriculum offerings. Recommendations regarding training have been provided by Yukelson (1986) and Wiese and Weiss (1987). A collaborative relationship with the sport psychologist can enhance the counseling function of the sports medicine specialist and provide greater quality of care for the athlete.

Building Rapport and Communicating Effectively

Rapport building and communication are the foundation of a good thera-peutic relationship. Rapport, the feeling of being comfortable or in harmony with another person, is usually established when one person communicates a sense of interest or caring for the other. Communication is the process of sending and receiving information. As a counselor, the sports medicine specialist usually must be a good listener or receiver, allowing the athlete to do most of the sending. Active listening and matching sensory language are two techniques that enhance listening skills by helping the sender know that he or she is being understood. A third method, utilization, is a means of encouraging the athlete's involvement in the therapeutic process and setting up positive expectations regarding outcome.

Active Listening. Active listening was originally developed by Carl Rogers (1951) as a counseling tool to help the client stay tuned into his or her feelings while sensing that the listener understands those feelings. It requires the listener to be an active partner in the communication process by "feeding back" her or his understanding of the message just received from the "sender" for verification. The therapeutic benefits of being listened to in this manner are well documented and can form the foundation of a helping relationship (Rogers, 1951; Gordon, 1970). An excellent presentation of this active listening process is provided by Gor-don (1970).

It is important that the sports medicine specialist pay particular atten-tion to staying in the athlete's time orientation when paraphrasing or doing active listening. For example, if the athlete says, "I'm never going to get this cast off" (future orientation), then the paraphrase could be "you're really wondering if this break will ever heal" (future orientation). By using such language, the sports medicine specialist communicates to the athlete that he or she is not trying to change the athlete's feelings (i.e., "you may feel this way now but wait until tomorrow and you will feel better") but is legitimately interested in accepting the athlete and under-standing the athlete's feelings.

A useful mnemonic for assessing the athlete's emotional response to injury is ALPS: Ask how the athlete is doing; Listen for clues about feelings; Paraphrase feelings; Stay in the athlete's time orientation. This procedure encourages the athlete to provide the "feeling data" that the specialist can use to understand the athlete's emotions.

Matching Sensory Language. Matching sensory language is a process in neurolinguistic programming (NLP) that is designed to build a common bond between sender and receiver, thus increasing a sense of rapport. NLP is a model for communication designed by Richard Bandler and John Grinder based upon their observation of master therapists. A main tenet of NLP is that people store and process information using one of three sensory modalities (seeing, hearing, feeling) as a primary channel. NLP assumes that through choice of language a person's preferred sensory frame of reference is revealed. For example, a person who uses phrases like "get the picture," "see to it," or "in view of" most likely processes information in a predominantly visual way. Phrases such as "loud and clear," "manner of speaking," or "rings a bell" typify the descriptive statements of a person whose primary channel is auditory. Finally, a person whose primary modality is kinesthetic (feeling) uses such phrases as "come to grips with it," "tickles my fancy," or "sharp as a tack."

In matching sensory language, the listener identifies the sender's primary modality and then responds with feedback using phrases from the same modality. This encourages a sender to be free and expressive in his or her communication style, thus facilitating the building of rapport.

Utilization Techniques.   By refraining from trying to change the athlete's viewpoint immediately, the sports medicine specialist communicates acceptance of the athlete's feelings as valid. This does not necessarily imply agreement with the athlete's beliefs or attitudes. By creating this atmosphere of acceptance (i.e., what you are doing/feeling/saying now is right for you now), the sports medicine specialist sets the stage for employing utilization technique. This technique was developed by Milton Erickson (Rossi, 1980) and was described by Stephen Gilligan (1987) as follows:

> Accepting behavior allows it to be therapeutically *utilized*. To do this, the therapist generally conveys to the client that "What you are doing right now is exactly that which will allow you to do (X)." The therapist assumes that the (specified) desired state will follow naturally from the present state, and thus generates communicational strategies based on aspects of the client's reality (e.g., present behavior, beliefs, limits, assets, memories). (p. 92)

Thus, the utilization technique is a process of pacing change in the athlete's behaviors and feelings by first feeding back information about his or her present state and then leading the athlete toward a desired state or feeling. The specialist does this by suggesting that the desired change is consistent with the athlete's present state. The following conversation between the athlete and the sports medicine specialist (SMS) demonstrates this approach:

Athlete: This exercise really kills me!

SMS: Yeah, it's a real pain!

Athlete: You said it, and I can't believe it's only 8 lb. I used to handle 90 lb with ease.

SMS: It really is blowing your mind that you are at this level.

Athlete: It sure is, and what really bugs me is that it seems like I've been at this level forever.

SMS: And you really don't know how quickly you are going to get stronger.

In this example, the sports medicine specialist utilizes the athlete's need to see improvement to suggest the possibility that the athlete is going to get stronger. The suggestion is made in a way that does not contradict the athlete's beliefs, because he or she really doesn't know how quickly strength will return. At the same time we can assume that the athlete is aware of having become stronger while recovering from prior illness or injury. Another thing to note in this example is the pacing of the indirect suggestion, which was interjected after the specialist provided direct feedback, did not suggest change.

Another example of the utilization technique employed with a healthy athlete follows:

Athlete: I'm learning some relaxation techniques to help me prepare myself mentally for the game.

SMS (While taping the athlete's ankle): Sounds like you are into something new.

Athlete: Yeah, I'm pretty turned on to this new stuff. Can't you feel my leg is more relaxed?

SMS (While holding the athlete's leg): Your leg sure does feel heavier and your arms are very still.

Athlete: I'm feeling pretty relaxed already.

SMS: You are feeling relaxed.

Athlete: Yeah.

SMS: And you can relax as deeply as you need to, to get yourself mentally ready.

In this scenario, the sports medicine specialist paces feedback not only by listening to the athlete's statements but also by observing the athlete's body posture and position. Employing the utilization technique is an ongoing process of observing, accepting, and utilizing the athlete's verbal and physical responses.

Pacing the athlete's behavior or feelings produces a sense of trust and understanding only when done sensitively and naturally. Mimicking a behavior or repeating an athlete's exact words will generally produce discomfort and undermine rapport, under which conditions an athlete will usually not accept a "leading" statement regarding change. It may be helpful to remember that pacing and feedback are common behaviors in which people engage naturally when they are engrossed in conversation.

Gilligan (1987) described three factors that can account for lack of success with utilization techniques:

> First, sufficient rapport may not be present: the client perhaps doesn't trust or feel in tune with the therapist, and consequently will not follow suggestions by the latter. Second, leading communications may specify some experience or behavior(s) too different from the present state; thus, the client may be willing but unable to oblige the therapist. Hence, a series of intermediary steps generally need to be sequenced. Third, the specified state may be inconsistent with the client's experience, values, or beliefs. In such cases, the client may be able but unwilling to follow directives. (p. 94)

Sports medicine specialists are faced daily with demands by both healthy and injured athletes that require specialists to attend to minds as well as muscle. By training in active listening, matching sensory language, and utilization technique, sports medicine specialists can better "get in touch with" (or "give an ear to" or "get a picture of") their natural abilities to use these methods.

Concluding Comments

The roles of the physician and sports medicine specialist in the psychological management of both healthy and injured athletes are of great importance. A psychologically sensitive approach to the injured athlete enhances trust, builds confidence, and minimizes distress. The degree to which this also expedites recovery is an interesting but unanswered question. The sports medicine specialist and physician have long assumed the role of counselor on a broad range of health issues including psychological problems. A collaborative interaction between the psychologist, the sports medicine specialist, and the physician enhances the effectiveness of patient management, especially with challenging patients. This is one more, albeit indirect, way in which the psychologist can contribute to the well-being of the injured athlete. The increasing prevalence of a team approach to treatment and the growing presence of the sport psychologist help make this collaboration a reality.

16
CHAPTER

Referral and Coordination of Care

John Heil

Bringing psychological considerations into medical treatment is essential, but it alone is not enough. Treatment providers must also be prepared to make timely and effective psychological referral, and to integrate coach, parent, and significant others into the treatment plan. This is accomplished most easily where ongoing working relationships exist among the core members of the sports medicine team—the physician, the sports medicine specialist, the sport psychologist, and the clinical psychologist. The way in which referral is introduced (by the physician or other member of the sports medicine team) will influence the likelihood of follow-through and the ultimate effectiveness of treatment. The athlete who is mentally prepared for and receptive to psychological treatment will experience greater gains more quickly than one who is reluctant or resistant. Coordination of care is a natural extension of referral and is based on ongoing communication among members of the treatment team.

Coaches and parents have been described as members of the extended treatment team (see chapter 1), because they exert a great deal of influence on the athlete. The degree of influence is a function primarily of the nature of the sport environment and the age of the athlete. Coaches and parents are potentially important allies in diagnosis and treatment. In contrast, each may be a part of the presenting problem. Where the coach and parents are closely involved in treatment, the potential benefits are enhanced and the deleterious influences limited.

The benefits of a team approach are nowhere more evident than in the decision to return to play; multiple perspectives provide the most complete picture of the athlete's readiness. Treatment providers should consider medical status, recovery of performance ability, and mental readiness. Depending upon the specific circumstances, this may require input from the physician, sports medicine specialist, psychologist, and coach, as well as from the athlete. With children it may also be necessary to consult with parents.

The importance of the athlete's desire to compete in the face of medical risk is increasingly recognized. Whereas in the past physicians typically had the last word in determining whether athletes would be allowed to participate in sports, the final say is now increasingly placed with athletes.

In the team approach to treatment, it is implicit that information is shared among health care providers. Because of the important input that the coach and parents can provide in both diagnosis and treatment, they need to be part of the information loop as well. However, the larger the treatment team, the more complex issues of confidentiality become. What kind of information will be shared and with whom needs to be clarified in the early phases of the treatment process, and the rules must be followed conscientiously.

The Referral Process

Psychological referral is a process that includes preparation, actual referral, and follow-up with the athlete and psychologist. An initial hurdle to overcome in psychological referral is athletes' lack of understanding of what psychologists do and the psychological stigma of referral (Linder, Pillow, & Reno, 1989; Ogilvie, 1977). Although the stigma of the past is rapidly diminishing, misconceptions linger, and many people see psychology solely as a means for treating mental illness. It is more accurate to think of psychology as an applied science of behavior change designed to improve performance in health and in illness.

The approach taken in the management of medical problems in general, and in the psychology of sport injury as well, is skill based and goal oriented. Often specific behaviors or problems are targeted for an intervention that unfolds relatively quickly. This approach reflects the cognitive behavioral tradition, which has served as a foundation of sport psychology.

Although many physicians will refer for depression and anxiety as well as substance abuse problems, they are much less likely to do so for persistent pain or compliance problems (Brewer, Van Raalte, & Linder, 1989a). This is unfortunate, because pain and compliance problems are common in the treatment of injury, and tested psychological approaches are available.

Psychological intervention is essential where significant adjustment problems arise with injury. However, there is also a role for psychology with routine injury, as a natural extension of the performance-enhancement approaches that are gaining increasing popularity in sport. Continued practice of psychological skills (concentration, goal setting, mental rehearsal) can proceed unimpaired by injury, and the downtime caused by injury can provide the athlete with extra time to work on the development of these skills. It makes sense for the athlete to do so, given the stress of injury and the stress management potential of the mental training techniques. Regular practice of mental training helps maintain a performance-enhancement orientation through injury and helps prepare the athlete psychologically for return to play.

A growing body of research suggests that psychological factors influence the speed of recovery from injury and illllness (Georgia Psychological Association, 1991). Remarkable recovery in sport has been linked to motivation, attitude, and social support (Duda et al., 1989; Fisher et al., 1988; Ievleva & Orlick, 1991).

Making Referral

Timely, well-planned referral to a psychologist is an important element in overall patient care. With injury, referral may be initiated by the physician, sports medicine specialist, or coach, although for optimal effectiveness referral should be endorsed by the physician. There are two strategies for referral. One is reactive and related to evident psychological difficulties, and the other is more proactive and preventive, aimed at optimizing speed of recovery and limiting potential rehabilitation problems. Reactive referral represents a more traditional pattern of referral for depression, anxiety, drug use, and eating disorders. Proactive referral is more performance oriented and recognizes the importance of quick return to play; it is indicated where rehabilitation proceeds more slowly than expected, where personality conflicts arise between treatment providers and patient, where compliance or pain problems are present, or where return to play fails. Referral should also be considered routinely when rehabilitation is long or complicated.

Referral is most effective when treated as a psychological process in itself that includes preparation and follow-up. Preparation begins with a clear and candid statement of the reasons for referral. This statement is most effective when it not only assures the patient of continuing concern and support but also implies an understanding of and support for psychological treatment. Some athletes will interpret referral to a psychologist as implication that they are "head cases" or that they are suspected of imagining or faking their injuries. Others may feel that they are being abandoned. As a consequence, special effort should be made to reassure the athlete that referral does not imply lack of respect, failure by the athlete, suspicion that illness or injury is imagined, or rejection by the physician or other referral source.

When explaining to the athlete the reason for referral, the physician or other referral source should emphasize the performance-enhancement potential of sport psychology and the inherently stressful nature of injury. The purpose of treatment can be described as helping to apply the mental skills of sport performance to rehabilitation in order to speed recovery. Further explanation is needed where the athlete shows signs of psychological difficulty in dealing with injury. Simply stating that psychological treatment will help with problems with pain (or sleep, or "feeling on edge") is often sufficient. Describing previous referrals and success associated with them is reassuring and encourages follow-through by the athlete.

Following an explanation of the reason for referral, a brief description of what is involved in working with a psychologist can be provided. It can be indicated that the psychologist will initially ask about injury, sport performance, and general life situation and will then initiate mental training along with recommendations for applying these techniques to rehabilitation. It should also be noted that this is an opportunity for the ahtletes to speak to someone confidentially about worries and concerns associated with injury or other life situations. This helps mentally prepare the athlete by letting him or her know what to expect, and it also expresses understanding and support of psychological treatment.

After the athlete is prepared for referral, the most simple way to assure follow-through is to immediately schedule an appointment for the athlete with the psychologist. By also scheduling a follow-up with the athlete soon after she or he meets with the psychologist, the physician, sports medicine specialist, or coach can limit the athlete's fear of abandonment and rejection. This also provides an opportunity to review the athlete's experience with the psychologist, facilitating coordination of care and reinforcing the psychological treatment plan.

How vigorously referral should be recommended will be influenced by the severity and urgency of the problem. Evident decompensation, significant depression, and persistent suicidal ideation demand prompt referral. In less pressing situations, or where the athlete wishes to defer an appointment, it is beneficial to suggest that the athlete attempt some coping measure to see if the situation improves—and that if it does not, referral will again be considered. Although strong encouragement is helpful, the athlete who is well motivated and ready for psychological treatment will gain the greatest benefits.

Coordination of Care

Without systematic and consistent effort at communication among treatment providers, there is no true team approach. Referral and follow-up, as described in the preceding section, are the foundations of coordinated care among health professionals. Finding the extra time required for this as well as integrating treatment providers' differing perspectives are challenges inherent in the team approach. However, the general parameters of treatment responsibility, confidentiality, and decision making are relatively well established as part of routine professional practice. Coordination of care thus relies on ongoing communication among treatment providers.

Parents and coaches should work together with the sports medicine team for the good of the athlete. Sometimes teammates and other family members also need to be involved. Most typically, this involves providing support to help the athlete cope with the loss associated with severe injury. Recommendations for the physician and sports medicine specialist regarding psychological management of the athlete have been described in chapter 15. The following sections look at the roles to be played by coaches and parents.

The Coach

The coach is an exceptionally influential person in an athlete's life. Often a special bond, rooted in effective communication, develops between athlete and coach. This is illustrated in my recollection of a conversation with some fellow track and field athletes at Lehigh University about our coach, John Covert. It was an interesting moment of discovery as we all came to the realization of a common link we had with our coach. We were each generally oblivious to crowd noise at large meets yet we were consistently able to hear encouragement and advice from him. The coach typically plays a variety of roles in sport. In highly competitive environments, he or she is a key figure in a large cast of characters (LeUnes & Nation, 1989). The coach supervises the assistant coaches and the support staff (who oversee equipment and facilities) and collaborates with the sports medicine team. He or she must answer to the team or sport organization owners or school administrators as well as to parents, fans, and the media. The coach also participates in the activities of local and national sport governing bodies (see Figure 16.1).

In *Sports in America* (1976), James Michener quoted Frank Cush, then head football coach at Arizona State University: "My job is to win football games. I've got to put people in the stadium, make money for the university, keep the alumni happy, give the school a winning reputation. If I don't win I'm gone" (p. 324). Although the presssures to win as well as the intensity and diversity of responsibilities will vary by level of competition, the coach is always the team leader.

Injury Management. The coach is typically involved in decisions about injury and return to play and must sometimes make decisions without the

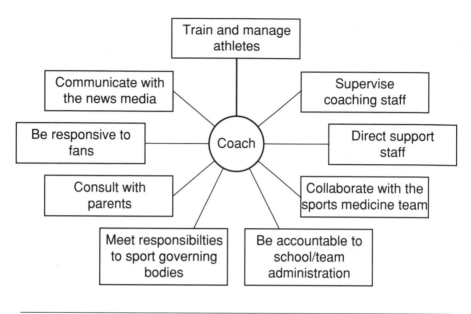

Figure 16.1 Roles of the coach.

opportunity for medical consultation. The following example illustrates how difficult the decision to play with minor injury can be and how damaging a poor decision can be to the athlete. The first time I saw Rick run he looked imposing, just as I expected he would, considering the numerous state and regional championships he had won as a high school distance runner. Then he reached back for his thigh, his gait becoming uncertain and awkward. In the years we competed together as collegiate runners, I would see him reach for his leg more times than I could count.

Toward the end of high school he had suffered a minor hamstring injury but continued to train and race in spite of flare-ups. Soon Rick began to miss training sessions but still competed in races. Unfortunately, he was talented and competitive enough to continue to win without training. He gradually fell into a pattern of racing and exacerbating his injury, then using the interim training periods to recuperate. In the process, he established an injury syndrome from which he never fully recovered. His college career was unfulfilled in light of the promise of his high school performance.

The circumstances of his injury—a relatively mild injury occurring in a situation without ready medical support—left his coach with the decision of what to do. In retrospect, it is clear that Rick should have been held out of practice and competition and allowed to recover fully. To this extent, he was a victim of poor coaching. Rick was also a victim of the risk-taking attitude that permeates sport and shapes the expectations of coach and player alike. He was not forced to race; he wanted to.

Daily, coaches make decisions like the one involving Rick, especially at the lower competitive rungs of sport, where medical care is less readily available. In addition, coaches' philosophies regarding risk taking, training intensity, and playing with pain shape athlete's attitudes and behaviors—and influence injury risk.

In the management of the injured athlete the coach has contributions to make in diagnosis and treatment. The coach knows the athlete and the demands of sport. The coach's perspective on the biomechanics of effective performance complements the sports medicine specialist's perspective on the biomechanics of safe performance. The coach can provide insight into the elements of training that may contribute to overuse injury and can often describe the circumstances of acute injury. The coach may be able to identify certain minor injuries through their impact on performance and can offer insight into the psychological impact of injury on the athlete. He or she can also create a supportive environment, facilitate ongoing team involvement for the injured athlete, and assist with the goal-setting and mental-training components of the rehabilitation program. When the athlete returns to play, it is the coach who best understands what is ultimately required for a successful performance.

Coach's Injury Checklist.   Because sport is such a sensitive barometer of psychological and physical well-being, the coach has a special perspective on the athlete. As an applied psychologist of sorts, the coach usually draws upon common sense and personal experience in recognizing and managing problems with the psychology of sport performance. The Coach's Injury Checklist (Heil, 1989) is designed to guide the coach in assessing the athlete's psychological adjustment to injury (see Figure 16.2). It functions analogously to the Sports Medicine Injury Checklist (presented in chapter 9).

The checklist is composed of two sections labeled "look" and "listen." The "look" section focuses on behaviors suggestive of adjustment problems that the coach may note through careful observation. It directs the coach in the systematic assessment of situational (e.g., reinjury, mental errors) and personal (e.g., fear, withdrawal, pain) factors that signal difficulty in adaptation. The "listen" section identifies key issues about which the coach may ask the athlete. These issues focus on concerns not readily observable that may interfere with recovery (e.g., worry regarding recovery, or inability to identify realistic goals or other life problems).

By using the checklist as a guide to inquiry and discovery, the coach can identify problems with adjustment to injury. As a general rule, the more factors noted, the greater the problem. However, the checklist is designed to be more than an exercise in information gathering. Conversation with the athlete should also function as an expression of concern for his or her well-being. Where it is necessary to ask the athlete specific questions, the coach should do this privately and unhurriedly; the interaction should be

Coach's Injury Checklist

Look

Situational:

____ Poor compliance with rehabilitation (exercise, medication, activity restrictions)

____ Rehabilitation setbacks

____ Reinjury following return to play

____ Mental errors following return to play

____ Failure to perform up to physical ability

Personal:

____ Loss (shows sadness or apathy; withdraws from team or coach; expresses guilt about letting team down)

____ Threat (often is nervous or uptight; shows outright fear at times; balks or is hesitant in key situations)

____ Overconfidence (acts unconcerned about injury; exaggerates past or future accomplishments)

____ Pain (complains or shows signs of physical discomfort)

Listen

____ Life problems? (sport, home, school, friends)

____ Physical problems? (headache, sleep, or stomach problems, or other worries about health)

____ Goals for performance? (unable to identify realistic goals)

____ Worry about injury? (uncertain regarding full recovery; concerned about making up for lost time; worried about teammates' or coach's reaction to injury)

Figure 16.2   Coach's Injury Checklist.

a cooperative effort between the coach and the athlete to solve injury-related problems. The coach may wish to relay his or her impressions to the sports medicine specialist or the physician. Where adjustment problems are evident, referral to a psychologist is suggested.

Parents

Parental attitudes and expectations influence children's performances and their enjoyment of sports (Hellstedt, 1988). Parents have an especially important role to play in injury prevention and management (Rotella & Heil, 1991). Parents are legally responsible for minor children and as a consequence are expected to participate in making treatment decisions. Although the scope and intensity of parental involvement decrease as an athlete ages, parents continue to play an important role into an athlete's early adulthood. The parents have special knowledge of the child athlete—just as the coach does—and can provide useful information regarding subtle changes in behavior. Parents should also be enlisted to help assure an athlete's compliance with medical regimens. Consequently, it is important to consider parents as part of the treatment team for practical as well as ethical reasons.

Problems With Parents.   The growing trend toward professionalism in youth sports can be seen at the lowest levels of competition, where some coaches and parents bring big-league attitudes to sandlot play. The intensity of emotion that parents display at youth sport events graphically illustrates the degree to which they can become caught up in their children's performances. Tennis standout Chris Evert has stated "I've never felt the pressure, not at Wimbledon, not at the U.S. Open, no where that I went through in junior tennis. . . . I still get chills thinking about it" (McDermott, 1982, p. 84). Nick Bollettieri, who runs a tennis academy for junior players, has commented that with greater sums of money at stake in professional tennis, parental striving and the pressure parents place on children have become more intense (McDermott, 1982). Similar concerns have been voiced about children's sport at all levels, observations that underscore the need for a balanced perspective on sport. The Bill of Rights for Young Athletes (Martens & Seefeldt, 1978) provides a useful set of guidelines for parents and youth sport coaches (see Table 16.1).

Well-intentioned parents can undermine a child's performance and health when their own vicarious needs for success take precedence. Expressions of disappointment by parents can exacerbate the emotional impact of injury on a child. Parental pressure can even precipitate stress-related medical conditions in children, most typically as gastrointestinal and dermatological problems (Adler, Bongar, & Katz, 1982; American Academy of Pediatrics Committee on Sports Medicine, 1983). Unrealistic expectations regarding playing with pain can cause relatively minor injuries to be worsened (Lord & Kozar, 1989). The potentially enduring impact of injury on a developing body is cause for special concern.

Injury can be as emotionally disruptive to parents as it is to children. As a consequence, in some cases parent management should be part of the overall treatment plan. Treatment providers may need to allay parents' anxieties, to counsel them regarding the impact of their behavior on their children, and to help them understand how to safeguard their children's health. The American Academy of Pediatrics publication *Sports Medicine:*

Table 16.1
Bill of Rights for Young Athletes

The right to participate in sports.

The right to participate at a level commensurate with each child's developmental level.

The right to have qualified adult leadership.

The right to participate in safe and healthy environments.

The right to share in the leadership and decision making of sport participation.

The right to play as a child and not as an adult.

The right to proper preparation for participation in sports.

The right to an equal opportunity to strive for success.

The right to be treated with dignity.

The right to have fun in sports.

Health Care for Young Athletes (1983) provides recommendations for counseling parents on a variety of issues related to children's health and well-being in sports.

Parents and Safe Sport. Because youth sport coaches are typically drawn from the community, coach and parent are often the same person. Even in the absence of formal coaching duties, parents are often actively involved in sport with their children.

   Educating parents about safe sport serves children in a variety of ways, including

1. injury prevention,
2. improved sport performance,
3. development of appropriate risk-taking attitudes, and
4. prevention of psychological casualties.

Of primary concern and of most direct relevance is the goal of decreasing the frequency and severity of injury. However, many of the practices that help prevent injury also lead to improved performance. Providing children with equipment that is scaled down to their size (e.g., bats, rackets, balls) allows them to use the equipment in the way that it is designed to be used. When equipment is too large or heavy, children will attempt to compensate physically and in the process can develop habits that are detrimental to both performance and safety. Less readily evident than physical injury are the psychological casualties of sport, which include the psychological trauma of injury, dropout due to lack of opportunity for participation, and burnout caused by competitive pressure.

Demonstrating safety consciousness sets a good example for children. Each time an athlete chooses to compete, he or she takes a chance on experiencing the thrill of victory or the agony of defeat. As children mature, they gain independence and access to increasingly risky sport activities. The way in which they choose to take chances will ultimately influence not only the likelihood of injury but also competitive success.

Preparticipation medical screenings and youth sport coaching seminars provide excellent opportunities for parent education. Specialized training programs (such as the American Coaching Effectiveness Program) and publications are available for the interested parent.

In *Parenting Your Superstar*, Rotella and Bunker (1987) presented a number of useful suggestions for preventing injury and enhancing the psychological benefits of sport participation. These and other suggestions for safe sport are summarized in Table 16.2.

Confidentiality

Confidentiality is essential for an effective treatment relationship and must be established as a priority. However, in the team treatment situation, practitioners must balance open, honest communication and protection of the athlete's privacy. The larger the treatment team and the greater the public interest in the sport, the more complex this process becomes. Treatment providers should discuss the limits of confidentiality and the benefits of coordination of care with the athlete and should arrange a communication plan that is acceptable to treatment providers, athlete, coach, and parents (if appropriate). To clarify how this arrangement will work, it is helpful if early in the treatment process treatment providers present to the athlete examples of the type of information that may be disclosed and to whom. Before reporting to other members of the treatment team following evaluation of the athlete, a practitioner can review the nature of the report with the athlete, discuss the athlete's feelings about it, and explain the specific reasons for sharing information. This process can be repeated as often as necessary during treatment.

Although rarely an issue in clinical or performance-enhancement interventions, confidentiality should and must be broken in some circumstances. These include circumstances in which there is significant danger to the athlete (as in suicidal intent), the athlete offers a significant danger to another, and there is evidence of child abuse.

Where a school or other sport organization refers the athlete for evaluation, the school or organization may expect to receive results of the evaluation. If so, the athlete should know this prior to the evaluation and should

Table 16.2
Safe Sport: Recommendations for Parents

1. Provide proper safety equipment, ensuring adequate quality and good fit of mouthpieces, helmets, padding, etc.
2. Match sports equipment to the size and strength of the child. Compensating for equipment that is too large or heavy leads to bad habits as well as injury.
3. Be sure the environment is safe. Arrange to repair or avoid safety hazards.
4. Limit the physical demands of practice and competition to help limit injuries. Be aware that fatigue increases injury risk.
5. Control the emotional intensity of practice and competition. A situation that is too intense can lead to poor judgment and excessive risk-taking behavior.
6. In contact sports, match children on the basis of age and physical size. This is most important at younger ages.
7. Modify rules to maintain safety with younger athletes. For example, limit innings pitched in baseball and body checking in ice hockey.
8. Modify rules to maintain interest and enthusiasm. This will limit dropout and burnout.
9. Be cautious but open-minded about mixing boys and girls in sport. Before sexual maturation, there are few true limitations.
10. Encourage healthy, well-balanced eating and discourage extreme weight control measures.
11. Have water or other fluids available, especially in warm weather. Encourage athletes to drink small amounts often.
12. Pay careful attention to your child's physical well-being. Have persistent aches and pains checked medically.
13. Be sure your child has regular medical examinations. Check with your family doctor or pediatrician about this.
14. Have an injury emergency plan. Know which medical facilities to use and how to contact family members.

agree to a release of information. Unfortunately, arrangements such as this can complicate the establishment of an effective treatment relationship, especially for psychological treatment.

In high-visibility sports where there is media involvement, the issue of confidentiality is further compounded. This is due in part to the enhanced reputations of clinicians who work with well-known athletes. A treatment provider should not even acknowledge that treatment of an athlete is in progress unless the athlete provides permission to do so. The provider and the athlete can discuss the pros and cons of the disclosure of the treatment to those outside the treatment team and can arrange a solution.

Return to Play

The most potentially challenging and controversial situation in athletic injury is the question of when to return an athlete to play following injury. The concert of factors to be addressed in this decision underscores its complexity and marks it as an aspect of sports medicine that is unique relative to general medicine. The decision begins with the physician and the sports medicine specialist, who determine when the athlete is recovered sufficiently to safely return to play. However, satisfactory medical recovery does not guarantee that the athlete is ready to compete effectively. It is up to the coach to assess whether the athlete's performance skills are intact. Then the athlete's mental readiness must be determined; the athlete who is not psychologically prepared for return to play is not yet fully recovered. This question is addressed in some degree by the physician, the sports medicine specialist, and the coach, and the psychologist's input is also helpful. Even though an athlete may be deemed ready by the sports medicine team, in the final analysis, the choice is the athlete's.

Athletes frequently must choose whether to compete in the face of pain and injury risk. As a general rule, the athlete who doesn't feel ready to compete is probably not ready. To compel an athlete to play against his or her wishes is a risky proposition from a variety of perspectives. However, athletes will often want to return to play as soon as possible and may overestimate their physical and mental readiness. For this reason the input of the coach is essential. That athletes will often choose to compete despite significant risk attests to how powerfully driven they are for success. For those who succeed, the achievement is all the more significant. This triumph over adversity is at the very heart of sport.

Andy Mill, the top American downhill skier at the 1976 Olympics, was injured before his final run. Rather than withdraw from competition, he packed his foot in snow to deaden the pain and went on to race, finishing in sixth place. Most consider this the top performance by an American in the downhill event at that time. Twelve years later his story was highlighted in a magazine advertisement ("Once Every Four Years," 1988) in support of the 1988 Winter Olympic Games. The text of the advertisement emphasized the value of success despite pain and injury. Andy Mill's success affirms that he made the right choice and all is well. Of course, this will not always be the case.

In 1988, San Francisco Giant pitcher Dave Dravecky underwent surgery for removal of a cancerous tumor. After months of rehabilitation the decision of whether to compete arrived. His physician stated, "We presented the options to him. Not to go back was the safest option, but it did not give him the opportunity to try" ("Dravecky: Fracture Halts Comeback," 1989, p. 21). Dravecky's comeback was ended when he fractured his arm in the middle of a pitch—the possibility of which he was well aware. His physician, emphasizing the importance of playing to Dravecky despite the risk involved, commented, "I don't think any of us are really dissatisfied with the decision we made to let him go back and try" ("Dravecky: Fracture Halts Comeback," 1989, p. 21).

That the athlete return to play and be injured is not the only potentially regrettable outcome. Heisman trophy winner Ernie Davis was diagnosed with leukemia early in his professional football career. His initial reaction to his diagnosis was "Now I knew what I was battling and there was something to look foward to—football" (Nack, 1989, p. 144). Controversy arose over whether Davis could or should compete again. Based on the medical advice that coach Paul Brown received, he refused to let Davis play. He commented, "It would be difficult to put a guy in a game who you know doesn't have much time to live. It was one of the saddest things I experienced in all my years as a coach" (Nack, 1989, p. 144). In contrast, teammate John Brown focused on how important football was to Davis. He stated, "My one regret is that I didn't have the clout, the insight or the maturity to speak up and say, 'let him play.' That bothers me to this day" (Nack, 1989, p. 144).

Probably the thorniest of situations occurs when the athlete is ready mentally and from a performance perspective but is at significant risk for reinjury. In situations such as this, the timing of the injury is a critical element. An athlete is most likely to want to take a significant risk when not to do so involves missing a key competition, especially one that may be perceived as making or breaking an athlete's career. The story about Andy Mill epitomizes this. A contrasting scenario is reflected in the comments of New York Mets pitcher Dwight Gooden on his decision to sit out the remainder of the 1989 baseball season because of injury ("Mets' Gooden," 1989):

> I'm just going to call it a year. . . . The situation the team is in, there is no sense for me to take a chance. If we were one or two games out, I would pitch. I could pitch now, but I wouldn't be 100%. Now I figure I might as well wait until next year and be 100% going into spring training. (p. B5)

Bergman (1989) has offered a strategy for the timing of medical treatment that weighs the importance of competition to the athlete. He recommends that before a key competition medical conditions be overtreated and surgical conditions be undertreated. For example, he suggests that antibiotics be provided to an athlete with a sore throat before culture reports are returned from the lab. Procedures that cause the athlete more discomfort than the condition itself should be deferred until after competition, whereas those that will increase the athlete's level of comfort should be performed before the event.

Richard Strauss (1990) characterized the role of the sports medicine physician as falling somewhere between the role of the general practitioner and that of the military physician, whose job is keeping the most soldiers at the most guns for the most amount of time. Strauss suggested that athletes will seek physicians who will help them get back to competition as soon as possible. He endorsed collaboration between the athlete and the physician in weighing the relative costs of injury risk against those of missed competition. The athlete is best able to determine how important a competition is and how costly missing it will be.

The sudden death during competition of Hank Gathers, an outstanding collegiate basketball player, as a consequence of known cardiovascular disease has brought questions regarding the assumption of risk to the forefront of awareness (Munnings, 1990). In the past, decisions about treatment and medical eligibility for competition were left to physicians, but courts have increasingly recognized the rights of athletes and parents to make the final choice. This includes athletes with sport-related injuries, preexisting medical conditions, and disabilities. In 1983, the American Academy of Pediatrics listed medical conditions for which limitations on sport participation were indicated. An update of these guidelines (American Academy of Pediatrics, 1988) shows more liberal standards of participation and a trend toward cooperative decision making. This is in keeping with the growing recognition of the broadly based right to participation.

The question of return to play is likely to remain both complex and controversial. The collective goals of the sport and the athlete will not be served unless those involved in sport are willing to take carefully calcu lated risks regarding athlete safety. Unfortunately, the decision regarding return to play is increasingly complicated by legal developments regarding the assumption of risk that place responsibility for injury with the coach and sports medicine professional (Lubell, 1989a).

Concluding Comments

This chapter emphasizes the importance of timely and appropriate referral as well as coordination of care among the members of the sports medicine team. Referral is presented as a process that includes preparation of the athlete, the referral itself, and follow-up. In addition to the core team of health professionals, an extended treatment team is identified that includes the athlete, the coach, and the parent.

This broad-based team approach offers enhanced quality of care through greater breadth of services and improved continuity of care. It also fosters early intervention in problem situations, given that timely treatment improves outcomes. However, there are inherent challenges in such an approach to treatment. Communication between members and coordination of care require a greater outlay of time by all involved. The issue of shared decision making must be attended to with caution, especially regarding the decision to return to play. A true system of cooperation and collaboration in treatment is difficult to implement. In the end it is only reasonable that those who wish to provide treatment to a team (in this case, the athletic team) should be able to function as a team themselves.

VI
PART

Biomedical Issues

Pain management and drug use are sources of great concern and controversy in sport, as they are in society at large. Although these issues touch on many aspects of athletic performance, they are nowhere more common or potentially problematic than in injury. Generally, lay and professional audiences have a poor understanding of both pain management and drug use. Misconceptions and inaccurate information concerning pain and medication use are frequently at the heart of snarls in the treatment process. The goal of Part VI is to provide a detailed overview of these topics. This material, which is a concise review for the physician, will be challenging for the psychologist. However, to work effectively with the injured athlete, psychologists must understand the basic science of pain and medication use. Just as Part V presented psychological information useful for the physician and sports medicine specialist, this part provides medical information useful for the psychologist. By thus developing an interdisciplinary knowledge base, treatment providers facilitate a team-based approach to treatment.

Chapter 17, "The Biology of Pain," provides a comprehensive overview of the pain-processing, nociceptive system. The chapter reviews the anatomic and chemical substrates of pain and describes the complex system of regulating pathways that modulate the transmission of pain. The chapter identifies common persistent pain syndromes including myofascial pain and sympathetically maintained pain, syndromes that often go undiagnosed and can contribute to physical as well as psychological complications.

Chapter 18, "Medications in the Treatment of Pain and Injury," offers an overview of commonly used medicines including nonsteroidal anti-inflammatories, opioid analgesics, local anesthetics, topical analgesics, muscle relaxants, and other psychotropic agents. Concerns regarding drug interactions are noted, as is the possibility of obtaining a false-positive drug screen as a consequence of routine, appropriate medication use.

How well pain and medication use are managed is an important measure of overall quality of care. The complexity and challenge of these aspects of injury management are a function of the overlay of multiple psychological and physiological factors. As a consequence these are rich areas for collaborative interaction between medical and psychological professionals.

17
CHAPTER

The Biology of Pain

Perry G. Fine

Pain is a private experience, its meaning varies depending upon the situation, and it is expressed by communicated behaviors. As such, it cannot be precisely measured or objectively assayed. At best, it can be relatively scaled, qualified, described, and perhaps experimentally reproduced. And so the study of pain processes requires an understanding of biological and psychological mechanisms, their interdependence, and their influence over each other.

This chapter will lay the groundwork for an understanding of the various anatomical and physiochemical components that constitute the nociceptive pain system. What will be most readily apparent is the diversity and complexity of this system. The model presented is based on basic animal and human research (in particular, on skin nociceptors) and on clinical studies of analgesic medicines (and the reversal of their efficacy by naloxone), neuroablative procedures (surgical destruction of nerve tracks for pain relief), stimulation-produced analgesia (direct electrical stimulation of nociceptive pathways in the central nervous system), and neural blockade (chemical blocking of pain by injection of analgesic or anesthetic medications). For simplicity's sake, it is clinically appropriate to assume that what a person says "hurts" (in the physical sense) is "pain," and the bodily system responsible for painful sensations is the nociceptive system.

Anatomic Substrates

The basic processing units of the nervous system are cells called neurons, which function like microprocessing chips in a computer. The main transmission lines to and from neurons and end organs (e.g., muscle fibers) are axons. Some axons are covered by a myelin sheath, which allows for much more rapid transmission of electrical signals than occurs in unmyelinated fibers. Nerves are bundles of neurons that form the roadways of communication between the periphery and the central nervous system (CNS).

The Periphery

The perception of pain is initially triggered by the activation of specialized pain receptors, called nociceptors, in many different tissues in the body. Figure 17.1 illustrates some of the anatomic components involved in the peripheral transmission of pain information. Most of the information to date regarding the properties of these receptors comes from studies of skin nociceptors (Burgess & Perl, 1973). Two types of neurons are involved in transmitting pain sensations. A population of slow-conducting neurons with unmyelinated axons, C-fibers, signals dull, poorly localized, and oftentimes lingering pain. More well localized and sharp pain is transmitted via neurons with the faster myelinated A-delta axons (Torebjork & Ochoa, 1980). Likewise, two types of receptors have been identified as the major units responsible for initiating nociceptive transmission: high-threshold mechanoreceptors with A-delta axons, and C-fiber polymodal nociceptors.

Polymodal nociceptors are so named because of their responsiveness to thermal, chemical, and mechanical stimuli. They have a relatively small receptive field, and following activation they maintain firing for several seconds after cessation of the given stimulus. Also, after initial activation, these receptors have a lower threshold to firing when exposed to a subsequent stimulus. This property is known as *sensitization* and may explain the increased sensitivity to pain, known as *hyperalgesia*, that develops after trauma to the skin such as sunburn.

Sensitization may also be a key physiological feature in the development of certain chronic pain syndromes (Roberts, 1986). Under some circumstances, groups of peripheral receptors or neurons in the CNS may become so spontaneously reactive as a result of stimulation that they no longer require a pain-producing stimulus to fire. This results in the perception of pain when, in fact, there is no pain-producing stimulus or event.

In contrast, high-threshold mechanoreceptors rapidly signal strong mechanical stimuli and have relatively larger overlapping receptive fields. The means by which information from these receptive systems is integrated and interpreted is not fully understood. However, each of these

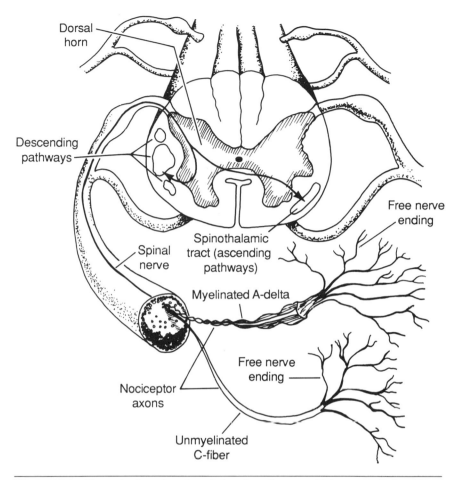

Figure 17.1   The spinal cord and peripheral nociceptors: Pain transmission fibers from the periphery enter the central nervous system via the dorsal root and synapse within the dorsal horns of the spinal cord.

specialized sets of neurons ultimately projects to termination points within the dorsal horn of the spinal cord. The dorsal horn, with its ascending and descending pathways is part of the central nervous system, which will be the focus of the following sections of this chapter.

The Central Nervous System

The central nervous system consists of the brain, the brain stem, and the spinal cord. These three large components are incredibly complex aggregates of discrete subcomponents, some of which are shown in Figure

17.2. Figure 17.2a shows diagrammatically how a pain signal ascends from first-order neurons in the spinal cord, and travels through spinal and brain-stem nuclei to the brain via the divisions of the spinothalamic tract. Figure 17.2b depicts the route whereby inhibitory impulses descend from the brain and travel through the brain-stem nuclei to arrive at sensory neurons in the dorsal horns, blocking (and thus regulating) ascending pain signals. Following sections discuss the roles played by some of these discrete CNS areas.

The Dorsal Horns. Although there are several spinal pain-processing centers, those in the dorsal horn merit special attention. Nociceptive information that reaches the dorsal horn region of the spinal cord is influenced by concurrent neuronal activity within the spinal cord (including that originating from non-pain-producing stimuli) as well as by descending pathways originating in the brain. That is, both local and remote influences combine to modulate the pain signal that originates in the periphery. As such, the dorsal horn region can be thought of as a neurosensory switching station, a concept that is the essence of the gate control theory of Melzack and Wall (1965). Though specific details of their original construct have been revised, the basic theory has withstood scrutiny. The gate control theory contends that neural mechanisms in the dorsal horns of the spinal cord that are activated by non-pain-producing peripheral nerve inputs serve to increase or decrease the flow of pain-producing impulses from the site of injury to processing centers in the CNS. This gating effect can inhibit pain signals before they reach those cortical areas in the brain that

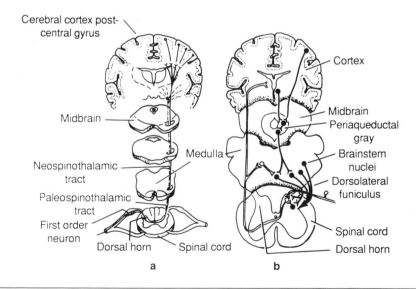

Figure 17.2 The central nervous system: ascending (a) and descending (b) pathways of pain.

register pain as a specific perception (see Figure 17.2). For example, a person can reduce the discomfort from stubbing a toe by rubbing the area around it. This tactile mechanical stimulation gates (or blocks) the nociceptive impulses. The theory proposes that at virtually all levels where sensory neurons interconnect (synapse), from spinal cord to cerebral cortex, sensory modulation can occur. That is, the "gate" can open or close, depending upon the state of concurrent input from multiple pain pathways (see Figure 17.3). The efficacy of seemingly diverse therapeutic modalities such as vibration, ultrasound, diathermy, transcutaneous nerve stimulation, and even acupuncture may have, to some extent, a common mechanism of action based upon this "gating" phenomenon. As applied to sport, pain due to injury or extreme exertion may thus be transiently "gated" by continued physical activity.

The neurons of the dorsal horn region of the spinal cord are grouped in several laminae or layers (depicted by dashed lines in Figure 17.3) according to their properties and functions (Perl, 1980; Rexed, 1952). For example, much attention has been paid to a population of cells within one of the middle laminae that is referred to as multireceptive or wide-dynamic-range neurons (Mayer, Price, & Becker, 1975). This is due to

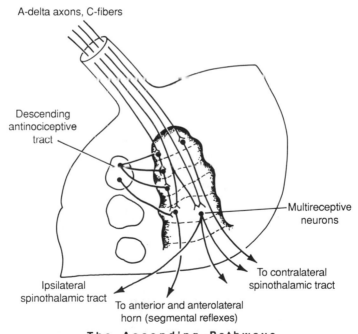

A-delta axons, C-fibers

Descending antinociceptive tract

Multireceptive neurons

Ipsilateral spinothalamic tract

To contralateral spinothalamic tract

To anterior and anterolateral horn (segmental reflexes)

The Ascending Pathways

Figure 17.3   The dorsal horn "spinal gate": A schematic illustration of synaptic connections in the dorsal horn laminae and formation of ascending nociceptive pathways and the descending antinociceptive (inhibitory) pathways.

these cells' differing firing rates in response to touch or to thermal, mechanical, or noxious stimuli. These neurons, like the peripheral receptors, may be subject to sensitization and as such have been implicated in the maintenance of certain chronic pain states (Roberts, 1986). Therefore, strategies that either prevent these neurons from becoming sensitized or that reverse this sensitization process are important in the prevention and management of persistent pain syndromes. The use of regional anesthesia for surgery, to block noxious signals from reaching the spinal cord, instead of general anesthesia is an example of such a strategy.

Ascending Pathways. There are several ascending nociceptive tracts that transmit painful sensations from the spinal cord to the brain (M.C. Smith, 1976). The spinothalamic tract, the most important pathway, has two divisions, the more laterally located neospinothalamic tract and the anterior paleospinothalamic tract (see Figure 17.2a).

The neospinothalamic tract is considered to be the more prominent pathway, serving a sensory-discriminative role. Thus, descriptors such as *pinching, burning,* or *sharp* might be used to describe pain sensations transmitted and perceived via this pathway. The neospinothalamic tract terminates in discrete areas within the thalamus (Mehler, 1967). Receiving neurons within the thalamus send projections to the sensory cortex in a direct and highly organized fashion.

In contrast, the paleospinothalamic tract is a more diffuse, polysynaptic, and indirect pathway that seems to be involved in the motivational and affective components of the pain response. Descriptors like *irritating, frustrating,* and *agonizing* may be generated as a result of pain perceptions evoked through this pathway. The paleospinothalamic tract is also responsible for triggering both somatic and autonomic reflexes in addition to activating inhibitory systems (Bowsher, 1976; Mayer & Price, 1976). In essence, the somatic and autonomic reflexes result in the body's preparedness for the so-called fight-or-flight responses. The inhibitory systems serve as a feedback loop that activates descending pathways that in turn tone down the initial pain signal. This is like a thermostat that regulates the activity of a furnace in order to maintain a certain temperature.

Multiple inputs (from the midbrain reticular formation, thalamus, hypothalamus, limbic sites, and basal ganglia) converge and ultimately reach the cortex as widely diffuse projections that activate brain centers subserving motivation, mood, and memory. So, the perception of a sensation (noxious or pleasant) is rarely isolated from an emotional response. In most acute pain situations, the contribution from this portion of the nociceptive system is short-lived and self-limiting. However, if there is continued stimulation of these pathways with maintained activation of brain centers that modulate cognitive and emotional status, significant behavioral changes may occur. This is often manifested as sleep disturbance, alterations in libido and appetite, and frank depression. So, a person may start with a discrete ankle injury and localized pain, and over time if the problem is uncorrected end up with her or his whole being "hurting." We need always to keep in mind the context of injury, because pain is so much a sensation with meaning. Knowledge of these pathways helps explain how this is so.

Regulating Pathways.   The study of ecology has shown us that built-in checks and balances are common in nature. The same is true in humans wherein the process of internal regulation by feedback systems promotes homeostasis, and thus survival. Melzack and Wall (1965) described such a regulatory system with their well-known gate control theory.

The existence of a descending (regulating) inhibitory system was first demonstrated through experiments whereby researchers reduced pain responses by stimulating certain areas of the brain (stimulation-produced analgesia) (Mayer, Wolfe, Akil, Carder, & Liebeskind 1971; Reynolds, 1969). Stimulation-produced analgesia has been found to be due, at least in part, to the release of endogenous opioids, which activates descending inhibitory pathways, blocking the transmission of nociceptive signals on the way to perceptual centers in the brain.

Pathways that originate at multiple brain sites (including the cortex, hypothalamus, amygdala, and brain stem) converge upon the midbrain region known as the periaqueductal gray (PAG). Fibers from the PAG project to the medulla, and form a descending tract known as the dorsolateral funiculus. This descending system ultimately projects to the dorsal horn, inhibiting the transmission of nociceptive impulses (Basbaum & Fields, 1978; Beitz, 1982; Mayer & Price, 1976) (see Figure 17.2b).

The onset of pain itself also activates this descending inhibitory system, forming a negative feedback loop. There is some evidence that physical or emotional stress can also activate this system, influencing phenomena such as "runner's high" and the placebo effect (Levine, Gordon, & Fields, 1978; Sachs, 1984). These phenomena are widely noted but poorly understood, and advances in knowledge about them have been limited by the tendency of researchers to explain them using simplistic models of pain perception.

Chemical Substrates

The nervous system is essentially electrochemically powered. Electrical signals are usually generated by the interaction of chemicals, known as neurotransmitters, with specific receptor sites on the neurons. One can think of the neurotransmitter as a key and the receptor site as a lock wherein there is a specificity of fit and effect. As a certain key fits into and unlocks a door, a certain neurotransmitter fits into a receptor site and activates a series of biochemical events. An ever-increasing number of pain-processing neurotransmitter substances are being identified. Definitive conclusions regarding the functions of most of these substances in the pain system are presently limited (Hokfelt et al., 1983). However, at least two types of chemical neurotransmitters, the endorphins and serotonin, are definitely involved in mediating pain. These are activated by noxious stimulation, which in turn activates the descending (regulatory) efferent pathways, which inhibit pain transmission (Basbaum & Fields, 1978), shown in Figure 17.2b.

The endorphins and their receptor sites have been identified throughout the brain, the brain stem, and various laminae within the dorsal horns of the spinal cord. Since the first endorphins were isolated (Hughes et al., 1975), a growing number of endogenously produced opioidlike substances have been identified. These compounds, as well as naturally occurring (e.g., morphine) and synthetically derived (e.g., Demerol) substances, act at specific receptor sites on neurons. These receptor sites, in turn, have been defined by their affinity for different types of endogenous opiates and the resultant spectrum of physiological effects they mediate (Pasternak, 1988; Yaksh, 1983; Zukin & Zukin, 1981).

Serotonin is found in appreciable concentrations in neurons within the brain stem in the medulla and in superficial layers of the spinal cord dorsal horns. Experiments show that blocking or depleting this neurotransmitter reduces the efficacy of opioid analgesics for pain relief and diminishes the amount of pain relief produced by experimentally stimulating specific brain regions (Yaksh, 1979).

Norepinephrine is a neurotransmitter that is usually associated with responses to stressful situations. Depending upon where it is injected or released, norepinephrine can enhance or inhibit nociceptive transmission and hence the perception of pain (Basbaum, Moss, & Glazer, 1983; Hammond, Levy, & Proudfit, 1980). Clonidine, which works by blocking the release of norepinephrine, has analgesic properties when applied to the spinal cord (Yaksh & Reddy, 1981). It can also block opiate withdrawal reactions when given systemically (Gold, Pottash, Sweeny, & Kreber, 1980). In the periphery, norepinephrine may enhance nociception and appears to be a mediator of "sympathetically maintained pain" (Scadding, 1981). This name is given to a set of painful conditions that seem to be at least partially perpetuated by input from the sympathetic nervous system. This condition is described in detail in a subsequent section.

One of the better characterized neurotransmitters involved in initiating painful sensations is substance P, which is present in the periphery at the source of painful sensations, in the dorsal horn of the spinal cord, and in other spinal sensory processing centers. Substance P is released by noxious stimuli and is inhibited by endogenous opiates (Henry, 1976). A host of other chemical substances act as neurotransmitters involved in the activation and suppression of the pain system. Many seem to have more than one function within the body, which causes a great deal of consternation over the way this system, and the whole organism, developed. Because many of these compounds are found within single neurons, it is easy to appreciate the difficulty of sorting out the interactions of this complex system.

Persistent Pain

Myofascial pain and sympathetically maintained pain syndromes may evolve as consequences of injury, causing increased pain in the immediate postinjury period and pain that persists beyond routine healing time. Although the causes for the perpetuation of such pain in the absence of ongoing tissue damage remain enigmatic, understanding of the causes and treatment of persistent pain syndromes is growing. It behooves those in sports medicine to recognize these syndromes early in order to support confidently return to play and to avoid any preventable disability. When these pain syndromes go undiagnosed and untreated, they may result in conflict between treatment providers (who suspect poor motivation for recovery) and athletes (who fear they are not receiving proper treatment). Athletes who are subject to recurrent injury are at increased risk for persistent pain syndromes.

Myofascial Pain

The myofascial pain syndrome is characterized by trigger points (localized areas of hyperirritability) that produce generally consistent patterns of referred pain (pain felt at a site away from the trigger point) and by associated musculoskeletal dysfunction (Fine & Petty, 1986). Myofascial trigger points (MTPs) originate in skeletal muscle or its investing fascia. Their compression via physical activity, passive muscular guarding, or direct palpation will generate a characteristic pattern of referred pain in a location often distant from the MTP. As a result of this persistently generated pain, the affected body area may feel weak, stiff, and immobile (Travell & Simons, 1983). It is postulated that the ongoing pain generated by these trigger points results from an aberrant reflex arc that is maintained by hyperactive peripheral receptors (within muscle or fascia) and sensitized neurons within the dorsal horns of the spinal cord (Fine, Milano, & Hare, 1988).

Myofascial trigger point pain is extremely common, and, though most prevalent in adults, it has been described in children (Fine, 1987). The most commonly affected areas are those that support weight and maintain posture such as the neck, shoulders, and low back. Many surveys have shown that up to 50% of seemingly asymptomatic young adults can be found to have latent MTPs. These restrict range of motion of affected muscle groups, and though they do not cause spontaneous pain, when palpated they cause localized and referred pain.

In the acute stage, a specific injury or overactivity usually accounts for the pain. In the absence of perpetuating factors, spontaneous healing may occur or an active painful MTP may revert to a latent state. Reactivation of latent MTPs by even minor exertional stress, mild injury, or psychomotor tension elicited by emotional distress accounts for recurrent episodes of pain and dysfunction (i.e., weakness, stiffness, and decreased mobility) over a period of months or years. Even relatively modest dysfunction in strength and mobility may interfere with the biomechanics of skill execution, undermining sport performance. Furthermore, chronic muscular guarding of painful areas can lead to the development of secondary MTPs in areas remote from the original injury, especially when the athlete fears reinjury.

Athletes who markedly decrease their levels of fitness and muscle tone often develop this syndrome (based on unpublished observations by the author and personal communication with other pain clinic clinicians). Perhaps this reduction of muscle tone activates latent multiple trigger points that have developed as a result of years of heavy use and actual abuse (i.e., contact sports, overtraining). Athletes who experience periods of prolonged enforced inactivity, as in cases of hospitalization and surgery, are particularly at risk. The vigorous program of physical activity beginning with the immediate postsurgery (or postinjury) period advocated by Steadman would appear to limit the activation of trigger points and help explain the remarkable recovery he has noted in athletes (Steadman, 1980, 1981). Similarly, many athletes note a reduction in "baseline" pain and stiffness with resumption of regular workouts following injury. This phenomenon may also be due to the release of endorphins that activate the internal pain-reduction system, as previously described (Fine, Milano, & Hare, 1988). It makes sense that warm-up, stretching, toning, and "cooldown" may prevent the development of MTPs associated with muscle strain. It is plausible that a psychological state that promotes muscular relaxation might also prevent pain by promoting greater muscular resiliency.

Specific therapies for the treatment of MTPs include ice and massage, stretching after the application of a vapocoolant spray, or, if necessary, trigger point injections with local anesthetic. "Stretch-and-spray" is usually a specialized technique applied by a trained therapist, and trigger point injections should be done only by a skilled physician. Muscular relaxation, biofeedback, and other mental training techniques may help reduce myofascial pain by reducing baseline tension in affected muscles. (See the section on muscular guarding in chapter 13 for guidelines on the use of these methods with injured athletes.)

In summary, myofascial pain syndromes represent a readily identifiable yet often overlooked source of both acute and persistent pain. Inattention or misdiagnosis can be quite costly, leading to delayed return to play and fear of reinjury as well as unnecessary medical interventions and tests, analgesic misuse, and long-term disability. After eliminating other treatable sources of pain, the practitioner should identify and aggressively treat MTPs with remobilization and activation types of physical therapy and trigger point injections if necessary.

Sympathetically Maintained Pain

Sympathetically maintained pain (SMP) refers to a group of syndromes characterized by persistent pain that is relieved by sympathetic blockade of the affected body part. Sympathetic blockade is the procedure of inactivating the sympathetic nervous system by chemical means, usually by injecting a local anesthetic in proximity to the sympathetic nerves. The term "sympathetically maintained pain" was coined by Roberts in order to consolidate the pathogenesis of certain poorly understood chronic pain syndromes under the umbrella of a unifying hypothetical mechanism (Roberts, 1986).

The two most common syndromes that appear to be, at least in part, mediated or maintained by sympathetic nervous system activity are causalgia and reflex sympathetic dystrophy (RSD). Causalgia consists of spontaneous burning pain, usually with the physical finding of markedly increased pain caused by light touching or gentle mechanical stimulation. Causalgia has been described most frequently in an arm or leg after nerve injury. Signs of excessive sympathetic nervous system discharge (e.g., cool, clammy skin), plus atrophy of skin, changes in texture and growth of hair, and depletion of underlying bone, can occur as the syndrome progresses. RSD is defined as continuous pain in a portion of an extremity, following even minor trauma, that does not involve apparent nerve injury. RSD may also progress with the same signs of sympathetic hyperactivity and physical changes that characterize causalgia.

The hallmark of SMP, then, is spontaneous pain and skin hypersensitivity that can lead to a severely dysfunctional and impaired extremity. The clinician diagnoses SMP using history and clinical findings and cooorobrates this diagnosis with results obtained from blocking the sympathetic nervous system. Once the diagnosis is confirmed, the clinician may need to undertake a series of sympathetic blocks and remobilize the affected part with physical therapy and oftentimes behavioral therapy interventions (e.g., relaxation and other mental training techniques) to alleviate and prevent relapse of the syndrome (Fine, 1988). Mental training techniques help improve pain tolerance and may ultimately reduce pain via their effect on the sympathetic nervous system.

It is presently held that the common mechanism underlying the development of SMP is an initiating traumatic event. This trauma, with its activation of peripheral nociceptors, sensitizes pain-receiving neurons within the dorsal horns of the spinal cord. Then, even after tissue has healed and nociceptive input has ceased, these neurons remain conditioned to fire either spontaneously or after sensory stimulation that would not ordinarily produce pain. The activity of these neurons is inadvertently "perceived" as a painful sensation. Even under normal conditions the sympathetic nervous system facilitates firing of peripheral receptors, which then converge on these sensitized spinal neurons, causing them to generate pain signals to otherwise non-pain-producing stimuli. Following this hypothesis, anything that enhances sympathetic nervous system activity (e.g., stress, anxiety, pain itself) will reinforce this reflex arc.

It is postulated in presently considered theories that sympathetic blockade breaks this vicious cycle and allows the function of all the components to return to normal. Therapies aimed at stress management and remobilization of the usually immobilized arm or leg help prevent the regeneration of the abnormal reflex arc. It is a mystery why certain people develop SMP at certain times and under various conditions. Though an "at risk" population has not been well defined, it appears that early aggressive therapy provides the best results for reversing the syndrome and preventing major disability.

Concluding Comments

The sensation and perception of pain are mediated by an immeasurably complex system that is further complicated by the fact that in the final analysis pain is a totally subjective experience.

Nonetheless, an understanding of the basic substrates of this system has led to great improvements in the management of both acute and chronic pain problems. It has also led to a growing appreciation of the relationship between pain and mood. It is my hope that this chapter has helped to illustrate, albeit simplisticially, the biological elements of the pain system. It is worthwhile to consider the thoughts of one of the pioneers in this field, William Noordenbos, who states, "Representations of tracts and the description of their function are really simplified models of the true state of affairs. Such representation is an absolute necessity; otherwise, neurophysiology cannot be taught at all" (Noordenbos, 1984, p. xiv). I would add that an appreciation of the emotional and biological interplay of the pain experience will help all members of the sports medicine team more effectively treat athletes.

18
CHAPTER

Medications in the Treatment of Pain and Injury

Arthur G. Lipman

Medicines are tools to be used wisely, lest they do more harm than good. Common overuse injuries rarely require medication; rather, education, correction of training errors, and mental training approaches to pain management (see chapter 11) are indicated. In the treatment of traumatic injury, relatively short-term medication regimens are indicated. In contrast to primary injuries, chronic injury syndromes call for a different medication strategy, implemented with careful attention to psychological factors. Although relatively infrequent, chronic injury syndromes merit careful attention not only because of their debilitating effects but also because of the complications often caused by inappropriate use of medications, surgery, and other procedures.

This chapter provides an overview of medications commonly used in pain and injury and offers general guidelines for their use. Recommendations for managing drug use problems are presented in chapter 15. For information on the use of performance-enhancement and recreational drugs see Tricker and Cook (1990) and Wadler and Hainline (1989).

Rational Drug Therapy

Rational therapeutics mandates that before any medication is used, the following must be assured.

1. There is a clear and appropriate indication for using the medication.
2. The potential benefit of using a particular medication for a particular patient is greater than the potential risk of using it.

A clear and appropriate indication for a particular medication might be a diagnosis, for example streptococcal pharyngitis, for which both an antibiotic and analgesic are indicated. However, even in this case caution must be exercised because of sport governing bodies' guidelines on the use of analgesic and other psychoactive medicines. In athletic performance, situational anxiety related to injury is a case in which there probably is no clear indication for pharmacological intervention.

If the benefits of using a particular drug do not clearly outweigh the risks, then use of the drug is irrational. Athletes are prone to be risk takers and may attempt continued play even when injured (Bergandi, 1985; Groves, 1989). Given the option of using a drug with a questionable or even an unfavorable risk/benefit ratio, the highly competitive athlete might choose to use it to the detriment of his or her well-being. The burden of responsibility that this places on professionals who advise athletes is readily evident.

Overuse and Underuse of Medications

Much, perhaps most, of the drug misuse that takes place in our society is due to overuse. Few patients overuse medications intentionally; rather, they take drugs because of unrealistic or exaggerated expectations of what drugs can do for them. When planning therapy for a patient with injury or when counseling such a patient, the practitioner should ensure that the patient has appropriate expectations of drug therapy. There is not "a pill for every ill," as many people believe. The treatment of choice for pain depends upon the cause of the pain and whether it is acute or chronic. If the etiology of the pain cannot be corrected, symptomatic drug therapy may provide only limited success.

Although many people overuse medications, others are very reluctant to take medications for any reason. Unrealistically negative expectations of medication use and a "macho" attitude that pain should be borne bravely contribute to this problem. Acute pain that is not successfully managed early may lead to a chronic pain syndrome, which is far more difficult and expensive to treat than the acute pain that precipitated it. Therefore, patients for whom analgesics and other symptomatic medications are indicated should be thoroughly educated and counseled about their medications. These patients should be told why medications were prescribed, how they should be taken, and what outcomes might be expected, including frequent side effects.

Acute Versus Chronic Pain

Pain is not a generic entity. Rather, pain may be classified as acute, chronic non-malignant, or chronic malignant (National Institutes of Health Consensus Development Conference, 1986). The third category includes pain due to a variety of progressive diseases and is not relevant to this chapter. But athletes often experience both acute and chronic benign pain, and these should be clearly differentiated.

Acute pain due to trauma usually resolves rapidly—within a period of hours to weeks. Adequate analgesic therapy should be initiated as soon as possible if healing is to occur as rapidly as possible. When a person remains in pain, the sympathetic (fight-or-flight) response of the autonomic nervous system remains stimulated. This leads to peripheral vasoconstriction (which may reduce the blood flow to injured tissues), muscle spasm (which may exacerbate the pain), and muscle bracing or guarding (Cousins & Phillips, 1985). The increased autonomic activity causes increased norepinephrine release, which may sensitize pain receptors. The net result is that the patient experiences more pain than necessary, resulting in an increased analgesic requirement and concomitant increased risk of adverse drug reactions (Acute Pain Management Guideline Panel, 1992).

Aggressive, early pharmacological management of pain due to trauma or surgery normally leads to a more rapid and successful resolution of the patient's discomfort. (See chapter 12 for related psychological approaches to acute pain.) Unfortunately, many patients may not receive adequate analgesia initially due to their physicians' fears of inducing drug dependence or depressing respiration. Even when their physicians prescribe analgesics optimally, many patients refuse to take them due to their own inappropriate fears. Several of the commonly held myths about analgesics—especially opioid analgesics—are discussed and refuted in the section on opioid analgesics.

Acute pain and the drugs used to manage it are commonly categorized as mild, moderate, or severe. Aspirin, acetaminophen (e.g., Tylenol), and the other nonsteroidal anti-inflammatory drugs (e.g., ibuprofen—Motrin, Advil) are in the mild class. Weak opioids with or without aspirin or acetaminophen, for example codeine or oxycodone (in Percodan, Percocet, Tylenol 3), are used to treat moderate pain; the stronger opioid analgesics, for example morphine or meperidine (Demerol), are used in severe pain. Most commonly, with appropriate drug use, severe pain becomes moderate within a few hours to a few days, moderate pain becomes mild in a like period of time, and the analgesics are tapered accordingly.

Carefully devised treatment strategies can maximize treatment efficacy. A common cause of the anxiety seen with severe pain is associated with the return of the pain every time a dose of analgesic loses its effect. This is an indication for regularly scheduled or time-contingent dosing rather than dosing as needed (prn). Time-contingent dosing prevents the patient from continually reexperiencing severe pain. Both the caregivers and the patient must understand that prevention of cyclical recurrence of pain reduces the associated anxiety, thus reducing the dose requirement and the concomitant risk of dose-related adverse drug reactions. Furthermore, time-contingent dosing may reduce drug-seeking behavior and is probably the only appropriate dosing regimen for a patient with a prior history of substance abuse. Because repeated prn dosing increases the level of narcotic analgesic used to achieve pain relief, the likelihood of toxicity and other medication side effects is increased. The blood level curves for appropriate time-contingent dosing, as well as for too-seldom or prn dosing (in which the pain is allowed to return), are illustrated in Figure 18.1.

Chronic pain is far more complex. As duration of the pain extends from hours to days, anxiety about the pain increases. Commonly, when the pain continues for days, depression occurs. As the pain continues for weeks, interpersonal functioning is adversely affected, which is commonly manifested in anger, hostility, and withdrawal from social contacts. In order to treat this chronic pain symptom complex effectively, the treatment provider must appreciate the breadth of its scope and the mutually reciprocal nature of pain, anxiety, and depression. Because chronic pain has multiple dimensions, it requires interdisciplinary management, including input from physicians, psychologists, and other health professionals. (See chapter 13 for more information.) A key member of the chronic pain treatment team is a professional who is very familiar with the pharmacology and pharmacokinetics of analgesic and psychotropic drugs.

Drug Use in Pain Management

The uses of nonsteroidal anti-inflammatory drugs (NSAIDs) and opioid analgesics are presented in the following sections. There is also a brief review of local anesthetics, topical analgesics, muscle relaxants, and psychotropic agents.

Nonsteroidal Anti-Inflammatory Drugs

The NSAIDs are potent and effective analgesics, anti-inflammatory agents, and antipyretics (fever-reducing drugs). Aspirin is the prototypical NSAID and is usually the agent of choice unless it is contraindicated due to drug interaction potential, allergy, peptic ulcer disease, or a preexisting bleeding disorder.

Many people think of aspirin as a relatively ineffective drug due to its ready availability. In fact, it is a potent medication that has been shown in controlled studies to be as effective as codeine alone (Moertel, Ahmann,

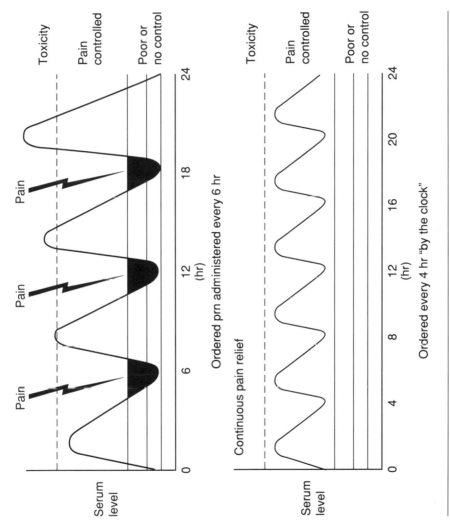

Figure 18.1 Dose-response curves for an analgesic with 4-hr duration of action.

Taylor, & Schwartau, 1974). But patients' beliefs about drugs do influence their efficacy. One third of patients who are given placebos will experience an analgesic effect, in which there is an elevated level of endogenous pain-relieving substances within their central nervous systems (Fields, 1987). Therefore, if a patient does not believe that aspirin is effective, an alternative drug should be used.

Acetaminophen is usually the simple analgesic alternative to aspirin. But acetaminophen has no peripheral anti-inflammatory activity, and most athletic injuries have a significant inflammatory component. Ibuprofen is the first of the newer NSAIDs to become available without a prescription; others should follow soon. All of the newer NSAIDs have both analgesic and anti-inflammatory activity. These include Naprosyn, Anaprox, Feldene, Clinoril, Dolobid, Indocin, Orudis, and others. Generic ibuprofen (e.g., Advil, Nuprin) is the drug of choice because it is inexpensive and available without a prescription.

The NSAIDs are generally safe drugs. The most common dangerous side effect is exacerbation of peptic ulcer disease in patients with a history of the problem. The NSAIDs also can cause or exacerbate renal toxicity in patients so disposed by preexisting kidney or other medical problems. Use of diuretics or excessive perspiration can cause dehydration and increase the toxic effects of these drugs on the kidneys. This is an especially important consideration in sports in which diuretics, laxatives, and other measures are used to induce dehydration (American College of Sports Medicine, 1976, 1983).

Opioid Analgesics

The opioids, sometimes referred to as narcotics or opiates, are the most potent analgesics available today. These drugs act by occupying and activating opioid receptors in the central nervous system, thus reducing pain perception centrally.

Codeine is the prototypical weak opioid; propoxyphene (found in Darvon) is another example. These are effective analgesics for moderate pain, especially when combined with an NSAID. However, propoxyphene and some others offer no clear advantage over NSAIDs alone. Morphine is the prototypical strong opioid. Several other opioids (e.g., Demerol, methadone) can provide the same level of analgesia if administered appropriately. There is potentiation between the strong opioids and NSAIDs (Weingart, Sorkness, & Earhart, 1985).

All of the opioids present some risk of causing dependence, tolerance, and respiratory depression. However, these risks are commonly overestimated in the management of acute pain, resulting in less than optimal pain treatment. In a study of 11,882 patients who received opioid analgesics for medical purposes and who were monitored for addiction, researchers found that in patients with no previous history of substance abuse, there were only four cases of addiction (Porter & Jick, 1980). Dependence on properly used opioids is rare. In contrast, the risks of the long-term use of opioids in the management of chronic pain are all too frequently underestimated or ignored. Opioids are seldom indicated in chronic non-malignant pain.

When athletes receive opioids for pain due to acute injuries, there is the risk that they may not allow their injuries to heal fully before resuming vigorous physical activity. This can result in ongoing pain, for which athletes may continue to take the opioids inappropriately, creating a mutually exacerbating cycle of pain and injury. There is concern that as this cycle becomes apparent and their physicians refuse to continue to prescribe the drugs, the athlete may seek other alternatives, including illegal activities, to obtain the medications. Identifying athletes who may be at high risk for such abuses is an important task for health professionals and advisers who counsel athletes.

Local Anesthetics

Injectable local anesthetics (e.g., lidocaine, bupivacaine) can be very useful for temporary treatment of localized pain. Pain may subside within 30 min to several hours. However, these anesthetics do not treat the underlying disorder. Athletes have been known to use local anesthetics to anesthetize painful areas prior to competition, a very dangerous practice that can lead to severe injury. Local anesthetics are also very effective in myofascial pain syndrome, for which trigger point injections are used to treat foci of irritability in muscles. (See chapter 17 for more extensive information on this condition and its treatment.)

Topical Analgesics

Liniment, balms, and other topical preparations have been used by athletes for many years and are available over the counter. What are here referred to collectively as topical (or external) analgesics can be categorized according to their analgesic (reduction of pain), anesthetic (reduction of sensation), antipruritic (reduction of itching), or counterirritant effects. Analgesics, anesthetics, and antipruritics act locally by decreasing cutaneous nerve impulses. In contrast, counterirritants work by stimulating cutaneous receptors, gaining their therapeutic effect most probably by closing the spinal gate to noxious stimuli. Counterirritants result in a feeling of warmth and may produce some muscle relaxation. Some counterirritants (e.g., menthol) also have some local anesthetic effect.

Most topical analgesics typically contain varying combinations of ingredients from different classes of counterirritants. Generally, counterirritants should be used no longer than 7 days if symptoms of pain and soreness persist. Continued or repeated use of any topical medication may lead to sensitization. Redness, rash, or itching that does not resolve rapidly is an indication of an allergic reaction. Heat, massage, and stretching can be valuable adjuncts to topical analgesic medications. However, many athletes respond well to these physical measures alone.

Dimethyl sulfoxide (DMSO) is a topical analgesic that has potent nerve-blocking, anti-inflammatory, vasodilating, muscle-relaxing, and diuretic properties. It also inhibits cholinesterase, which can have a profound effect on autonomic nervous system function. It is a clear colorless liquid that is rapidly absorbed through the skin. Pharmaceutical-grade DMSO is available as Rimso-50; it is also commercially available in a variety of forms not intended for human use. Because DMSO is a very potent solvent, it is absorbed rapidly through the skin into the systemic circulation, carrying with it dissolved impurities, which can be very dangerous. DMSO should not be used as a topical analgesic except in the pharmaceutical-grade formulation in approved, controlled scientific studies. Use of non-pharmaceutical-grade DMSO is very dangerous and should be firmly discouraged.

Muscle Relaxants

Muscle relaxants can occasionally be useful as adjuncts in the short-term treatment of muscle spasm following traumatic injury. However, these drugs do cloud awareness and thinking and can cause dependence. They should be used only for a few days to a week in most cases and should be avoided when high levels of mental alertness are required. If an athlete requires a muscle relaxant, that muscle should not be put under stress. Consequently, the athlete should not compete or train while taking this class of medication. Varieties of muscle relaxants are available such as carisoprodol (e.g., Soma), chlorzoxazone (e.g., Paraflex), methocarbamol (e.g., Robaxin), orphenadrine (e.g., Norflex), and chlorphenesin (e.g., Maolate). The benzodiazepines (e.g., Valium) are also potent muscle relaxants.

Other Psychotropic Agents

Athletic competition can provoke anxiety, especially when injury is involved. Anxiolytic medications are often prescribed inappropriately in the management of injury, especially where there is enduring pain or sleep disturbance. All of the antianxiety agents that are available have the potential to depress the higher central nervous system functions. They may reduce muscular coordination and response time and therefore may increase the risk of exacerbation of injury in athletes who perform under their influence. Additionally, these drugs have the potential for inducing dependence. Several of the benzodiazepines, most notably triazolam (Halcion), can cause anterograde amnesia for a short period of time. Some of the older drugs used for this purpose, such as meprobamate, are sedative-hypnotics, markedly reduce central nervous system function and carry a high risk of dependence. Mental skills training is a preferable approach for managing anxiety in injured athletes.

The tricyclic antidepressants are very useful in the treatment of nerve injury–related pain (e.g., deafferentation pain). Relatively low doses (one third to one half of the antidepressant doses) are often effective in 5 days or less (in contrast to the 2 or more weeks required for an antidepressant effect). This class of medication is also effective in the management of sleep disturbance related to a wide variety of chronic pain problems. However, these drugs can have bothersome sedative and anticholinergic side effects (e.g., dry mouth, blurred vision, urinary retention, tachycardia). Relaxation training is recommended as an adjunct to medication use in pain-related sleep disturbance.

Drug Interactions and Other Unintended Effects

Many drugs have an inherent risk of interacting with other drugs including prescribed and over-the-counter medication as well as recreational drugs and dietary supplements. As the number of drugs a person takes increases arithmetically, the risk of interactions increases geometrically. Patients who are taking more than one drug or dietary supplement can have their medication profile screened by a competent pharmacist to minimize the risk of adverse drug interactions.

The widespread use of a variety of ergogenic and recreational substances has led sport governing bodies to ban their use. Because banned substances are essentially illegal, their use by an athlete (whether appropriate or inappropriate medically) can lead to disqualification and other penalties. Because of the broad range of substances banned, and because drug testing often identifies metabolites (i.e., products of chemical breakdown) that may be common to both banned and allowable substances, many medications used in general medical treatment may lead to positive drug tests. This can complicate routine medical management of athletes, in particular in regard to respiratory and cardiovascular disorders. It is also noteworthy that some medications prescribed for general medical purposes may be ergolytic or performance inhibiting (Strauss, 1987). Performance problems with anxiolytics and muscle relaxants were noted previously.

The Psychologist's Role

Because of the pervasiveness of noncompliance (including various forms of underuse and overuse), all health professionals, including the psychologist, can share in monitoring (and encouraging) athletes' use of medications as prescribed and noting side effects and therapeutic efficacy. This information may be routinely communicated to the physician through copies of treatment notes. Perhaps the most important task for the psychologist is to monitor pain reported (and pain behavior observed) across time and situation as well as the psychological sequelae of pain. Inconsistency between self-report and behavior or inconsistency in behavior from one situation to another can be quite revealing. Thorough psychological assessment of the relative role of depression, anxiety, sleep disturbance, or other behavioral factors in complicating pain can be valuable as well. For example, sometimes medication prescribed for one symptom (e.g., opioid analgesics for pain) may also be used to treat another symptom (e.g., sleep) but less effectively. Timely identification of pain-related sleep disturbance allows an appropriate medication regimen (e.g., an antidepressant) to be instituted.

For some athletes appropriate medication use and routine recovery are not sufficient to maintain emotional equilibrium in the face of injury. With these athletes pain and psychological distress may come to operate in a mutually reinforcing cycle. For more information on the psychological management of pain, see sections in chapters 4, 11, 12, and 13.

Concluding Comments

The use of medications by injured athletes provides a special challenge to the prescriber, who needs to be aware of the unique pressures that shape the athlete's world. Many of the medications available for pain and injury may be perceived as ergogenic or performance-continuing and therefore may be deliberately but inappropriately sought by athletes.

Much misinformation about drug effects exists within the general community, and unrealistic expectations about drugs for treatment of pain and injury is a real problem. The use of drugs to continue performance without consideration of the potential consequences has been detrimental to many athletes. Inadequate management of acute pain has led to long-term difficulties for other athletes, and overuse of opioid analgesics and other psychoactive medications with chronic pain has led to problems as well. Today's medications are potent agents with the potential to do both good and harm, and all professionals and advisers who interact with athletes regarding drug use should emphasize this.

19
CHAPTER

Sport Injury and Psychology: Current Practices and Future Challenges

John Heil

Injury is a psychological and a physical challenge to the athlete. The psychology of sport injury is a health-oriented psychology of performance and a clinical psychology of disorder. It strives to limit suffering and loss that occur as consequences of injury and to ensure mental readiness for return to play. As a young discipline, the psychology of sport injury must face significant challenges if it is to continue to grow and to reach full utilization. The maturity of this discipline will be marked by an expanding scope of practice within sport and by the application of its knowledge base and methods to other performance-related problems.

The Scope of Practice

Although it is clear that sport psychology and sports medicine need to look beyond the competitive athlete, the question of "how far" remains. In considering this question, I am reminded of a humorous story told by Ernest Johnson (1987), who reported treating a college president for "tennis elbow" that presumably resulted from handshaking following a major football bowl victory. Is this a sport injury? What about others who play their roles on the sidelines? It seems an inherently good idea to include the coach; the profound stresses of coaching (especially where it is true vocational pursuit) are well recognized and presumably render the individual at risk for a variety of disorders (Pacelli, 1990). Cheerleaders should also be included. As this activity has evolved from a simple dancelike routine to a pseudogymnastic event, injury (including catastrophic injury) has become increasingly common.

The psychology of sport injury, like sports medicine, stands to be criticized for being an elite science that is oriented toward a relatively privileged few and that neglects the population at large. This is hardly a fair characterization. The sheer number of those involved worldwide in sport argues against the elitist label (Goldstein, 1989; Tolpin & Bentkover, 1986). The argument further pales in light of the increasing evidence of the benefits of physical activity throughout the person's life span, in sickness and in health. Also to be considered is the significant economic impact of sport injuries (Tolpin & Bentkover, 1986) and, conversely, of the illnesses that occur as consequences of inactivity.

Sport psychology and sports medicine are not for sport alone (Sheehan, 1990; Strauss, 1989) but more precisely for the athlete. Athleticism is the province of all who must precisely execute physical skills under demanding conditions. Performing artists, such as dancers and musicians, most certainly deserve inclusion in this category, as perhaps do the craftspersons and production workers who labor to produce quality products under time constraints. Sports medicine and behavioral medicine have already made significant contributions to the management of both acute and chronic occupational injury. It is increasingly common for the injured athlete and the work-injured patient to find themselves rehabilitating side by side at the growing number of sports medicine and rehabilitation centers. The newly coined designation of the rehabilitating injured worker as an "industrial athlete" further extends the picture of athleticism.

The psychology of sport injury stands to make an important contribution to a variety of medical problems. The possibilities for the application of goal setting and mental training in the management of spinal cord injury (Asken & Goodling, 1986) and malignant disease (Unestahl, 1985) have been demonstrated. The psychology of sport injury also offers promise in the treatment of disorders of diminished performance. This includes a variety of maladies that have in common a pervasive disruption of performance with significant psychological concomitants in the absence of definitive organic pathology. Collectively, these disorders of diminished performance are increasingly impacting health in industrialized nations. Overtraining syndrome, burnout, myofascial pain disorder, and chronic pain have been discussed in this text. Chronic fatigue syndrome (Holmes et al., 1988) and fibromyalgia syndrome (Goldenberg, 1987) also merit inclusion in this category.

Principles for Practice

The psychology of sport injury is built on a set of principles that evolve from a synthesis of sport psychology, behavioral medicine, and sports medicine. These are summarized next.

- Managing injury effectively (i.e., avoiding it initially and recovering well following occurrence) is an aspect of the game that the athlete must play well in order to succeed.
- Injury rehabilitation is a performance task, the effectiveness of which relies on much the same skills as used in sport performance.
- Just as relatively small changes in behavior in sport can significantly impact performance, so do small changes in behavior significantly impact rehabilitation.
- Speedy, effective return to play depends not only on physical function but also on psychological status. The athlete whose injury is physically healed but who is not mentally ready to return to play is not yet recovered.
- The goals of treatment are to reduce the psychological impact of injury, to help the athlete maintain a performance-oriented mental set, and to speed readiness for return to play. This implies benefits from intervention, even in the absence of evident adjustment problems.
- A multidisciplinary team that simultaneously addresses medical and psychological issues offers the best quality of care.
- Optimal injury management requires a proactive program that incorporates a psychological approach to routine rehabilitation as well as early identification and treatment of adjustment problems.
- The pillars of a psychological approach to rehabilitation are education, goal setting, mental training, and social support.
- Severe injury and adjustment problems demand specialized treatment approaches. When these are delivered to the athlete in a timely fashion, the impact of injury is reduced.
- Optimal treatment evolves from a therapeutic relationship in which the athlete feels an alliance with treatment providers. This implies that the athlete takes an active role in rehabilitation and decision making.
- Treatment effectiveness is enhanced when the athlete senses the alliance of treatment providers with one another. This evolves from coordination of care.
- Treatment providers must be sensitive to the prevailing sport milieu. For example, similar injuries to a Little Leaguer and to a big league baseball player typically have different meanings as problems and merit different approaches to treatment.

- Risk taking is an inherent part of sport. It is often an important motive for participation, and is a fundamental right and responsibility of the athlete; facts upon which treatment decisions must be based.
- Treatment providers need to balance their typically cautious and conservative approaches with the athlete's desires. Thus treatment providers must understand the cost to the athlete of being withheld from competition.

Challenges

The psychology of sport injury is young even in comparison to the relatively youthful disciplines from which it evolves. It must face significant challenges before it can come to maturity. Most fundamental is the need for greater understanding and credibility in the fields of sport and medicine. Like sports medicine, the psychology of sport injury needs continuing development of a base of theory, research, and practice that is sensitive to the distinct needs of the athlete. At the same time, it is important to demonstrate that sports medicine and sport psychology are not simply elite specialties for the privileged few but can contribute to the health and well-being of other populations.

Psychology is slowly coming to be recognized as an applied science of behavior change, in contrast to a general treatment for people who are mentally ill. Although psychology has made great gains in acceptance, this long-standing struggle goes on. In spite of the widely held notion that sport is some large percent mental, sport psychology has made relatively modest inroads in sport (Linder et al., 1989; Ogilvie, 1977). Although the psychology of sport injury has made significant inroads in medicine, the practical aspects of how and when to refer patients to psychologists need to be better understood (Brewer et al., 1989a). Fundamental to the acceptance of psychologists as treatment providers in the medical arena is an appreciation of the subtlety and complexity of mind-body interactions and of how they function in sport performance and in injury. Education of those in sport and medicine in these fundamental issues must be a priority for all who practice psychology.

The issue of credibility for sport psychology reflects more pervasive underlying issues of professional identity. As a profession, sport psychology has experienced both significant victories and significant losses. For the most part, the losses have come at the hands of those who have been quick to move through a window of opportunity—much to the frustration of those trained in the practice of sport psychology.

Sport psychology has drawn heavily on previously established practices in clinical psychology. As these have been modified to suit the special needs of athletes, sport psychology has begun to evolve its own distinct set of principles and practices. The maturity of sport psychology will be marked by its contributions, in turn, to the disciplines from which it evolved. The same can also be said for the psychology of sport injury.

Many of the greatest personal losses and victories in sport are played out quietly in the battle with injury. The psychology of sport injury is designed to help the athlete perform in this arena of rehabilitation. It is distinct from a more broadly based psychology of injury, because professionals who treat sport injury must be sensitive and responsive to the prevailing attitudes and pressures of the world of sport. In many ways, the psychology of sport injury carries the important issues of individualized treatment and personal responsibility to new levels. In so doing, it stands to make an important contribution to health care that reaches well beyond the world of sport.

References

Achterberg, J., & Lawlis, G.F. (1978). *Imagery of cancer*. Champaign, IL: Institute for Personality and Ability Testing.

Acute pain management guideline panel. (1992, February). *Acute pain management: Operative or medical procedures and trauma: Clinical practice guidelines*. Rockville, MD: United States Department of Health and Human Services, Public Health Service, Agency for Health Care Policy and Research.

Adams, S.H., Adrian, M.J., & Bayless, M.A. (1987). *Catastrophic injuries in sports: Avoidance strategies* (2nd ed.). Indianapolis: Benchmark Press.

Adler, R., Bongar, B., & Katz, E.R. (1982). Psychogenic abdominal pain and parental pressure in childhood athletics. *Psychosomatics*, **23**(11), 1185-1186.

Agras, W.S. (1987). *Eating disorders*. New York: Pergamon Press.

Allen, R.J. (1983). *Human stress: Its nature and control*. Minneapolis: Burgess International.

American Academy of Pediatrics. (1988). Recommendations for participation in competitive sports. *The Physician and Sports Medicine*, **16**(5), 165-167.

American Academy of Pediatrics Committee on Sports Medicine. (1983). *Sports medicine: Health care for young athletes*. Evanston, IL: Author.

American College of Physicians. (1986). *Eating Disorders: Anorexia nervosa and bulimia*. Philadelphia: Author.

American College of Sports Medicine. (1976). Physicians stand on weight loss in wrestlers. *Medicine and Science in Sports and Exercise*, **8**(2), xi-xiii.

American College of Sports Medicine. (1982). The use of alcohol in sports. *Medicine and Science in Sports and Exercise*, **14**(6), ix-xi.

American College of Sports Medicine. (1983). Physicians stand on proper and improper weight loss programs. *Medicine and Science in Sports and Exercise*, **15**(1), ix-xiii.

American College of Sports Medicine. (1987a). Physicians stand on blood doping as an ergogenic aid. *Medicine and Science in Sports and Exercise*, **19**(5), 540-543.

American College of Sports Medicine. (1987b). Physicians stand on the use of anabolic-androgenic steroids in sports. *Medicine and Science in Sports and Exercise*, **19**(5), 534-539.

American Psychiatric Association. (1987). *Diagnostic and statistical manual of mental disorders* (3rd ed., rev.). Washington, DC: Author.

Andersen, M.B., & Williams, J.M. (1988). A model of stress and athletic injury: Prediction and prevention. *Journal of Sport and Exercise Psychology*, **10**, 294-306.

Andersen, M.B., & Williams, J.M. (1989, March). *Peripheral vision narrowing during stress: Possible mechanisms behind stress injury relationships.* Paper presented at the meeting of the Society for Behavioral Medicine, San Francisco.

Anderson, K.O., & Masur, F.T. (1983). Psychological preparation for invasive medical and dental procedures. *Journal of Behavioral Medicine*, **6**(1), 1-40.

Anderson, W.A., & McKeag, D.B. (1985). *The substance use and abuse habits of college student-athletes* (Report No. 2). Mission, KS: The National Collegiate Athletic Association.

Anderson, W.A., & McKeag, D.B. (1989). *Replication of the national study of the substance use and abuse habits of college student-athletes*. Mission, KS: The National Collegiate Athletic Association.

Anshel, M.H. (1987). Psychological inventories used in sport psychology research. *The Sport Psychologist*, **1**, 331-349.

Antonovsky, A. (1985). The sense of coherence as a determinant of health. In J.D. Matarazzo, S.M. Weiss, J.A. Herd, & N.E. Miller (Eds.), *Behavioral health: A handbook of health enhancement and disease prevention* (pp. 37-50). New York: Wiley.

Asken, M.J. (1989). Sport psychology and the physically disabled athlete: Interview with Michael D. Goodling, OTR/L. *The Sport Psychologist*, **3**, 166-176.

Asken, M.J., & Goodling, M.D. (1986). The use of sport psychology techniques in rehabilitation medicine: A pilot study—case report. *International Journal of Sport Psychology*, **17**, 156-161.

Association for the Advancement of Behavior Therapy. (1990, September). *Fact sheet on chronic pain*. New York: Author. (Available from the Association for the Advancement of Behavior Therapy, 15 West 36th St., New York, New York 10018)

Astle, S.J. (1986). The experience of loss in athletes. *Journal of Sportsmedicine and Physical Fitness: A Quarterly Review*, **26**, 279-284.

Baekeland, F. (1970). Exercise deprivation: Sleep and psychological reactions. *Archives in General Psychiatry*, **22**, 365-369.

Baldick, R. (1985). *The duel*. London: Chapman & Hall.

Barron, G.L., Noakes, T.D., Levy, W., Smith, C., & Millar, R.P. (1985). Hypothalamic dysfunction in overtrained athletes. *Journal of Clinical Endocrinology and Metabolism*, **60**(4), 803-806.

Basbaum, A.I., & Fields, H.L. (1978). Endogenous pain control mechanisms: Review and hypothesis. *Annals of Neurology*, **4**, 451-462.

Basbaum, A.I., Moss, M.S., & Glazer, E.J. (1983). Opiate and stimulation-produced analgesia: The contribution of the monoamines. *Advances in Pain Research and Therapy*, **5**, 475-479.

Beck, A.T., & Emery, G. (1985). *Anxiety disorders and phobias: A cognitive perspective*. New York: Basic Books.

Beck, A.T., Rush, A.J., Shaw, B.P., & Emery, G. (1979). *Cognitive therapy of depression*. New York: Guilford Press.

Beecher, H.K. (1946). Pain in men wounded in battle. *Annals of Surgery*, **123**(1), 96-105.

Beecher, H.K. (1956). Relationship of significance of wound to pain experienced. *Journal of the American Medical Association*, **161**(17), 1609-1613.

Behavioral medicine [Special issue]. (1982). *Journal of Consulting and Clinical Psychology*, **50**(6).

Beitz, A.J. (1982). The organization of afferent projections to the midbrain periaqueductal gray of the rat. *Neuroscience*, **7**, 133-259.

Bergandi, T.A. (1985). Psychological variables relating to the incidences of athletic injury. *International Journal of Sport Psychology*, **16**, 141-149.

Bergman, R.T. (1989). When to treat elective surgical conditions in the competing athlete. *The Physician and Sportsmedicine*, **17**(4), 181-182, 187.

Bishop, B. (1978). *The running saga of Walter Stack*. Millbrae, CA: Celestial Arts.

The black athlete [Special issue]. (1991, August 5). *Sports Illustrated*.

Blackwell, B., & McCullagh, P. (1990). The relationship of athletic training to life stress, competitive anxiety, and coping resources. *Athletic Training*, **25**, 23-27.

Blanchard, E.B. (1982). Behavioral medicine: Past, present and future. *Journal of Consulting and Clinical Psychology*, **50**(6), 795-796.

Booth, W. (1987, August 21). Arthritis Institute tackles sports. *Science*, **237**, 846-847.

Borg, G.A.V., & Ottoson, D. (Eds.). (1986). *The perception of exertion and physical work*. New York: Macmillan.

Bortz, W.M. (1984). The disuse syndrome [Commentary]. *The Western Journal of Medicine*, **141**, 691-694.

Botterill, C. (1982). Retirement and detraining: What "endings" tell us about "beginnings." In T. Orlick, J.T. Partington, & J.H. Salmela (Eds.), *Mental training for coaches and athletes* (pp. 164-166). Ottawa: Sport in Perspective.

Bowsher, D. (1976). Role of the reticular formation in response to noxious stimulation. *Pain*, **2**, 361-378.

Bradley, B. (1976). *Life on the run*. New York: Bantam Books.

Bramwell, S.T., Masuda, M., Wagner, N.N., & Holmes, T.H. (1975). Psychosocial factors in athletic injuries: Development and application of the social and athletic readjustment rating scale (SARRS). *Journal of Human Stress*, **1**, 6-20.

Braverman, M. (1977). Validity of psychotraumatic reactions. *Journal of Forensic Sciences*, **22**, 654-662.

Brena, S.F., & Chapman, S.L. (1982). Chronic pain: An algorithm for management. *Postgraduate Medicine*, **1**, 111-117.

Brewer, B.W., Van Raalte, J.L., & Linder, D.E. (1989a, September). *Role of the sport psychologist in treating injured athletes: A survey of sports medicine providers*. Paper presented at the annual meeting of the Association for the Advancement of Applied Sport Psychology, Seattle, WA.

Brewer, B.W., Van Raalte, J.L., & Linder, D.E. (1989b, June). *Effects of pain on motor performance*. Paper presented at the 1989 North American Society for the Psychology of Sport and Physical Activity Conference, Kent, OH.

Bridges, J.K. (1987). Try comprehensive case management to curb chronicity during rehabilitation. *Back Pain Monitor*, **5**(11) 145-147.

Browne, M.A., & Mahoney, M.J. (1984). Sport psychology. *Annual Review of Psychology*, **35**, 605-625.

Brownell, K.D., Marlatt, G.A., Lichtenstein, E., & Wilson, G.T. (1986). Understanding and preventing relapse. *American Psychologist*, **41**(7), 765-782.

Bump, L.A. (1989). *American Coaching Effectiveness Program, Level II: Sport Psychology Study Guide*. Champaign, IL: Human Kinetics.

Bunker, L., Williams, J.M., & Zinsser, N. (1993). Cognitive techniques for improving performance and building confidence. In J.M. Williams (Ed.), *Applied sport psychology: Personal growth to peak performance* (2nd ed.). Palo Alto, CA: Mayfield.

Burckes-Miller, M.E., & Black, D.R. (1989). Male and female college athletes: Use of anorexia nervosa and bulimia nervosa weight loss methods. *Proceedings of the First IOC World Congress on Sport Sciences*. Colorado Springs, CO: International Olympic Committee Medical Commission.

Burgess, P.R., & Perl, E.R. (1973). Cutaneous mechanoreceptors and nociceptors. In A. Iggo (Ed.), *Handbook of sensory physiology* (Vol. 2, pp. 29-78). Berlin: Springer Verlag.

Carron, A.V. (1984). *Motivation: Implications for coaching and teaching*. London, ON: Pear Creative.

Casson, I.R., Siegel, O., Sham, R., Campbell, E.A., Tarlau, M., & DiDomenico, A. (1984). Brain damage in modern boxers. *The Journal of the American Medical Association*, **251**(20), 2663-2667.

Cataldi, A. (1987, December 24). Tim Kerr turns to family in a season that never was. *The Philadelphia Inquirer*, pp. D1-D3.

Cautela, J.R. (1983). The self-control triad: Description and clinical applications. *Behavior Modification*, **7**(3), 299-315.

Chambers, W.N. (1963). Emotional factors complicating industrial injuries. *Journal of Occupational Medicine*, **5**(12), 568-574.

Chapman, C.R., Casey, K.L., Dubner, R., Foley, K.M., Gracely, R.H., & Reading, A.E. (1985). Pain measurement: An overview. *Pain*, **22**, 1-30.

Chapman, C.R., & Turner, J.A. (1986). Psychological control of acute pain in medical settings. *Journal of Pain and Symptom Management*, **1**(1), 9-20.

Christophersen, E.R. (1989). Injury control. *American Psychologist*, **44**(2), 237-241.

Cinque, C. (1989). Mickey Mantle: Still grappling with old knee injuries. *The Physician and Sportsmedicine*, **17**(6), 170-172, 174.

Clain, M.R., & Hershman, E.B. (1989). Overuse injuries in children and adolescents. *The Physician and Sportsmedicine*, **17**(9), 111-112, 115-116, 119-120, 122-123.

Clanin, D.R., Davison, D.M., & Plastino, J.G. (1986). Injury patterns in university dance students. In C.G. Shell (Ed.), *The dancer as athlete* (pp. 195-199). Champaign, IL: Human Kinetics.

Clarke, K.S. (1989). Epidemiology of neurologic injuries in sports. In B.D. Gordan, P. Tsairis, & R.F. Warren (Eds.), *Sports neurology* (pp. 63-74). Rockville, MD: Aspen.

Coakley, J.J. (1986). *Sport in society: Issues and controversies*. St. Louis, Mosby.

Coddington, R.D., & Troxell, J.R. (1980). The effect of emotional factors on football injury rates: A pilot study. *Journal of Human Stress*, **6**(4), 3-5.

Cohen, F., & Lazarus, R.S. (1979). Coping with the stresses of illness. In G.C. Stone, F. Cohen, N.E. Adler, & Associates, *Health psychology: A handbook* (pp. 217-255). San Francisco: Josey Bass.

Compas, B.E., Davis, G.E., Forsythe, C.J., & Wagner, B. (1987). Assessment of major and daily stressful events during adolescence: The adolescent perceived events scale. *Journal of Consulting and Clinical Psychology*, **55**, 534-541.

Costill, D.L. (1986). *Inside running* (pp. 123-132). Indianapolis: Benchmark Press.

Cousins, M.J., & Phillips, G.D. (Eds.). (1985). Acute pain management. *Clinics in Critical Care Medicine Series: Volume 8*. New York: Churchill.

Couturie, B., & Else, J. (Directors), & Couturie, B., Else, J., & Witte, K. (Producers). (1986). *Disposable heroes* [Videotape]. Los Angeles: Active Home Video.

Creed, F. (1985). Life events and physical illness [Invited review]. *Journal of Psychosomatic Research*, **29**, 113-123.

Cross, M.J., Pinczewski, L.A., & Bokor, D.J. (1989). Acute knee injury in a rock musician: A case conference. *The Physician and Sportsmedicine,* **17**(7), 79-82.

Crossman, J., & Jamieson, J. (1985). Differences in perceptions of seriousness and disrupting effects of athletic injury as viewed by athletes and their trainer. *Perceptual and Motor Skills,* **61,** 1131-1134.

Crue, B.L. (1985). Multidisciplinary pain treatment programs: Current status. *The Clinical Journal of Pain,* **1,** 31-38.

Cryan, P.O., & Alles, E.F. (1983). The relationship between stress and football injuries. *Journal of Sportsmedicine and Physical Fitness,* **23,** 52-58.

Cummings, N.A. (1985, May). *Saving health care dollars through psychological service.* Paper presented at a meeting cosponsored by Honorable D.K. Inouye, Honorable M. Baucus, and The American Psychological Association, Washington, DC.

Dalhauser, M., & Thomas, M.B. (1979). Visual disembedding and locus of control as variables associated with high school football injuries. *Perceptual and Motor Skills,* **49,** 254.

Damron, C.F., Hoerner, E.F., & Shaw, J.L. (1986). Injury surveillance systems for sports. In P.E. Vinger & E.F. Hoerner (Eds.), *Sports injuries: The unthwarted epidemic* (2nd ed., pp. 1-22). Littleton, MA: PSG.

Danish, S. (1986). Psychological aspects in the care and treatment of athletic injuries. In P.E. Vinger & E.F. Hoerner (Eds.), *Sports injuries: The unthwarted epidemic* (2nd ed., pp. 345-353). Littleton, MA: PSG.

Davis, J.O. (1991). Sports injuries and stress management: An opportunity for research. *The Sport Psychologist,* **5,** 175-182.

Dean, J.E., Whelan, J.P., & Meyers, A.W. (1990). *An incredibly quick way to assess mood states: The incredibly short POMS.* Paper presented at the annual meeting of the Association for the Advancement of Applied Sport Psychology, San Antonio, TX.

Derevenco, P., Florea, E., Derevenco, V., Anghel, I., & Simu, Z. (1967). Einige physiologishe aspekte des uebertrainings [Some physiological aspects of overtraining]. *Sportarzt und Sportmedizin,* **18,** 151-161.

Dishman, R.K. (1987). Psychological aids to performance. In R.H. Strauss (Ed.), *Drugs and performance in sports* (pp. 121-146). Philadelphia: Saunders.

Dishman, R.K. (Ed.). (1988). *Exercise adherence: Its impact on public health.* Champaign, IL: Human Kinetics.

Dlin, B.M. (1985). Psychobiology and treatment of anniversary reactions. *Psychosomatics,* **26**(6), 505-508, 510-512, 520.

Dravecky: Fracture halts comeback. (1989). *The Physician and Sportsmedicine,* **17**(10), 21-22.

Druckman, D., & Bjork, R.A. (Eds.). (1991). *In the mind's eye: Enhancing human performance.* Washington, DC: National Academy Press.

Duda, J.L., Smart, A.E., & Tappe, M.K. (1989). Predictors of adherence in the rehabilitation of athletic injuries: An application of personal investment theory. *Journal of Sport and Exercise Psychology*, **11**(4), 367-381.

Eichman, W.J. (1978). Profile of mood states. In O.K. Buros (Ed.), *The eighth mental measurements yearbook*. Lincoln: University of Nebraska Press.

Eichner, E.R. (1989). Chronic fatigue syndrome: How vulnerable are athletes? *The Physician and Sportsmedicine*, **17**(6), 157-160.

Eldridge, W.D. (1983). The importance of psychotherapy for athletic-related orthopedic injuries among adults. *Comprehensive Psychiatry*, **24**(3), 271-277.

Ellingson, K. (1981). *2500-mile walk: An oldtimer on the Pacific Crest Trail*. San Francisco: Alchemy Books.

Everett, J.J., Smoll, F.L., & Smith, R.E. (1990, September). Football players' recall of self-protection information: Implications for behavioral compliance. Paper presented at the annual meeting of Association for the Advancement of Applied Sport Psychology, San Antonio, TX.

Farley, F. (1990, May). The type T personality with some implications for practice. *The California Psychologist*, p. 29.

Fender, L.K. (1989). Athlete burnout: Potential for research and intervention strategies. *The Sport Psychologist*, **3**, 63-71.

Feigley, D.A. (1988, October). *Coping with fear in high level gymnastics*. Paper presented at the annual meeting of the Association for the Advancement of Applied Sport Psychology, Nashua, NH.

Fernandez, E., & Turk, D.C. (1986, August). *Overall and relative efficacy of cognitive strategies in attenuating pain*. Paper presented at the 94th annual convention of the American Psychological Association, Washington, DC.

Fernando, C.K., & Basmajian, J.V. (1978). Biofeedback in physical medicine and rehabilitation: Task force report of the Biofeedback Society of America. *Biofeedback and Self-Regulation*, **3**(4), 435-455.

Feuerstein, M., Labbe, E.E., & Kuczmeirczyk, A.R. (1986). *Health psychology: A psychobiological perspective*. New York: Plenum Press.

Fine, P.G. (1987). Myofascial trigger point pain in children. *Journal of Pediatrics*, **111**, 547-548.

Fine, P.G. (1988). The pharmacological management of sympathetically maintained pain. *Hospital Formulary*, **23**, 796-808.

Fine, P.G., Milano, R.A., & Hare, B.D. (1988). The effects of myofascial trigger point injections are naloxone reversible. *Pain*, **32**, 15-20.

Fine, P.G., & Petty, W.C. (1986). Myofascial trigger point pain: Diagnosis and treatment. *Current Reviews in Clinical Anesthesia*, **7**, 34-39.

Fisher, A.C., Domm, N.A., & Wuest, D.A. (1988). Adherence to sports-injury rehabilitation programs. *The Physician and Sportsmedicine*, **16**(7), 47-51.

Flint, F. (1991, October). *Modeling influences on self-perceptions and adherence in athletic injury rehabilitation*. Paper presented at the annual meeting of the Association for the Advancement of Applied Sport Psychology, Savannah, GA.

Ford, C.B. (1983). *The somatisizing disorders: Illness as a way of life*. New York: Elsevier Biomedical.

Fordyce, W.E. (1976). *Behavioral methods for chronic pain and illness*. St. Louis: Mosby.

Fordyce, W.E. (1979). Use of the MMPI in the assessment of chronic pain. In J. Butcher, G. Dahlstrom, M. Gynther, & W. Schofield (Eds.), *Clinical notes on the MMPI* (pp. 2-13). Nutley, NJ: Roche Psychiatric Service Institute.

Fordyce, W.E. (1988). Pain and suffering: A reappraisal. *American Psychologist*, **43**(4), 276-283.

Fordyce, W.E., Brockway, J.A., Bergman, J.A., & Spengler, D. (1986). Acute back pain: A control-group comparison of behavioral versus traditional management methods. *Journal of Behavioral Medicine*, **9**(2), 127-140.

Fordyce, W.E., Fowler, R.S., Lehmann, J.F., & DeLateur, B.J. (1978, August 15). 10 steps to help patients with chronic pain. *Patient Care*, p. 263.

Friedman, H.S., & Booth-Kewley, S. (1987). The "disease-prone personality": A meta-analytic view of the construct. *American Psychologist*, **42**(6), 539-555.

Froehlich, J., Simon, G., Schmidt, A., Hitschhold, T., & Bierther, M. (1987). Infektanfalligkeit von sportlern nach gabe von immunglobulinen [Disposition to infections of athletes during treatment with immunoglobulins]. In H. Rieckert (Ed.), *Sportmedizin—Kursbestimmung* (pp. 29-33). Berlin: Springer.

Furney, S.R., & Patton, B. (1985, Winter). An examination of health counseling practices of athletic trainers. *Athletic Training*, **20**, 294-297.

Garrick, J.G. (1989). Anterior knee pain (chondromalacia patellae). *The Physician and Sportsmedicine*, **17**(1), 75-76, 81-84.

Gayuna, S.T., & Hoerner, E.F. (1986). The role of the trainer. In P.E. Vinger & E.F. Hoerner (Eds.), *Sports injuries: The unthwarted epidemic* (2nd ed., pp. 354-372). Littleton, MA: PSG.

Gauron, E.F., & Bowers, W.A. (1986). Pain control techniques in college-age athletes. *Psychological Reports*, **59**, 1163-1169.

Georgia Psychological Association. (1991). *Health care costs are skyrocketing. Can this trend be slowed. . .?: Psychologists can be part of the solution*. Atlanta, GA: Author. (Available from the Georgia Psychological Association, 1170 Fourteenth Place, Atlanta, GA 30309)

Gilligan, S. (1987). *Therapeutic trances*. New York: Brunner/Mazel.

Gipson, M., Blake, D., & Foster, M. (1989, October). *Behavioral medicine for health professionals involved in international sport*. Paper presented at the first International Olympic Committee World Congress on Sport Sciences, Colorado Springs, CO.

Glasser, W. (1976). *Positive addiction*. New York: Harper & Row.

Gold, M.S., Pottash, A.C., Sweeny, D.R., & Kreber, H.D. (1980). Opiate withdrawal using clonidine. *Journal of the American Medical Association*, **243**, 343-346.

Goldenberg, D.L. (1987). Fibromyalgia syndrome. *Journal of the American Medical Association*, **257**(20), 2782-2787.

Goldsmith, B. (1985, October 13). "The first thing I had to conquer was fear": The story of concert pianist Byron Janis. *Parade Magazine*, pp. 4-6.

Goldstein, D. (1989). Clinical applications for exercise. *The Physician and Sportsmedicine*, **17**(8), 83, 86, 89-90, 93.

Gordon, T. (1970). *Parent effectiveness training*. New York: Wyden.

Gould, D. (1987). Understanding attrition in children's sport. In D. Gould & M.R. Weiss (Eds.), *Advances in pediatric sport sciences: Behavioral issues* (Vol. 2, pp. 61-85). Champaign, IL: Human Kinetics.

Gregg, E., & Rejeski, W.J. (1990). Social psychologic dysfunction associated with anabolic steroid abuse: A review. *The Sport Psychologist*, **4**(3), 275-284.

Groves, D. (1989). Pro football: Do players pay with their health? *The Physician and Sportsmedicine*, **17**(1), 168-174, 177.

Grunert, B.K., Devine, C.A., Matloub, H.S., Sanger, J.R., & Yousif, N.J. (1988). Flashbacks after traumatic hand injuries: Prognostic indicators. *Journal of Hand Surgery*, **13a**(1), 125-127.

Hall, R.C.W., Gruzenski, W.P., & Popkin, M.K. (1979). Differential diagnosis of somatopsychic disorders. *Psychosomatics*, **20**(6), 381-389.

Hamel, R. (1992). AIDS: Assessing the risk among athletes. *The Physician and Sportsmedicine*, **20**(2), 139-140, 142, 145-146.

Hammond, D.L., Levy, R.A., & Proudfit, H.K. (1980). Hypoalgesia induced by microinjection of a norepinephrine antagonist in the raphe magnus: Reversal by intrathecal administration of a serotonin antagonist. *Brain Research*, **201**, 475-479.

Hankins, P., Gipson, M., Foster, M., Yaffe, D., & O'Carroll, D. (1989, October). *Psychosocial factors in sports injury diagnosis and rehabilitation: The case of women's intercollegiate volleyball*. Paper presented at the first International Olympic Committee World Congress on Sport Sciences, Colorado Springs, CO.

Hardy, C.J., Prentice, W.E., Kirsanoff, M.T., Richman, J.M., & Rosenfeld, L.B. (1987, June). Life stress, social support, and athletic injury: In search of relationships. In J.M. Williams (Chair), *Psychological factors in injury occurrence*. Symposium conducted at the meeting of the North American Society for the Psychology of Sport and Physical Activity, Vancouver, BC.

Harre, D. (Ed.) (1979). *Trainingslehre* [Textbook of Training]. Berlin: Sportverlag.

Harris, D.V., & Harris, B.L. (1984). *The athlete's guide to sport psychology: Mental skills for physical people.* Champaign, IL: Leisure Press.

Harris, D.V., & Williams, J.M. (in press). Relaxation and energizing techniques for regulation of arousal. In J.M. Williams (Ed.), *Applied sport psychology: Personal growth to peak performance* (2nd ed.). Palo Alto, CA: Mayfield.

Hathaway, S.R., & McKinley, J.C. (1989). *Minnesota Multiphasic Personality Inventory—2* [Manual]. Minneapolis: University of Minnesota Press.

Haycock, C.E. (1986). Women in sports. In P.E. Vinger & E.F. Hoerner (Eds.), *Sports injuries: The unthwarted epidemic* (2nd ed., pp. 77-80). Littleton, MA: PSG.

Hays, K.F. (1990, September). *Negative addiction: When bad things happen to good sports.* Paper presented at the meeting of the Association for the Advancement of Applied Sport Psychology, San Antonio, TX.

Head, H., & Holmes, G. (1911). Sensory disturbances from cerebral lesions. *Brain,* **34,** 102-254.

Heil, J. (1984). Imagery for sport: Theory, research and practice. In W.F. Straub & J.M. Williams (Eds.), *Cognitive sport psychology* (pp. 245-252). Lansing, NY: Sport Science Associates.

Heil, J. (1986, September). *From the hospital bed: Consultation and intervention with the seriously injured athlete.* Paper presented at the annual meeting of the Association for the Advancement of Applied Sport Psychology, Jekyll Island, GA.

Heil, J. (Chair) (1987, April). *Pain and injuries of athletes: The sports medicine team, injury and the psychological care of athletes.* Symposium conducted at the American Alliance of Health, Physical Education, Recreation and Dance National Convention and Exposition, Las Vegas.

Heil, J. (1988, October). *Early identification and intervention with injured athletes at risk for failed rehabiliation.* Workshop conducted at the annual meeting of the Association for the Advancement of Applied Sport Psychology, Nashua, NH.

Heil, J. (1989, June). *Pain management in athletes.* Workshop conducted at the University of Virginia Sport Psychology Conference, Charlottesville.

Heil, J. (1990, October). *Association and dissociation: Clarifying the concept.* Paper presented at the annual meeting of the Association for the Advancement of Applied Sport Psychology, San Antonio, TX.

Heil, J. (1992, June). The thrill of victory!: Risk-taking attitudes in sport. *ASTM Standardization News,* **20**(6), 60-62.

Heil, J., & Lanahan, R. (1992, October). *The HIV positive/athlete with AIDS: Performance and confidentiality issues.* Paper presented at the annual meeting of the Association for the Advancement of Applied Sport Psychology, Colorado Springs, Colorado.

Heil, J., & Russell, S. (1987, July). *Psychological approaches to the management of pain in athletic injury.* Paper presented at the United States Olympic Training Center Festival, 1987 Conference on Sports Medicine and Sport Science, Chapel Hill, NC.

Hellstedt, J.C. (1988). Kids, parents and sports: Some questions and answers. *The Physician and Sportsmedicine,* **16**(4), 59-60, 62, 64, 69-71.

Hendler, N., Mollett, A., Talo, S., & Levin, S. (1988). A comparison between the Minnesota Multiphasic Personality Inventory and the "Mensana Clinic Back Pain Test" for validating the complaint of chronic back pain. *Journal of Occupational Medicine,* **30**(2), 98-102.

Henry, J.L. (1976). Effects of substance P on functionally identified units in cat spinal cord. *Brain Research,* **114**, 439-451.

Henschen, K.P. (1986). Athletic staleness and burnout: Diagnosis, prevention and treatment. In J.M. Williams (Ed.), *Applied sport psychology: Personal growth to peak experience* (pp. 327-342). Palo Alto, CA: Mayfield.

Henschen, K.P., & Heil, J. (1992). A retrospective study of the effect of an athlete's sudden death on teammates. *Omega,* **25**(3), 217-223.

Hokfelt, T., Skirboll, L., Lunberg, J.M., Dalsgaard, C.-J., Johansson, O., Pernow, B., & Jancso, G. (1983). Neuropeptides and pain pathways. In J.J. Bonica (Ed.), *Advances in pain research and therapy* (pp. 227-246). New York: Raven.

Holmes, G.P., Kaplan, J.E., Gantz, N.M., Komaroff, A.L., Schonberger, L.B., Straus, S.E., Jones, J.F., Dubois, R.E., Cunningham-Rundles, C., Pahwa, S., Tosato, G., Zegans, L.S., Purtilo, D.T., Brown, N., Schooley, R.T., & Brus, I. (1988). Chronic fatigue syndrome: A working case definition. *Annals of Internal Medicine,* **108**, 387-389.

Holmes, T.II. (1970). Psychological screening (1969, February). In *Football injuries: Papers presented at a workshop* (sponsored by the Subcommittee on Athletic Injuries, Committee on the Skeletal System, Division of Medical Sciences, National Research Council, pp. 211-214). Washington, DC: National Academy of Sciences.

Holmes, T.H., & Rahe, R.H. (1967). The social readjustment rating scale. *Journal of Psychosomatic Research,* **11**, 213-218.

Hudson, P.B. (1988). Pre-participation screening of Special Olympics athletes. *The Physician and Sportsmedicine,* **16**(4), 101-104.

Hughes, J., Smith, T.W., Kosterlitz, H.W., Fothergill, L.A., Morgan, B.A., & Morris, H.R. (1975). Identification of two related pentapeptides from the brain with potent opiate agonist activity. *Nature,* **258**, 577-579.

Hyams, J. (1979). *Zen in the martial arts.* Los Angeles: Tarcher.

Ievleva, L. (1988). *Psychological factors in knee and ankle injury recovery: An exploratory study.* Unpublished master's thesis, University of Ottawa, Ottawa, ON.

Ievleva, L., & Orlick, T. (1991). Mental links to enhanced healing: An exploratory study. *The Sport Psychologist,* **5**(1), 25-40.

Injury statistics groups. (1991). *The Physician and Sportsmedicine*, **19**(1), 116-118.

International Association for the Study of Pain Subcommittee on Taxonomy. (1986). Classification of chronic pain: Descriptions of chronic pain syndromes and definitions of pain terms. In H. Merskey (Ed.), *Pain: The Journal of the International Association for the Study of Pain*, (Suppl. 3), S1-S226.

Israel, S. (1967). Das akute entlastungssyndrom des leistungssportlers [The acute exercise-abstinence syndrome of competitive athletes]. *Sportarzt und Sportmedizin*, **18**, 185-190.

Israel, S. (1976). Zur problematik des uebertrainings aus internistischer und leistungsphysiologischer sicht [The problem of overtraining from the perspective of internal medicine and exercise physiology]. *Medizin und Sport*, **16**, 1-12.

Iversen, G.E. (1990). Behind schedule: Psychosocial aspects of delayed puberty in the competitive female gymnast. *The Sport Psychologist*, **4**(2), 155-167.

Jacobs, D.T. (1991). *Patient communication for first responders and EMS personnel: The first hour of trauma*. Englewood Cliffs, NJ: Brady.

Jaremko, M.E., Silbert, L., & Mann, T. (1981). The differential ability of athletes and non-athletes to cope with two types of pain: A radical behavioral model. *The Psychological Record*, **31**, 265-275.

Johnson, E.W. (1987, July). *Pain management in sport injuries*. The Burroughs Welcome Lecture presented at the United States Olympic Festival—1987 Congress on Sports Medicine and Science, Chapel Hill, NC.

Johnson, R.J. (1991). Help your athletes heal themselves. *The Physician and Sportsmedicine*, **19**(5), 107-108, 110.

Johnston, D., & Mannell, R.C. (1980). The effects of experimentally created team norms on pain perception. In P. Klavora & K.A.W. Wipper (Eds.), *Psychological and sociological factors in sport* (pp. 306-314). Toronto: School of Physical and Health Education, University of Toronto.

Kabat-Zinn, J. (1982). An outpatient program in behavioral medicine for chronic pain patients based on the practice of mindfulness meditation: Theoretical considerations and preliminary results. *General Hospital Psychiatry*, **4**, 313-347.

Kahneman, D. (1973). *Attention and effort*. Englewood Cliffs, NJ: Prentice Hall.

Kanner, A.D., Coyne, J.C., Schaefer, C., & Lazarus, R.S. (1981). Comparison of two modes of stress management: Daily hassles and uplifts versus major life events. *Journal of Behavioral Medicine*, **4**(1), 1-39.

Kardiner, A. (1959). Traumatic neuroses of war. In S. Arietia (Ed.), *American handbook of psychiatry* (Vol. 1, pp. 246-257). New York: Basic Books.

Karofsky, P.S. (1990). Death of a high school hockey player. *The Physician and Sportsmedicine*, **18**(2), 99-100, 102-103.

Keefe, F.J., & Block, A.R. (1982). Development of an observation method in assessing pain behavior in chronic low back pain patients. *Behavior Therapy*, **13**, 363-375.

Kerlan, R. (1978). *Health and fitness through physical activity*. New York: Wiley.

Kerr, G., & Minden, H. (1988). Psychological factors related to the occurrence of athletic injuries. *Journal of Sport and Exercise Psychology*, **10**, 167-173.

Kiesler, S., & Finholt, T. (1988). The mystery of RSI. *American Psychologist*, **43**(12), 1004-1015.

Kindermann, W. (1986). Das uebertraining—ausdruck einer vegetativen fehlsteuerung [Overtraining—expression of a disturbed autonomic regulation]. *Deutsche Zeitschrift für Sportmedizin, 37*, 238-245.

Kindermann, W. (1988). Metabolic and hormonal reactions in overtraining. *Seminars in Orthopaedics*, **3**(4), 207-216.

Kizilos, P.J. (1989). In pro hockey getting out may be smarter than playing hurt. *The Physician and Sportsmedicine*, **17**(3), 215-216, 218.

Knapp, D.N. (1988). Behavior management techniques and exercise promotion. In R.K. Dishman (Ed.), *Exercise adherence: Its impact on public health* (pp. 203-236). Champaign, IL: Human Kinetics.

Kobasa, S.C. (1979). Stressful life events, personality and health: An inquiry into hardiness. *Journal of Personality and Social Psychology*, **37**, 1-11.

Koesters, E., & Heil, J. (1986). Athlete and artist: Search for a common ground. In L.-E. Unestahl (Ed.), *Sport psychology: In theory and practice* (pp. 190-195). Orebro, Sweden: Veje.

Koplan, J.P., Siscovick, D.S., & Goldbaum, G.M. (1985). The risks of exercise: A public health view of injuries and hazards. *Public Health Reports*, **100**, 189-195.

Kraus, J.F., & Conroy, C. (1984). Mortality and morbidity from injuries in sports and recreation. *Annual Review of Public Health*, **5**, 163-192.

Kreiner-Phillips, K. (1990, January). Psyche up for skiing. *Ski Canada*, pp. 111, 114.

Kroll, W. (1970). Current strategies and problems in personality assessment of athletes. In L.E. Smith (Ed.), *Psychology of motor learning* (pp. 349-371). Chicago: Athletic Institute.

Kubler-Ross, E. (1969). *On death and dying*. New York: Macmillan.

Kuipers, H., & Keizer, H.A. (1988). Overtraining in elite athletes. Review and directions for the future. *Sports Medicine*, **6**, 79-92.

LaMott, E.E., & Petlichkoff, L.M. (1990, September). *Psychological factors and the injured athlete: Is there a relationship?* Paper presented at the annual meeting of the Association for the Advancement of Applied Sport Psychology, San Antonio, TX.

Landry, G.L. (1989). *AIDS in sport*. Champaign, IL: Human Kinetics.

Langley, J. (1984). Injury control—psychosocial considerations. *Journal of Child Psychology and Psychiatry*, **25**(3), 349-356.

Layman, D.P., & Morris, A. (1986, June). *Addiction and injury in runners: Is there a mind-body connection?* Paper presented at the meeting of the North American Society for the Psychology of Sport and Physical Activity, Scottsdale, AZ.

Lehmann, M., Dickhuth, H.H., Gendrisch, G., Lazar, W., Thum, M., Aramendi, J.F., Hounker, M., Jakob, E., Durr, H., Stockhausen, W., Wieland, H., & Keul, J. (1990). Training—over-training: A prospective, experimental study with experienced middle and long distance runners. *Deutsche Zeitschriff für Sportmedizin*, **41**.

Lerch, S.H. (1979). *Adjustment to early retirement: A case of professional baseball players.* Unpublished doctoral dissertation, Purdue University, Lafayette, IN.

LeUnes, A.D., Hayward, S.A., & Daiss, S. (1988). Annotated bibliography of the Profile of Mood States in sport. *Journal of Sport Behavior*, **11**, 213-219.

LeUnes, A.D., & Nation, J.R. (1989). *Sport psychology: An introduction.* Chicago: Nelson-Hall.

Levine, J.D., Gordon, N.C., & Fields, H.L. (1978). The mechanism of placebo analgesia. *Lancet*, **2**, 654-657.

Linder, D.E., Pillow, D.R., & Reno, R.R. (1989). Shrinking jocks: Derogation of athletes who consult a sport psychologist. *Journal of Sport and Exercise Psychology*, **11**(3), 270-280.

Lipowski, Z.J. (1969). Psychosocial aspects of disease. *Annals of Internal Medicine*, **71**, 1197-1206.

Little, J.C. (1969). The athlete's neuroses—A deprivation crisis. *Acta Psychiatrica Scandinavica*, **45**, 187-197.

Lloyd, T., Trianthafyllou, S.T., Baker, E.R., Houts, P.S., Whiteside, J.A., Kalenak, A., & Stumpf, P.G. (1986). Women athletes with menstrual irregularity have increased musculoskeletal injuries. *Medicine and Science in Sports and Exercise*, **18**(4), 374-379.

Locke, E.A., & Latham, G.P. (1985). The application of goal-setting to sports. *Journal of Sport Psychology*, **7**, 205-222.

Loeser, J. (1982). Concepts of pain. In M. Stanton-Hicks & R.A. Boas (Eds.), *Chronic low back pain*, New York: Raven.

Loeser, J. (1991, February). *Pain management: Past and current status including the role of the anesthesiologist.* Paper presented at the 36th Annual Postgraduate Course in Anesthesiology, Snowbird, UT.

Lord, R.H., & Kozar, B. (1989). Pain tolerance in the presence of others: Implications for youth sports. *The Physician and Sportsmedicine*, **17**(10), 71-72, 77.

Lubell, A. (1989a). Chronic brain injury in boxers: Is it avoidable? *The Physician and Sportsmedicine*, **17**(11), 126-128, 130, 132.

Lubell, A. (1989b). Does steroid abuse cause—or excuse—violence? *The Physician and Sportsmedicine,* **17**(2), 176-185.

Lusk, J.T. (in press). *30 Scripts for Relaxation, Imagery, and Inner Healing* (Vol. 2). Duluth, MN: Whole Person Press.

Lybbert, M.R., & Laycock, L.R. (1987). Medicolegal aspects of youth athletic participation. *Syllabus: Sportsmedicine seminar—1987.* Salt Lake City, UT: The University of Utah Medical Center, Departments of Orthopaedics and Pediatrics.

Macera, C.A., Pate, R.R., Powell, K.E., Jackson, K.L., Kendric, J.S., & Craven, T.E. (1989). Predicting lower-extremity injuries among habitual runners. *Archives of Internal Medicine,* **149**, 2565-2568.

Mahoney, M.J., Gabriel, T.J., & Perkins, T.S. (1987). Psychological skills and exceptional athletic performance. *The Sport Psychologist,* **1**(3), 181-199.

Maliszewski, M. (1990). Injuries in boxing: Evaluations and policy decisions. *The Sport Psychologist,* **4**, 55-62.

Martens, R. (1977). *Sport Competition Anxiety Test.* Champaign, IL: Human Kinetics.

Martens, R. (Ed.) (1978). *Joy and sadness in children's sports.* Champaign, IL: Human Kinetics.

Martens, R. (1987). *Coaches guide to sport psychology.* Champaign, IL: Human Kinetics.

Martens, R. (1989). *American Coaching Effectiveness Program, Level II: Sport psychology.* Champaign, IL: Human Kinetics.

Martens, R., Burton, D., Vealey, R.S., Bump, L.A., & Smith, D. (1982). *Cognitive and somatic dimensions of competitive anxiety.* Paper presented at the annual meeting of the North American Society for the Psychology of Sport and Physical Activity, University of Maryland, College Park.

Martens, R., & Landers, D.M. (1969). Coaction effects on a muscular endurance task. *The Research Quarterly,* **40**(4), 733-737.

Martens, R., & Seefeldt, V. (1978). Bill of rights for young athletes. In R. Martens (Ed.), *Joy and sadness in children's sports* (p. 360). Champaign, IL: Human Kinetics.

Martland, H.S. (1928). Punch drunk. *The Journal of the American Medical Association,* **91**, 1103-1107.

Masters, K.S., & Lambert, N.J. (1989). The relations between cognitive coping strategies, reasons for running, injury, and performance of marathon runners. *Journal of Sport and Exercise Psychology,* **11**(2), 161-170.

Mathews, A. (1978). Fear reduction research and clinical phobias. *Psychological Bulletin,* **85**(2), 390-404.

Mavissakalian, M. & Barlow, D. (Eds.). (1981). *Phobia: Psychological and pharmacological treatment.* New York: Guilford Press.

Mayer, D.J., & Price, D.D. (1976). Central nervous system mechanisms of analgesia. *Pain: The Journal of the International Association for the Study of Pain*, **2**, 379-404.

Mayer, D.J., Price, D.D., & Becker, D.P. (1975). Neurophysiological characterization of the anterolateral spinal cord neurons contributing to pain perception in man. *Pain: The Journal of the International Association for the Study of Pain*, **1**, 51-58.

Mayer, D.J., Wolfe, T.L., Akil, H., Carder, B., & Liebeskind, J.C. (1971). Analgesia from electrical stimulation in the brain stem of the rat. *Science*, **174**, 1351-1354.

McCabe, P., & Schneiderman, N.S. (1984). Psychophysiological reactions to stress. In N.S. Schneiderman & J.J. Tapp (Eds.), *Behavioral medicine: The biopsychosocial approach*. Hillsdale, NJ: Erlbaum.

McCarthy, P. (1989). Managing bursitis in the athlete: An overview. *The Physician and Sportsmedicine*, **17**(11), 115-118, 120, 122, 125.

McDermott, B. (1982, November). The glitter has gone. *Sports Illustrated*, pp. 83-96.

McDonald, S.A., & Hardy, C.J. (1990). Affective response patterns of the injured athlete: An exploratory analysis. *The Sport Psychologist*, **4**(3), 261-274.

McGrath, P.A. (1990). *Pain in children: Nature, assessment & treatment*. New York: Guilford Press.

McNair, D.N., Lorr, M., & Droppleman, L.F. (1971). *Profile of Mood States*. San Diego: Educational and Industrial Testing Services.

Mehler, W.R. (1967). The anatomy of the so-called "pain tract" in man: An analysis of the source and distribution of the ascending fibers of the fasciculous anterolateralis. In J.D. French & R.W. Porter (Eds.), *Basic research in paraplegia* (pp. 26-55). Springfield, IL: Charles C Thomas.

Meichenbaum, D. (1976). Cognitive factors in biofeedback therapy. *Biofeedback and self-regulation*, **1**(2), 201-216.

Meichenbaum, D. (1985). *Stress inoculation training*. New York: Pergamon Press.

Meichenbaum, D., & Turk, D.C. (1987). *Facilitating treatment adherence: A practitioner's guidebook*. New York: Plenum Press.

Melzack, R. (1961). The perception of pain. *Scientific American*, **204**, 41-49.

Melzack, R. (1975). The McGill pain questionnaire: Major properties and scoring methods. *Pain: The Journal of the International Association for the Study of Pain*, **1**, 277-299.

Melzack, R., & Wall, P.D. (1965). Pain mechanisms: A new theory. *Science*, **150**, 971-979.

Mets' Gooden calls it a year. (1989, September 24). *Roanoke Times & World-News*, p. B-5.

Michener, J.A. (1976). *Sports in America*. Greenwich, CT: Fawcett.

Mies, H. (1957). Erschoepfung und uebermuedung [Exhaustion and over-tiredness]. *Sportmedizin*, **8**, 13-17.

Miller, L.H., & Smith, A.D. (1982, December). Stress audit questionnaire. *Bostonia: In-depth*, pp. 39-54.

Miller, R.R., Feingold, A., & Paxinos, J. (1970). Propoxyphene hydrochloride: A critical review. *Journal of the American Medical Association*, **213**, 996-1006.

Millon, T., Green, C.J., & Meagher, R.B. (1982). *Millon Behavioral Health Inventory Manual* (3rd ed.). Minneapolis: NCS Interpretive Scoring Systems.

Moertel, C., Ahmann, D.L., Taylor, W.F., & Schwartau, N. (1974). Relief of pain by oral medications. *Journal of the American Medical Association*, **229**, 55-59.

Monahan, T. (1987). Sport psychology: A crisis of identity? *The Physician and Sportsmedicine*, **15**(9), 202-212.

Monahan, T. (1988). Perceived exertion: An old exercise tool finds new applications. *The Physician and Sportsmedicine*, **16**(10), 174-176, 178-179.

Monroe, S.M. (1983). Major and minor life events as predictors of psychological distress: Further issues and findings. *Journal of Behavioral Medicine*, **6**(2), 189-205.

Morgan, W.P. (1978, April). The mind of the marathoner. *Psychology Today*, pp. 38-40, 43, 45-46, 49.

Morgan, W.P. (1979). Negative addiction in runners. *The Physician and Sportsmedicine*, **7**(2), 57-63, 67-69.

Morgan, W.P., Brown, D.R., Raglin, J.S., O'Conner, P.J., & Ellickson, K.A. (1987). Psychological monitoring of overtraining and staleness. *British Journal of Sports Medicine*, **21**(3), 107-114.

Morgan, W.P., & O'Conner, P.J. (1988). Exercise and mental health. In R.K. Dishman (Ed.), *Exercise adherence: Its impact on public health* (pp. 91-121). Champaign, IL: Human Kinetics.

Morgan, W.P., & Pollock, M.L. (1977). Psychological characterization of the elite distance runner. *Annals of the New York Academy of Science*, **301**, 382-403.

Mueller, F.O., & Blyth, C.S. (1987). *National Center for Catastrophic Sports Injury Research: Fifth Annual Report, 1982-1987*. Chapel Hill: University of North Carolina.

Mueller, F.O., & Cantu, R.C. (1990). *National Center for Catastrophic Sports Injury Research: Eighth Annual Report, 1982-1990*. Chapel Hill: University of North Carolina.

Mumford, E., Schlesinger, H.J., & Glass, G.V. (1982). The effects of psychological intervention on recovery from surgery and heart attacks: A review of the literature. *American Journal of Public Health*, **72**, 141-151.

Munnings, F. (1987). What is sportsmedicine? [Editorial]. *The Physician and Sportsmedicine*, **15**(1), 41.

Munnings, F. (1990). The death of Hank Gathers: A legacy of confusion. *The Physician and Sportsmedicine*, **18**(5), 97-102.

Murphy, S.M., Fleck, J.J., Dudley, G., & Callister, R. (1990). Psychological and performance concomitants of increased volume training in elite athletes. *Journal of Applied Sport Psychology*, **2**(1), 34-50.

Muse, M. (1985). Stress related, posttraumatic chronic pain syndrome: Criteria for diagnosis, and preliminary report on prevalence. *Pain: The Journal of the International Association for the Study of Pain*, **23**, 295-300.

Nack, W. (1989, September 4). A life cut short. *Sports Illustrated*, pp. 136-146.

Nash, H.O. (1987). Elite child-athletes: How much does victory cost? *The Physician and Sportsmedicine*, **15**(8), 128-133.

National Institutes of Health Consensus Development Conference. (1986). The integrated approach to the management of pain. *Journal of Pain and Symptom Management*, **2**, 35-44.

Neisler, N.M., Bean, M.H., Pittington, J., Thompson, W.R., Johnson, J.T., & Smith, J.L. (1989). Alteration of lymphocyte subsets and endocrine response during 42 days of competitive swim training. *Medicine and Science in Sports and Exercise*, **27**(2) (Suppl.), 110.

Nicholas, J.A. (1976). Risk factors, sportsmedicine and the orthopaedic system: An overview. *Journal of Sportsmedicine*, **3**(5), 243-259.

Nideffer, R.M. (1976). Test of Attentional and Interpersonal Style. *Journal of Personality and Social Psychology*, **34**, 394-404.

Nideffer, R.M. (1981). *The ethics and practice of applied sport psychology*. Ithaca, NY: Mouvement.

Nideffer, R.M. (1983). The injured athlete: Psychological factors in treatment. *Orthopaedic Clinics of North America*, **14**(2), 373-385.

Nideffer, R.M. (1990). Use of the Test of Attentional and Interpersonal Style (TAIS) in sport. *The Sport Psychologist*, **2**(3), 285-300.

Nims, J.F. (Ed.) (1983). *Western wind: An introduction to poetry* (2nd ed.). New York: Random House.

Noordenbos, W. (1984). Prologue. In R. Melzack & P.D. Wall (Eds.), *Textbook of pain* (pp. xi-xv). New York: Churchill Livingstone.

Nowlin, T.B. (1974). *The relationship between experimental pain tolerance and personality traits among four athletic groups*. Unpublished doctoral dissertation. Greeley, CO: University of Northern Colorado.

Ogilvie, B.C. (1974, October). Stimulus addiction: The sweet psychic jolt of danger. *Psychology Today*, pp. 88, 93-94.

Ogilvie, B.C. (1977). Walking the perilous path of the team psychologist. *The Physician and Sportsmedicine*, **5**(4), 63-68.

Ogilvie, B.C., & Tutko, T.A. (1966). *Problem athletes and how to handle them*. London: Pelham Books.

Okwumabua, T.M., Meyers, A.W., Schleser, R., & Cooke, C.J. (1983). Cognitive strategies and running performance: An exploratory study. *Cognitive Therapy and Research*, **7**(4), 363-370.

Once every four years, someone does the impossible. (1988, January 31). *Parade Magazine*, p. 3.

Orlick, T. (1986). *Psyching for sport: Mental training for athletes*. Champaign, IL: Human Kinetics.

Orlick, T., & Partington, J. (1988). Mental links to excellence. *The Sport Psychologist*, **2**, 105-130.

Ostrow, A.C. (Ed.) (1990). *Directory of psychological tests in the sport and exercise sciences*. Morgantown, WV: Fitness Information Technology.

Overdose caused death of Matuszak. (1989, June 28). *The Washington Post*, p. F4.

Pacelli, L.C. (1990). Mike Ditka and stress or . . . The case of the exploding coach. *The Physician and Sportsmedicine*, **18**(2), 127-128, 130.

Pargman, D. (1986). *Preparing the injured athlete for resumption of performance*. Paper presented at the annual meeting of the Association for the Advancement of Applied Sports Psychology, Jekyll Island, GA.

Partington, J., & Orlick, T. (1987). The sport psychology consultant: Olympic coaches' views. *The Sport Psychologist*, **1**(2), 95-102.

Passer, M.W., & Seese, M.D. (1983). Life stress and athletic injury: Examination of positive versus negative events and three moderator variables. *Journal of Human Stress*, **9**, 11-16.

Pasternak, G.W. (1988). Multiple morphine and enkephalin receptors and the relief of pain. *Journal of the American Medical Association*, **259**, 1362-1367.

Pearson, R.E., & Petitpas, A.J. (1990, September/October). Transitions of athletes: Developmental and preventive perspectives. *Journal of Counseling & Development*, **69**, 7-10.

Pelletier, K.R. (1977). *Mind as healer, mind as slayer*. New York: Delta Books.

Pelletier, K.R. (1979). *Holistic medicine: From stress to optimal health*. New York: Delacorte & Delta.

Percy, E.C. (1986). The athletic alchemist: Drugs in sport. In P.E. Vinger & E.F. Hoerner (Eds.), *Sports injuries: The unthwarted epidemic* (2nd ed., pp. 281-285). Littleton, MA: PSG.

Perl, E.R. (1980). Afferent basis of nociception and pain. In J.J. Bonica (Ed.), *Pain* (Vol. 58). New York: Research Publications, Association for Research in Nervous and Mental Disease.

The petals are un-folding for Darryl Stingley again. (1982, August 22). *The Day* [New London, CT], p. C-6.

Peterson, K., Durtschi, S., & Murphy, S. (1990, September). *Cognitive patterns and conceptual schemes of elite distance runners during sub-maximum and maximum running effort*. Paper presented at the annual meeting of the Association for the Advancement of Applied Sport Psychology, San Antonio, TX.

Petipas, A., Danish, S., McKelvain, R., & Murphy, S. (1992). A career assistance program for elite athletes. *Journal of Counseling & Development*, **70**, 383-386.

Petrie, T.A. (in press). Psychosocial antecedents of athletic injury: The effects of life stress and social support on female collegiate gymnasts. *Behavioral Medicine.*

Petruzzello, S.J., Landers, D.M., & Salazar, W. (1991). Biofeedback and sport/exercise performance: Applications and limitations. *Behavior Therapy,* **22,** 379-392.

Pines, A.M., Aronson, E., & Kafry, D. (1981). *Burnout.* New York: Free Press.

Pomerleau, O.F. (1982). A discourse on behavioral medicine: Current status and future trends. *Journal of Consulting and Clinical Psychology,* **50**(6), 1030-1039.

Porter, J., & Jick, H. (1980). Addiction rare in patients treated with narcotics [Letter to the editor]. *New England Journal of Medicine,* **302,** 123.

Puhl, J.L., Brown, C.H., & Voy, R.O. (Eds.) (1988). *Sport science perspectives for women.* Champaign, IL: Human Kinetics.

Ransford, A.O., Cairns, D., & Mooney, V. (1976). The pain drawing as an aid to the psychologic evaluation of patients with low-back pain. *Spine,* **1**(2), 127-134.

Ravizza, K. (1988). Gaining entry with athletic personnel for season-long consulting. *The Sport Psychologist,* **2**(3), 243-254.

Reed, J.D. (1976, April 26). Week of disgrace on ice. *Sports Illustrated,* **44**(17), 22-25.

Reif, A.E. (1986). Risks and gains. In P.E. Vinger & E.F. Hoerner (Eds.), *Sports injuries: The unthwarted epidemic* (2nd ed., pp. 48-57). Littleton, MA: PSG.

Repeated stress fractures in an amenorrheic marathoner: A case conference. (1989). *The Physician and Sportsmedicine,* **17**(4), 65-66, 69-71.

Rettig, A.C. (1990). Scanning Sports. *The Physician and Sportsmedicine,* **18**(9), 19.

Rexed, B. (1952). The cytoarchitectonic organization of the spinal cord in the cat. *Journal of Comparative Neurology,* **96,** 415-495.

Reynolds, D.V. (1969). Surgery in the rat during electrical analgesia induced by focal brain stimulation. *Science,* **164,** 444-445.

Rians, C.B. (1990). *Principles and practices of sportsmedicine.* Unpublished manuscript.

Richman, J.M., Hardy, C.J., Rosenfeld, L.B., & Callanan, R.A.E. (1989). Strategies for enhancing social support networks in sport: A brainstorming experience. *Applied Sport Psychology,* **1,** 150-159.

Roberts, G. (1991). Working with various populations [Special theme issue]. *The Sport Psychologist,* **5**(4).

Roberts, W.J. (1986). A hypothesis on the physiological basis for causalgia and related pains. *Pain: The Journal of the International Association for the Study of Pain,* **24,** 297-311.

Rogers, C. (1951). *Client-centered therapy.* Boston: Houghton Mifflin.

Romano, J.N., Turner, J.A., & Sullivan, N.D. (1989, Winter). What are some basic guidelines for the primary care practitioner's management of chronic nonmalignant pain? *American Pain Society Newsletter*, p. 4.

Rosenfeld, L.B., Richman, J.N., & Hardy, C.J. (1989). Examining social support networks among athletes: Description and relationship to stress. *The Sport Psychologist*, **3**, 23-33.

Rossi, E. (Ed.) (1980). *The collected papers of Milton H. Erickson* (Vol. 4). New York: Irvington.

Rotella, R.J. (1982). Psychological care of the injured athlete. In D.N. Kulund (Ed.), *The injured athlete* (pp. 213-224). Philadelphia: Lippincott.

Rotella, R.J., & Bunker, L.K. (1987). *Parenting your superstar*. Champaign, IL: Leisure Press.

Rotella, R.J., & Heil, J. (1991). Psychological aspects of sports medicine. In B. Reider (Ed.), *Sports medicine: The school-age athlete*. Philadelphia: Saunders.

Rotella, R.J., & Heyman, S.R. (1986). Stress, injury and the psychological rehabilitation of athletes. In J.M. Williams (Ed.), *Applied sport psychology: Personal growth to peak performance* (pp. 343-364). Palo Alto, CA: Mayfield.

Rotter, J.B. (1966). Generalized expectancies for internal versus external locus of control of reinforcement. *Psychological Monographs*, **80**(Whole No. 609).

Rozek, M. (1985, February/March). Musicians and medicine: Is there a doctor in the house? *Symphony Magazine*, pp. 9-12.

Russell, S., Heil, J., & Milano, R. (1986, November). *The impact of aerobic exercise in the rehabilitation of chronic pain patients*. Paper presented at the annual meeting of the Association for the Advancement of Applied Sport Psychology, Jekyll Island, GA.

Ryan, A.J. (1973). Medical practices in sports. *Law and Contemporary Problems*, **38**(1), 99-111.

Ryan, A.J., Brown, R.L., Frederick, E.C., Falsetti, H.L., & Burke, E.R. (1983). Overtraining of athletes [Round table]. *The Physician and Sportsmedicine*, **11**(6), 93-100.

Ryan, E.D., & Foster, R.L. (1967). Athletic participation and perceptual augmentation and reduction. *Journal of Abnormal Psychology*, **6**, 472-476.

Ryan, E.D., & Kovacic, C.R. (1966). Pain tolerance and athletic participation. *Perceptual and Motor Skills*, **22**, 383-390.

Sachs, M.L. (1984). The runner's high. In M.L. Sachs & G.W. Buffone (Eds.), *Running as therapy* (pp. 273-283). Lincoln: University of Nebraska Press.

Sachs, M.L., & Henschen, K. (1988). Applied psychology forum. *AAASP Newsletter*, **3**(2), 8.

Saigh, P.A. (1992). *Post traumatic stress disorder: A behavioral approach to assessment and treatment*. New York: Macmillan.

Samples, P. (1987). Mind over muscle: Returning the injured athlete to play. *The Physician and Sportsmedicine*, **15**(10), 172, 174-175, 179-180.

Samples, P. (1989). Spinal cord injuries: The high cost of careless diving. *The Physician and Sportsmedicine*, **17**(7), 143-144, 147-148.

Sanderson, F.H. (1978). The psychological implications of injury. *British Journal of Sportsmedicine*, **12**(1), 41-43.

Sandweiss, J.H., & Wolf, S.L. (1985). *Biofeedback and sport science*. New York: Plenum Press.

Sarason, I.G., Sarason, B.R., & Pierce, G.R. (1990). Social support, personality, and performance. *Journal of Applied Sport Psychology*, **2**(2), 117-127.

Sass, R., & Crook, G. (1981). Accident proneness: Science of non-science? *International Journal of Health Sciences*, **11**(2), 175-190.

Scadding, J.W. (1981). Development of ongoing activity, mechanosensitivity and adrenaline sensitivity in severed peripheral nerve axons. *Experimental Neurology*, **73**, 345-364.

Schaap, D. (1984, July 8). The story of two young fighters, one of whom you will never know: And now . . . the winner. *Parade Magazine*, pp. 10-11.

Schacham, S. (1983). A shortened version of the Profile of Mood States. *Journal of Personality Assessment*, **47**, 305-306.

Schlesinger, H.J., Mumford, E., Glass, G.V., Patrick, C., & Sharfstein, S. (1983). Mental health treatment and medical care utilization in a fee-for-service system: Outpatient mental health treatment following the onset of a chronic disease. *American Journal of Mental Health*, **73**, 422-429.

Schmid, A., & Peper, E. (in press). Techniques for training concentration. In J.M. Williams (Ed.), *Applied sport psychology: Personal growth to peak performance* (2nd ed.). Palo Alto, CA: Mayfield.

Schomer, H.H. (1986). Mental strategies and the perception of effort of marathon runners. *International Journal of Sport Psychology*, **17**, 41-49.

Schomer, H.H. (1987). Mental strategy training programme for marathon runners. *International Journal of Sport Psychology*, **18**, 133-151.

Schwartz, M.S. (1987). *Biofeedback: A practitioner's guide*. New York: Guilford.

Scott, V., & Gijsbers, K. (1981). Pain perception in competitive swimmers. *British Medical Journal*, **283**, 91-93.

Selye, H. (1956). *The stress of life*. New York: McGraw-Hill.

Selzer, M.L., & Vinokur, A. (1974). Life events, subjective stress, and traffic accidents. *American Journal of Psychiatry*, **131**, 903-906.

Sheehan, G. (1990). Sports medicine renaissance. *The Physician and Sportsmedicine*, **18**(11), 26.

Shell, C.G. (Ed.). (1986). *The dancer as athlete*. Champaign, IL: Human Kinetics.

Shepard, J.G., & Pacelli, L.C. (1990). Why your patients shouldn't take aging sitting down. *The Physician and Sportsmedicine*, **18**(11), 83-84, 89-90.

Silva, J.M. (1989). *Sport performance phobias*. Paper presented at the annual meeting for the Association for the Advancement of Applied Sport Psychology, Seattle, WA.

Silva, J.M. (1990). An analysis of the training stress syndrome in competitive athletics. *Journal of Applied Sport Psychology*, **2**(1), 5-20.

Smith, A.M., Scott, S.G., O'Fallon, W.M., & Young, M.L. (1990). Emotional responses of athletes to injury. *Mayo Clinic Proceedings*, **65**, 38-50.

Smith, M.C. (1976). Retrograde cell changes in human spinal cord after anterolateral cordotomies: Location and identification after different periods of survival. *Advances in Pain Research and Therapy*, **1**, 91-98.

Smith, R.E. (1979). A cognitive affective approach to stress management for athletics. In C.H. Nadeau, W.R. Halliwell, K.M. Newell, & G.C. Roberts (Eds.), *Psychology of motor behavior and sport* (pp. 54-72). Champaign, IL: Human Kinetics.

Smith, R.E. (1986). Toward a cognitive-affective model of athletic burnout. *Journal of Sport Psychology*, **8**, 36-50.

Smith, R.E., Smoll, F.L., & Ptacek, J.T. (1990a). Conjunctive moderator variables in vulnerability and resiliency: Life stress, social support and coping skills, and adolescent sport injuries. *Journal of Personality and Social Psychology*, **58**, 360-370.

Smith, R.E., Smoll, F.L., & Ptacek, J.T. (1990b, September). *Sport and non-sport-related negative life events, sensation-seeking motivation, and athletic injuries*. Paper presented at the annual meeting of the Association for Advancement of Applied Sport Psychology, San Antonio, TX.

Smith, T.W., Aberger, E.W., Follick, M.J., & Ahern, D.K. (1986). Cognitive distortion and psychological distress in chronic low back pain. *Journal of Consulting and Clinical Psychology*, **54**(4), 573-575.

Smith, T.W., Follick, M.J., Ahern, D.K., & Adams, A. (1986). Cognitive distortion and disability in chronic low back pain. *Cognitive Therapy and Research*, **10**(2), 201-210.

Sologub, J.B. (1982). Elektroenzelphalographische untersuchungen ueber die entwicklung des trainingszustandes bei sportlern [Electroencephalographic examinations to monitor the training state of athletes]. In K. Tittel & L. Pickenhan (Eds.), *Anpassungsesrscheinungen und Sport Sportliche Belastung* [Signs of Adaptation and Physical Exercise] (pp. 27-44). Leipzig, Germany: Barth.

Sonstroem, R.J. (1988). Psychological models. In R.K. Dishman (Ed.), *Exercise adherence: Its impact on public health* (pp. 125-154). Champaign, IL: Human Kinetics.

Spengler, D.M., & Freeman, C.W. (1979, March/April). Patient selection for lumbar discectomy: An objective approach. *Spine*, **4**(2), 129-134.

Spolin, V. (1963). *Improvisation for the theater: A handbook of teaching and directing techniques.* Evanston, IL: Northwestern University Press.

Staats, T.E., & Reynolds, J.S. (1990, July). Tests help spot exaggerated back problems. *Back Pain Monitor,* pp. 103-106.

Stanish, W.D. (1984). Overuse injuries in athletes: A perspective. *Medicine and Science in Sports and Exercise,* **16,** 1-7.

Stanley, T.H., Ashburn, M.A., & Fine, P.G. (Eds.) (1991). *Anesthesiology and pain management.* Boston: Kluwer Academic

Steadman, J.R. (1980). Rehabilitation after knee ligament surgery. *The American Journal of Sports Medicine,* **8**(4), 294-296.

Steadman, J.R. (1981). Rehabilitation of tibial plafond fractures after stable internal fixation. *The American Journal of Sports Medicine,* **9**(1), 71-72.

Steadman, J.R. (1982). Rehabilitation of skiing injuries. *Clinics in Sportsmedicine,* **1**(2), 289-294.

Steckbeck, J.S. (1951). *Fabulous redmen: The Carlisle Indians and their famous football teams.* Harrisburg, PA: McFarland.

Stein, H. (1984, September). Brought to his knees. *Sport,* pp. 61, 63-67.

Sternbach, R.A. (1987). *Mastering pain: A 12-step program for coping with chronic pain.* New York: Putnam.

Stout, C.E. (1988). A clinician's guide to differential diagnosis between physical and psychiatric disorders. *Medical Psychotherapy,* **1,** 65-72.

Strauss, R.H. (1987). Effects of therapeutic drugs on sports performance. In R.H. Strauss (Ed.), *Drugs and performance in sport* (pp. 167-172). Philadelphia: Saunders.

Strauss, R.H. (1989). A new meaning for "playing hurt" [Editor's notes]. *The Physician and Sportsmedicine,* **17**(7), 3.

Strauss, R.H. (1990). Sports physicians caught between health and the pursuit of happiness. *The Physician and Sportsmedicine,* **18**(5), 26.

Stuart, J.C., & Brown, B.M. (1981). The relationship of stress and coping ability to incidence of diseases and accidents. *Journal of Psychosomatic Research,* **25,** 255-260.

Suinn, R.M. (1976, July). Body thinking: Psychology for Olympic champs. *Psychology Today,* pp. 38, 40-41.

Suinn, R.M. (1980). *Psychology in sports: Methods and applications.* Minneapolis: Burgess International Group Inc.

Svoboda, B., & Vanek, M. (1982). Retirement from high level competition. In T. Orlick, J.T. Partington, & J.H. Salmela (Eds.), *Mental training for coaches and athletes* (pp. 166-175). Ottawa, ON: Sport in Perspective.

Tatum, J., & Kushner, B. (1979). *They call me assassin.* New York: Everest House.

Taylor, G.J. (1984). Alexithymia: Concept, measurement, and implications for treatment. *American Journal of Psychiatry,* **141**(6), 725-732.

Taylor, S.E., Falke, R.L., Shoptaw, S.J., & Lichtman, R.R. (1986). Social support groups and the cancer patient. *Journal of Consulting and Clinical Psychology,* **54**(5), 608-615.

Teens' health: Injury rates are up. Why? What can you do about it? (1990, November). *Mayo Clinic Health Letter*, **8**(11), 7. (Available from 200 1st Street South West, Rochester, MN 55905)

Tharp, G.D., & Barnes, M.W. (1989). Reduction of immunoglobulin-A by swim training. *Medicine and Science in Sports and Exercise*, **21**(2) (Suppl.), 109.

Thompson, R.A. (1987). Management of the athlete with an eating disorder: Implications for the sport management team. *The Sport Psychologist*, **1**, 114-126.

Tolpin, H.G., & Bentkover, J.D. (1986). The economic costs of sport injuries. In P.E. Vinger & E.F. Hoerner (Eds.), *Sports injuries: The unthwarted epidemic* (2nd ed., pp. 37-47). Littleton, MA: PSG.

Torebjork, H.E., & Ochoa, J.L. (1980). Specific sensations evoked by activity in single identified sensory units in man. *Acta Physiologica Scandinavica*, **110**, 1445-1447.

Travell, J.G., & Simons, D.G. (1983). *Myofascial pain and dysfunction: The trigger point manual*. Baltimore/London: Williams & Wilkins.

Tricker, R., & Cook, D. (1990). Athletes at risk: Drugs in sport. Dubuque, IA: Brown.

Turk, D.C., Meichenbaum, D., & Genest, M. (1983). *Pain and behavioral medicine: A cognitive behavioral perspective*. New York: Guilford Press.

Unestahl, L.-E. (1982). *Better sport by I.M.T.—inner mental training*. Orebro, Sweden: Veje.

Unestahl, L.-E. (1985, April). *Mental aspects of peak performance*. Paper presented at the American Alliance for Health, Physical Education, Recreation and Dance National Convention and Exposition, Atlanta, GA.

United States Olympic Committee. (1987). *Sports nutrition: Eating disorders*. Colorado Springs, CO: Author.

Van Camp, S.P., & Boyer, J.L. (1989). Exercise guidelines for the elderly. *The Physician and Sportsmedicine*, **17**(5), 83-86, 88.

Wack, J.T., & Turk, D.C. (1984). Latent structures in strategies for coping with pain. *Health Psychology*, **3**, 27-43.

Waddell, G., McCulloch, J.A., Kummel, E., & Venner, R.M. (1980). Nonorganic physical signs in low-back pain. *Spine*, **5**(2), 117-125.

Wadler, G.I., & Hainline, B. (1989). *Drugs and the athlete*. Philadelphia: Davis.

Walker, J. (1971). Pain and distraction in athletes and non-athletes. *Perceptual and Motor Skills*, **33**, 1187-1190.

Wallston, B.S., Alagna, S.W., DeVellis, B.M., & DeVellis, R.F. (1983). Social support and physical health. *Health Psychology*, **2**(4), 367-391.

Ward, A., Taylor, P., & Rippe, J.N. (1991). How to tailor an exercise program. *The Physician and Sportsmedicine*, **19**(9), 64-66, 69-71, 73-74.

Weingart, W.A., Sorkness, C.A., & Earhart, R.H. (1985). Analgesia with oral narcotics and added ibuprofen in cancer patients. *Clinical Pharmacy*, **4**, 53-58.

Weltman, G., & Egstrom, G.H. (1966). Perceptual narrowing in novice divers. *Human Factors*, **8**, 499-506.

Wiese, D.M., & Weiss, M.R. (1987). Psychology rehabilitation and physical injury: Implications for the sportsmedicine team. *The Sport Psychologist*, **1**(4), 318-330.

Wiese, D.M., Weiss, M.R., & Yukelson, D.P. (1991). Sport psychology in the training room: A survey of athletic trainers. *The Sport Psychologist*, **5**(1), 15-24.

Williams, A.W., Ware, J.E., & Donald, C.A. (1981). A model of mental health, life events, and social supports applicable to general populations. *Journal of Health and Social Behavior*, **22**, 324-336.

Williams, J.M., Tonymon, P., & Andersen, M.B. (1990). Effects of life-event stress on anxiety and peripheral narrowing. *Journal of Behavioral Medicine*, **16**(4), 174-181.

Williams, J.M., Tonymon, P., & Andersen, M.B. (1991). The effects of stressors and coping resources on anxiety and peripheral narrowing. *Journal of Applied Sport Psychology*, **3**(2), 126-141.

Williams, J.M., Tonymon, P., & Wadsworth, W.A. (1986). Relationship of stress to injury in intercollegiate volleyball. *Journal of Human Stress*, **12**, 38-43.

Williams, J.M., & Roepke, N. (1992). Psychology of injury and injury rehabilitation. In R.N. Singer, M. Murphe, & L.K. Tennant (Eds.), *Handbook of research on sport psychology*. New York: Macmillan.

Williamson, D.A. (1990). *Assessment of eating disorders: Obesity, anorexia, and bulimia nervosa*. New York: Pergamon Press.

Wiltse, L.L., & Rocchio, P.D. (1975). Preoperative psychological tests as predictors of success of chemonucleolysis in the treatment of the low back syndrome. *Journal of Bone and Joint Surgery*, **57**, 478-483.

Wise, A., Jackson, D.W., & Rocchio, P. (1979). Preoperative psychologic testing as a predictor of success in injury: A preliminary report. *The American Journal of Sportsmedicine*, **7**(5), 287-292.

Wise, H.H., Fiebert, I.M., & Kates, J.L. (1984). EMG biofeedback as treatment for patellofemoral pain syndrome. *The Journal of Orthopaedic and Sports Physical Therapy*, **6**(2), 95-103.

Wittig, A.F. (1986, June). *Millon Behavioral Health Inventory (MBHI) indicants of rehabilitation adherence by injured athletes*. Paper presented at the North American Society for Psychology of Sport and Physical Activity Conference, Scottsdale, AZ.

Wolff, B.B. (1985). Ethnocultural factors influencing pain and illness behavior. *The Clinical Journal of Pain*, **1**, 23-30.

Wolpe, J.N., & Lazarus, A.A. (1968). *Behavior therapy techniques*. New York: Pergamon Press.

Yaffe, M. (1983). Sports injuries: Psychological aspects. *British Journal of Hospital Medicine*, **29**(3), 224, 226, 229-230, 232.

Yaksh, T.L. (1979). Direct evidence that spinal serotonin and noradrenalin terminals mediate the spinal antinociceptive effects of morphine in the periaqueductal gray. *Brain Research*, **160**, 180-185.

Yaksh, T.L. (1983). In vivo studies on spinal opiate receptor systems mediating antinociception. *Journal of Pharmacology and Experimental Therapeutics*, **226**, 303-316.

Yaksh, T.L., & Reddy, S.V.R. (1981). Studies in the primate on the analgesic effects associated with intrathecal action of opiates, alpha adrenergic agonists and baclofen. *Anesthesiology*, **54**, 451-467.

Yukelson, D. (1986). Psychology of sports and the injured athlete. In D.B. Benhardt (Ed.), *Clinics in physical therapy: Vol. 10. Sports physical therapy*. Livingston, NY: Churchill.

Zaichkowsky, L.D., & Fuchs, C.Z. (1988). Biofeedback applications in exercise and athletic performance. *Exercise and Sport Science Review*, **16**, 381-421.

Zemper, E.D. (1989). Injury rates in a national sample of college football teams. *The Physician and Sportsmedicine*, **17**(11), 100, 102, 105-108, 113.

Zuckerman, M. (1984). Experience and desire: A new format for sensation seeking scales. *Journal of Behavioral Assessment*, **6**, 101-114.

Zuckerman, M., Kolin, E.A., Price, L., & Zoob, I. (1964). Development of a sensation seeking scale. *Journal of Consulting Psychology*, **28**, 477-482.

Zukin, R.S., & Zukin, S.R. (1981). Multiple opiate receptors: Emerging concepts. *Life Science*, **29**, 2681-2690.

Index

Page numbers in italics refer to figures or tables.

A

Ability, in cognitive schema, 44, *44*-45

Absolutist/dichotomous thinking, 42, *43*, 43-44

Acceptance stage, 35, 36

Acetaminophen, 286

Achievement, level of, 121-122. *See also* Excellence, pursuit of

Achievement motivation, risks in, 54-55

Active listening, 246

Acute injury assessment protocols, 123-126, *124*, 132

Acute pain, medication for, 282, 283-284

Adams, S.H., 190-191

Adaptive stage in injury response, 36

Addiction, to sport activity, 202-204. *See also* Drug abuse

Adherence to treatment (compliance), 82, 196, 199-200

Adjustment to injury. *See* Response to injury, psychological

Adolescent Perceived Events Scale, 77

Adolescents, 77, 118, 119, 128, 221-223, 231, 259-260. *See also* High school football, injuries due to; Parents

Adrian, M.J., 190-191

Adults, developmental issues with, 119-123

Aerobic activity, 29, 31, 67, 213

Affective cycle of injury, 36-42, *37*

AIDS, 190, 191

Aids in Sport (Landry), 191

Alcohol use. *See* Drug abuse

American Academy of Pediatrics, 259-260, 265

American Coaching Effectiveness Program, 191

American College of Sports Medicine, 238

American Physical Therapy Association, 245

American Psychiatric Association, 206, 208-209

American Psychological Association, 185

Amnesia, 79, 288

Anabolic steroid use, 3, 78, 223-225, 231-232

Analgesics, opioid, 178, 283, *285*, 286-287

Analgesics, topical, 287-288

Anatomy, in biology of pain, 270-275, *271*, *272*, *273*

Andersen, Mark B., 49-57

Anesthetics, local, 278, 279, 287

Anesthetics, regional, 274

Anger. *See also* Mood disturbance
and culpability attributions, 81
in injury response models, 35, 36, 38

Anorexia nervosa, 69, 79, 204, 227

Anti-inflammatory drugs, 283, 284, 286

Ascending pathways, 272, *272*, *273*, 274-275

Ashe, Arthur, 190

Aspirin, 284, 286

Assessment, medical. *See* Assessment, of injury; Diagnosis, medical

Assessment, of injury